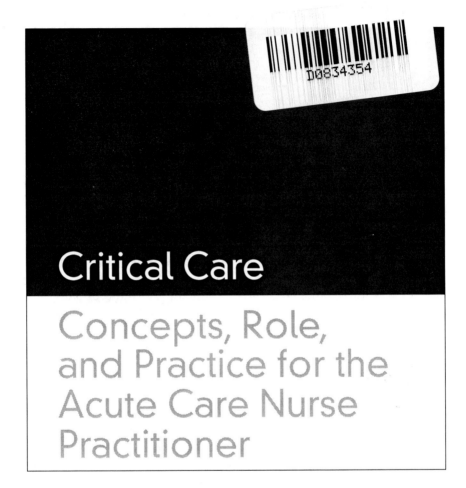

Critical Care

Concepts, Role, and Practice for the Acute Care Nurse Practitioner

Mary M. Wyckoff, PhD, MSN, ACNP, BC, FNP-BC, NNP, CCNS, CCRN, is the lead nurse practitioner in the Surgical Intensive Care Unit at Jackson Health System, Jackson Memorial Hospital, a 40-bed intensive, critical care unit in Miami, Florida. Dr. Wyckoff is an Assistant Professor at the University of Miami and provides education in the acute care nurse practitioner program. Dr. Wyckoff has presented nationally and internationally at multiple conferences. She is a national leader as an elected member of the Congress on Nursing Practice and Economics of the American Nursing Association (ANA). Dr. Wyckoff was the State of Florida Nurse Practitioner for the year 2008 and received her award at the American Academy of Nurse Practitioners (AANP).

Douglas Houghton, ARNP, MSN, CCRN, is a nurse practitioner in the Trauma Intensive Care Unit at Jackson Health System, Jackson Memorial Hospital, Miami, Florida. He has lectured and published nationally and internationally on infections and antibiotic use in the critically ill patient, end of life care, invasive procedures, and other clinical topics. He has published multiple clinical articles and several research studies in critical care. He has a master's degree in nursing and is currently in a post-Masters ACNP certificate program.

Carolyn T. LePage, PhD, ARNP, is a Family Nurse Practitioner and an Assistant Professor at Barry University, Division of Nursing in Miami Shores, Florida. Dr. LePage teaches in the acute and family nurse practitioner specializations and in the DNP and PhD programs. Dr. LePage completed her graduate and doctoral education from Barry University.

Critical Care

Concepts, Role, and Practice for the Acute Care Nurse Practitioner

- Mary M. Wyckoff, PhD, MSN, ACNP, BC, FNP-BC, NNP, CCNS, CCRN
- Douglas Houghton, MSN, ARNP, CCRN
- Carolyn T. LePage, PhD, ARNP

Editors

Springer Publishing Company, LLC
11 West 42nd Street
New York, NY 10036
www.springerpub.com

Acquisitions Editor: Allan Graubard
Cover Design: Steven Pisano
Composition: Six Red Marbles

E-book ISBN: 978-0-8261-3827-9

14 15/ 6 5

Library of Congress Cataloging-in-Publication Data

Critical care concepts, role, and practice for the acute care nurse practitioner / [edited by] Mary M. Wyckoff, Douglas Houghton, Carolyn T. LePage.
    p. ; cm.
  Includes bibliographical references.
  ISBN 978-0-8261-3826-2
1. Intensive care nursing. 2. Nurse practitioners. I. Wyckoff, Mary M. II. Houghton, Douglas. III. LePage, Carolyn T.
  [DNLM: 1. Critical Care—methods. 2. Critical Illness—nursing. 3. Acute Disease—nursing. WY 154 C9323 2009]
  RT120.I5C735 2009
  616.02'8—dc22

                                        2009018359

Printed in the United States of America by Gasch Printing.

Contents

Contributors

Doris Braddy, RN, BSN
Jackson Health System
Jackson Memorial Hospital
Miami, FL

Suzanne M. Burns, MSN, RRT, ACNP,
CCRN, FAAN, FCCM, FAANP
Professor of Nursing and APN 2
Director of PNSO Research Program
UVA Health System
Claude Moore Building
School of Nursing
University of Virginia
Charlottesville, VA

Filissa M. Caserta, MSN, ACNP-BC,
CNRN
Acute Care Nurse Practitioner
The Johns Hopkins Hospital
Baltimore, MD

Miguel A. Cobas, MD
Department of Anesthesia
University of Miami/Jackson Health
System, Jackson Memorial Hospital
Miami, FL

Joseph P. Corallo, MD
Trauma/Critical Care Fellow
University of Miami/Jackson Health
System, Jackson Memorial Hospital
Miami, FL

Marie S. Depew, MS, ACNP-BC, CNRN
Acute Care Nurse Practitioner
The Johns Hopkins Hospital
Baltimore, MD

Scott Gmora, MD
Trauma/Critical Care Fellow
University of Miami/Jackson Health
System, Jackson Memorial Hospital
Miami, FL

Ruth M. Kleinpell, PhD, RN, FAAN,
FAANP, FCCM
Director, Center for Clinical Research
and Scholarship
Rush University Medical Center
Professor, Rush University College of
Nursing
Nurse Practitioner, Our Lady of the
Resurrection Medical Center
Chicago, IL

Jennifer Lefton, MS, RD, CNSD
Clinical Dietitian
Washington Hospital Center
Washington, DC

John Mason, BSN, EMT-P, CEN, CFRN
Vascular Access Specialist
Jackson Health System
Jackson Memorial Hospital
Miami, FL

Barbara A. McLean, MN, RN, CCRN,
CCNS-NP, FCCM
Nurse Intensivist and Critical Care
Specialist
Clinical Faculty, Emory University
Atlanta, GA

Jennifer L. Moran, MS, ACNP-BC,
CNRN
Acute Care Nurse Practitioner
The Johns Hopkins Hospital
Baltimore, MD

Amanda J. Morehouse, MD
Trauma/Critical Care Fellow
University of Miami/Jackson Health
System, Jackson Memorial Hospital
Miami, FL

Nicholas Namias, MD, MBA, FACS,
FCCM
Professor, Clinical Surgery and
Anesthesiology
University of Miami
Miami, FL

Sean M. Quinn, MD
Department of Anesthesia
University of Miami/Jackson Health
System, Jackson Memorial Hospital
Miami, FL

Olga Quintana, ARNP, MSN
Jackson Health System,
Jackson Memorial Hospital
Miami, FL

Anna G. Small, Esq, ARNP, CNM
Associate, Health Law Practice Group
Broad and Cassel
Tallahassee, FL

Richard B. Silverman, MD
Assistant Professor, Anesthesia and
Critical Care Anesthesia
University of Miami
Intensivist, Cardiovascular
Intensive Care Unit and Director
of Anesthesiology
Jackson Memorial Hospital
Miami, FL

Akin Tekin, MD
Transplant Attending
University of Miami/Jackson Health
System, Jackson Memorial Hospital
Miami, FL

Robin Prater Varas, ARNP, BC, MSN
Jackson Health System,
Jackson Memorial Hospital
Miami, FL

Valerie Wells, MSN, ARNP, BC, CCRN
Jackson Health System
Jackson Memorial Hospital
Surgical Intensive Care Unit
Miami, FL

Preface

Loretta Ford, RN and Henry Silver, MD, founders of the first nurse practitioner (NP) program in 1965 at the University of Colorado, could have never envisioned the complex and independent role evolution of NP practice that has subsequently taken place. The nurse practitioner role was developed in response to a need for primary care providers in rural areas, with a focus on family health. The success of nurse practitioners in providing safe and effective health care in the United States is well documented in multiple objective studies. By far, the greatest testament to the value of nurse practitioners is the tremendous growth in our numbers and the continued diversification and advancement of NP practice during the past 40 years. As the health care system has become more complex and specialized the nurse practitioners' role has kept pace with or has surpassed that level of growth and has changed to meet the needs of patients within the system. The role continues to expand, with continually higher and more complex levels of education, certification, and specialization being expected or required for entry into practice.

The editors of this text provide firsthand testimony to the rapid evolution of the nurse practitioner role. Initially educated as family nurse practitioners in the early 90s, two of the editors work exclusively within the critical care environment in a relatively independent manner and have subsequently advanced their degrees to attain certification. Both provide care for extremely ill patients and perform complex invasive procedures on a regular basis. The role of nurse intensivist has become the de facto reality of their practice, and this unique and challenging role for the acute care nurse practitioner (ACNP) has become increasingly found in many health care settings in the United States, and to a lesser degree, abroad.

The educational preparation for entry into advanced practice positions continues to evolve and the Doctorate of Nursing Practice (DNP) degree has developed and progressed into a preferred entry level of practice. Disagreement exists within both the nursing and medical communities with regard to "appropriate" medical supervision and remains a highly debated political battle, with significant variations in legal statutes from state to state. Not surprisingly, there is sparse reference literature available to guide new NPs in this rapidly evolving intensivist role.

This text has been planned and developed with world-renowned authors to address this growing need and to provide such a reference. Nurse practitioners in the critical care environment deserve an authoritative resource for the care of critically ill patients, written by experts with diverse educational backgrounds and perspectives predominantly from within the discipline of nursing. The ACNP programs address the care of patients with urgent problems and those who may require hospitalization or other specialized care. However, critical care content within ACNP programs remains minimal. The expertise contained within this text will contribute to increasing and improving the critical care content, knowledge, and complexity within graduate education programs for ACNPs and for the practicing ACNP.

This text contains the insights and first-hand experience of clinicians actively working in critical care, many of whom are considered experts on a national and international level. The topics covered are not exhaustive; however, the editors believe that the subject matter chosen within these chapters will provide the basis for sound evidence-based care of most common health problems faced by individuals requiring critical care. The editors and authors anticipate that critical care nurse practitioners (both novice and expert) and ACNP students will find this text invaluable in guiding and improving their care of persons requiring critical care of all types. We are proud to present the reader with this first edition of a reference that we hope will become the standard for advanced practice nursing care and education within the critical care environment.

Acknowledgments

The coeditors would like to thank the people who have contributed to this pioneering book. Such a comprehensive work has required significant efforts of many professionals who are in high demand and are leading busy everyday lives.

Foremost, the editors would like to express their utmost appreciation and gratitude to the authors who have contributed chapters to this work. All of the contributors have demanding professional practices, and the editors understand and greatly appreciate the sacrifice of time and effort required to produce chapters that are clinically relevant, evidence-based, and reflect current practice standards.

We would also like to express appreciation to Springer Publishing Company Senior Editor Allan Graubard for having the vision to initiate this text and the patience to persevere through the publication process.

Finally, we would like to thank our family members and significant others for their patience, encouragement, and sacrifice of personal time during the writing and editing of this text. Those times can never be recovered. However, we hope that their recognition of the importance of this book and the impact that the book will have on the education of nurse practitioners will highlight the vital role that they have played in its successful completion.

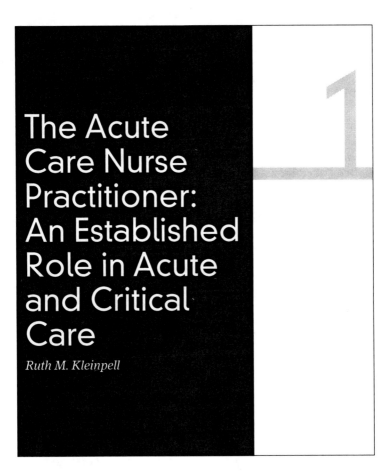

The Acute Care Nurse Practitioner: An Established Role in Acute and Critical Care

Ruth M. Kleinpell

Introduction

Nurse practitioners (NPs) are registered nurses with a master's and or Doctoral degrees, advanced licensure, certification, and function as independent practitioners who practice in various health care settings, including ambulatory, acute, critical, and long-term care (American Academy of Nurse Practitioners [AANP], 2006). Although the original focus of advanced practice nursing care was to provide health promotion and disease prevention services in primary care, an increasing number of NPs are working in acute care settings. This is related to the increased acuity levels of hospitalized patients and the need for expert practitioners to assist in managing patients with complex health conditions.

The acute care nurse practitioner (ACNP) role represents a unique opportunity for advanced practice in acute and critical care. According to the 2004 National Nurse Practitioner Sample Survey, approximately 4.5% of the NP population or more than 4,500 NPs are ACNPs (Goolsby, 2005). Since the formulation of the ACNP role, it has evolved into an established specialty area of NP practice.

Origins of the Acute Care Nurse Practitioner Role

The ACNP role evolved from the need to have an expert practitioner to provide care to patients with critical, acute illness as well as patients with critical, chronic illness. Driving forces in the evolution of the ACNP role included an increase in the severity of illness of hospitalized patients, reduction in hospital lengths of stay, increase in the aging population with chronic conditions, increase in demands for care, access to care issues, and changes in medical residency coverage in the hospital setting (Steel, 1997).

Similar to the evolution of the neonatal NP role in the late 1970s, the ACNP role developed in response to residency shortages in the intensive care unit (ICU) (Keeling & Bigbee, 2005). As medical education became more sensitive to the long hours required by interns and residents, the acute care facilities sought alternatives to promote ongoing effective care for their patients. The nurses who had expertise as primary providers were ideally suited to attain the additional knowledge and skills to meet the complex needs of these patients. Keane and Richmond (1993) were among the first to document the role of the inpatient NP in acute care, a role that was predominantly focused on patient care in the ICU and hospital setting.

There were several significant milestones in the development of the ACNP role. The formulation of annual conferences addressing the educational preparation of ACNPs was a crucial element to organize and unify the essential elements for this advanced practice specialty. In 1993, the transition began and existing bodies of nursing, including the American Nurses Association, American Association of Colleges of Nursing, American Association of Critical Care Nurses, and the state's Boards of Nursing, sought to address specific clinical practice issues. The first national certification and the publication of the ACNP scope and standards followed in 1995. The development of ACNP specialty competencies occurred in 2004, including research expectations and publications, highlighting the expansion and growth of the role. These developments substantiated the ACNP as a distinct specialty of advanced nursing practice. Exhibit 1.1 outlines some of the historical developments related to the ACNP role.

Exhibit

1.1 Historical Developments of the Acute Care Nurse Practitioner (ACNP) Role

Year	Event
1980s–1990	Literature reports and publications on inpatient nurse practitioner roles
1992–1993	Development of first ACNP educational programs
1993	First ACNP Consensus Conference held in Boston, with 40 attendees to discuss issues related to ACNP education and training
1993	Published reports on ACNP educational programs and curriculum
1994	Second ACNP Consensus Conference held in Cleveland, with 80 attendees to discuss issues related to ACNP education and training
1995	Scope of practice for the ACNP, published by the American Nurses and the American Association of Critical Care Nurses
1995	First National Certification for ACNP, offered by the American Nurses Credentialing Center
1995	Third Annual ACNP Consensus Conference held in Rochester New York, with more than 100 attendees
1996	Fourth Annual ACNP Consensus Conference held in Hartford, Connecticut
1997	Book published pertaining to ACNP role (*The Acute Care Nurse Practitioner.* Springer Publishing, 1997)
1997	Fifth Annual ACNP Consensus Conference held in Myrtle Beach, South Carolina

(continued)

Exhibit

1.1 Historical Developments of the Acute Care Nurse Practitioner (ACNP) Role *(continued)*

Year	Event
1998	Publication of first national survey on ACNP practice (Kleinpell, R. M., *AACN Clinical Issues*)
1998	Book published on ACNP practice issues (*Practice Issues for the Acute Care Nurse Practitioner.* Kleinpell, R. M., & Piano, M. R. Springer Publishing, 1998)
1998	Sixth Annual ACNP Consensus Conference held in Pittsburgh, Pennsylvania
1999	Publication of ACNP Certification Review Book (*Acute Care Nurse Practitioner Clinical Curriculum and Certification Review.* Gawlinski A, Hamwi, & D. Philadelphia: WB Saunders)
1999	Publication of ACNP practice book (*Principles of Practice for the Acute Care Nurse Practitioner.* Logan, P. Stamford: Appleton & Lange)
1999	Publication of ACNP Certification Review Questions Book (Miller, S. Health Leadership Associates)
1999	Seventh Annual ACNP Consensus Conference held in Portland, Oregon
1999	Publication of National Longitudinal Survey on ACNP practice: Year 1 (Kleinpell, R. AACN Clinical Issues)
2000	Eighth Annual ACNP Consensus Conference held in Chicago, Illinois
2001	Book published on ACNP practice guidelines (*Practice Guidelines for Acute Care Nurse Practitioners.* Barkley, T. W. & Myers C. M. Philadelphia: Saunders)
2001	Ninth Annual ACNP Consensus Conference held in Huntsville, Alabama
2001	Publication of National Longitudinal Survey on ACNP practice: Year 2 (Kleinpell, R. *AACN Clinical Issues*)
2002	Publication of certification review book (*Acute Care Nurse Practitioner Certification Examination Review Questions and Strategies.* Todd, B. Philadelphia: FA Davis)
2002	Tenth Annual Acute Care Nurse Practitioner Consensus Conference held in Charlottesville, Virginia (last educator conference)
2002	Acute Care Interest Group Forum established at the American Academy of Nurse Practitioners Conference

Year	Event
2003	Acute Care Track established at the annual American Academy of Nurse Practitioners Conference (transitioning of annual ACNP Conference to National Nurse Practitioner Association)
2004	Publication of the Acute Care Nurse Practitioner Competencies, National Panel for Acute Care Nurse Practitioner Competencies
2005	Publication of Acute care nurse practitioner practice: results of a 5-year longitudinal study. (Kleinpell, R. *American Journal of Critical Care*)
2005	Publication of nursing secrets series book on ACNP practice (*Acute Care Nurse Practitioner Secrets*. Todd BA. St Louis: Elsevier Mosby)
2005	Acute Care Column initiated in the *Journal of the American Academy of Nurse Practitioners*
2005	Acute Care Column initiated in the *Journal Nurse Practitioner*
2006	Publication of the revised ACNP Scope and Standards (*Scope and Standards of Practice for the Acute Care Nurse Practitioner*, American Association of Critical Care Nurses
2006	Publication on results of national survey of skills taught in ACNP programs (Kleinpell et al. *Nurse Practitioner*)
2007	Second National Certification Exam becomes available from the American Association of Critical Care Nurses
2008	Development and expansion of doctoral level (doctorate of nursing practice) ACNP programs

Acute Care Nurse Practitioner Role

ACNPs have evolved and refined the role. Practice is not limited to the confines of the ICU and acute inpatient settings. ACNPs care for patients who are critically ill, regardless of the practice setting (Howie-Esquivel & Fontaine, 2006). ACNPs are currently working in a wide variety of settings including hospitals, subacute care facilities, emergency departments, urgent care facilities, clinic settings, and various specialty practices. The ACNP's role has also evolved and now includes specialty tertiary care areas (e.g., interventional cardiology, interventional radiology, oncology, bone marrow transplant) and a growing number of specialty settings (e.g., the intensivist and hospitalist roles) (Kleinpell, et al., 2005).

Although the ACNP role is recognized as a specialty area of NP practice, specific competencies were developed to reflect the knowledge base and scope of practice of ACNPs (National Panel for Acute Care Nurse Practitioner Competencies, 2004). The competencies outline essential role components, including assessment and diagnosis of complex acute, critical, and chronic health conditions and implementation of interventions to support patients with deteriorating physiologic conditions, including the application of basic and advanced life support and other invasive interventions or procedures to promote physiologic stability (National Panel for Acute Care Nurse Practitioner Competencies, 2004) (Exhibit 1.2).

The scope of practice for ACNPs identifies that the performance of noninvasive and invasive diagnostic and therapeutic interventional measures such as, but not limited to, EKG interpretation, radiographic interpretation, respiratory support, hemodynamic monitoring, central line and tube insertion, and lumbar puncture are within the scope of ACNP practice (National Panel for Acute Care Nurse Practitioner Competencies, 2004). The acute care practice setting involves the care of patients with acute and critical care conditions with high acuity levels. The ACNP may perform diagnostic and therapeutic measures to manage these significant health issues (National Panel for Acute Care Nurse Practitioner Competencies, 2004; Becker et al., 2006). This is a unique aspect of ACNP practice that is based on education, training, and specialty certification. A national survey of ACNP educational programs validated that the majority (>55%) teach skills such as hemodynamic monitoring, suturing, central line insertion, and arterial puncture, which highlights the advanced skill set and training of ACNPs (Kleinpell et al., 2006).

The scope and standards of practice for the ACNP define the educational requirements needed for an ACNP. This enables advanced practice regulatory bodies to promote a universally comparable level of education. Graduates of ACNP programs should be able to comprehend and demonstrate advanced skills necessary to perform comprehensive health assessment, order and interpret diagnostic tests and procedures, use differential diagnosis, provide and evaluate outcomes of interventions for patients who are physiologically unstable, technologically dependent, and highly vulnerable for complications (American Association of Critical Care Nurses, 2006) (Table 1.1).

Exhibit

1.2   ACNP Specialty Competencies for Direct Clinical Practice

A. Assessment of Health Status

1. Assesses the patients with complex acute, critical, and chronic illness for urgent and emergent conditions, using both physiologically and technologically derived data, to evaluate for physiologic instability and potentially life-threatening conditions
2. Obtains and documents a health history for patients with complex acute, critical, and chronic illness
3. Performs and documents complete, system-focused, or symptom-specific physical examinations on patients with complex acute, critical, and chronic illness
4. Assess the need for and performs additional screening, based on initial assessment findings
5. Performs evaluations for substance use, violence, neglect and abuse, barriers to learning, and pain
6. Distinguishes between normal and abnormal developmental and age-related physiologic and behavioral changes in patients with complex acute, critical, and chronic illness
7. Assess for multiple interactive and synergistic effects of pharmacological agents, including over the counter preparations and alternative and complementary therapies, in patients with complex acute, critical, and chronic illness.
8. Assess the impact of an acute, critical and/or chronic illness or injury on the individual's: (a) health status (physical and mental), (b) functional status, including activity and mobility, (c) growth and development, (d) nutritional status, (e) sleep and rest patterns, (f) quality of life, (g) family, social, and educational relationships
9. Provides for the promotion of health and protection form disease by assessing for risks associated with the care of complex acute, critical, and chronic illness, such as physiologic risk, including but not limited to immobility, impaired nutrition and immunocompetence, fluid and electrolyte imbalance, invasive interventions, therapeutic modalities, and diagnostic tests
10. Prioritizes data collection, according to the patient's immediate condition or needs, as a continuous proves n acknowledgement of the dynamic nature of complex acute, critical, and chronic illness.
11. Assesses the needs of families and caregivers of patients with complex acute, critical, and chronic illness

(continued)

Exhibit

1.2 ACNP Specialty Competencies for Direct Clinical Practice *(continued)*

B. Diagnosis of Health Status

1. Diagnoses acute and chronic conditions that may result in rapid physiologic deterioration or life-threatening instability
2. Manages diagnostic tests through ordering, interpretation, performance, and supervision in the assessment of patients with complex acute, critical, and chronic illness
3. Utilizes specialty-based technical skills in the performance of diagnostic procedures to confirm or rule out health problems
4. Synthesizes data from various sources to make clinical judgments and decisions about appropriate recommendations and treatments
5. Prioritizes health problems during complex acute, critical, and chronic illness
6. Formulates differential diagnoses by priority considering multiple potential mechanisms causing complex acute, critical, and chronic illness states
7. Distinguishes complications of complex acute, critical, and chronic illness considering multisystem health problems
8. Distinguishes common mental health and substance use or addictive disorder/disease, such as anxiety, depression, and alcohol and drug use, in the presence of complex acute, critical, and chronic illness
9. Reformulates diagnoses by priority based on new or additional assessment data and the dynamic nature of complex acute, critical, and chronic illness

C. Plan of Care and Implementation of Treatment

1. Formulates a plan of care to address complex acute, critical, and chronic health care needs that (a) integrates knowledge of rapidly changing pathophysiology of acute and critical illness in the planning of care and implementation of treatment, (b) prescribes appropriate pharmacologic and nonpharmacologic treatment modalities, and (c) utilizes evidence-based practice in planning and implementing care.
2. Implements interventions to support the patient with a rapidly deteriorating physiologic condition, including the application of basic and advanced life support and other invasive interventions or procedures to regain physiologic stability.

3. Manages, through ordering, performance, interpretation, or supervision, (a) interventions that utilize technological devices to monitor and sustain physiologic function, (b) diagnostic strategies to monitor and sustain physiologic function and ensure patient safety, including but not limited to ECG interpretation, X-ray interpretation, respiratory support, hemodynamic monitoring, and nutritional support.
4. Performs therapeutic interventions to stabilize acute and critical health problems, such as suturing, wound debridement, tube and line insertion, and lumbar puncture.
5. Analyses the indications, contraindications, risk of complications, and cost–benefits of therapeutic interventions.
6. Manages the plan of care through evaluation, modification, and documentation according to the patient's response to therapy, changes in condition, and to therapeutic interventions to optimize patient's outcomes.
7. Manages the patient's response to life support strategies.
8. Manages pain and sedation for patients with complex acute, critical, and chronic illness. (a) Prescribes pharmacologic and nonpharmacologic interventions. (b) Monitor patient's response to sedation. (c) Evaluates patient's response to therapy and changes the plan of care accordingly.
9. Implements palliative and end-of-life care in collaboration with the family, patient (when possible), and other members of the multidisciplinary health care team.
10. Initiates appropriate referrals and performs consultations.
11. Assures that the plan of care is individualized, recognizing the dynamic nature of the patient's condition, reflecting the patient's and family's needs, and considering cost and quality benefits.
12. Coordinates interdisciplinary and intradisciplinary teams to develop or revise plans of care focused on patient and/or family concerns.
13. Incorporates health promotion, health protection and injury prevention measures into the plan of care within the context of the complex acute, critical, and chronic illness.
14. Facilitates the patient's transition between and within health care settings, such as admitting, transferring, and discharging patients.

Adapted from: National Panel for Acute Care Nurse Practitioner Competencies. (2004). *Acute Care Nurse Practitioner Competencies*. Washington, DC: National Organization of Nurse Practitioner Faculties.

1.1 Standards of Clinical Practice for the Acute Care Nurse Practitioner

Standards of ACNP Clinical Practice

Standard I: Assessment
The ACNP generates, collects, and integrates data from a wide variety of sources to make clinical judgments and decisions about indicated orders, procedures, and treatments.

Standard II: Diagnosis
The ACNP diagnoses and prioritizes actual or potential health care problems as the basis for designing interventions for the restoration of health or to meet a patient's goals.

Standard III: Outcome Identification
The ACNP assumes a leadership role in assuring that the patient and health care team identify expected outcomes of care as the basis for developing the interdisciplinary plan of care.

Standard IV: Planning
The ACNP develops a plan of care that prescribes interventions to attain expected outcomes for the patient with acute, critical, and complex needs.

Standard V: Implementation
The ACNP implements interventions identified in the interdisciplinary plan of care for the patient with acute, critical, and complex chronic illness

Standard VI: Evaluation
The ACNP evaluates the patient's progress toward attainment of expected outcomes.

Standards of ACNP Professional Performance

Standard I: Professional Practice
The ACNP evaluates his or her clinical practice in relation to institutional guidelines, professional practice standards, and relevant statutes and regulations.

Standard II: Education
The ACNP acquires and maintains current knowledge in advanced nursing practice.

Standard III: Collaboration
The ACNP collaborates with the patient, family, and other health care providers in patient care.

Standard IV: Ethics
The ACNP integrates ethical considerations into all areas of practice.

Standard V: Systems Management
The ACNP develops and participates in organizational systems and processes promoting optimal patient outcomes.

Standard VI: Resource Utilization
The ACNP considers factors related to safety, effectiveness, and cost in planning and delivering care.

Standard VII: Leadership
The ACNP provides leadership in the practice setting and the profession.

Standard VIII: Collegiality
The ACNP contributes to the professional development of peers, colleagues, and others.

Standard VII: Research
The ACNP continually explores scientific knowledge, identifies specific research priorities in practice, and strives to enhance knowledge and skills through participation in research studies and provision of evidence-based practice.

Standard IX: Quality of Practice
The ACNP systematically evaluates and enhances the quality and effectiveness of advanced nursing practice and care delivery across the continuum of acute care services.

Adapted from American Association of Critical Care Nurses (2006). *Scope and standards of practice for the acute care nurse practitioner.* Aliso Viejo, CA: Author.

Considerations for Acute Care Practice: Regulation

ACNP practice is regulated by individual state practice acts and ACNP scope and standards of practice. Regulatory authority over advanced practice is predominantly governed by the Board of Nursing within each state. The majority of states afford title protection for NP practice through the Board of Nursing with sole authority over NP practice and no statutory or regulatory requirements for physician collaboration, direction, or supervision (Phillips, 2007). Currently, in all but 6 of the 50 states, regulatory control of NP practice falls under the control of the Board of Nursing (American Academy of Nurse Practitioners, 2006). In five states (Florida, South Dakota, North Carolina, Virginia, and Massachusetts), NP practice is collaborative, regulated by both the Board of Nursing and Board of Medicine. Nurses in these states must enter into an agreement with a physician to fully engage in advanced practice. In two states (Illinois and Nebraska), NP practice is regulated by a separate advanced practice board (American Academy of Nurse Practitioners, 2006). Awareness of state practice regulations provides information regarding credentialing and privileging requirements and the need for specific physician "supervision." ACNP practice can include performance of invasive skills and implementation of life-sustaining therapies such as, but not limited to, chest tube insertion, arterial line placement, central line placement, intubation, percutaneous tracheostomy, percutaneous endoscopic gastric (PEG) tube placement, initiation and adjustment of mechanical ventilation, and interpretation of hemodynamic monitoring.

Collaborative practice agreements outlining the ACNP scope of practice are important for defining, enacting, and review of specific aspects of advanced nursing practice.

Considerations for ACNP Practice: Opportunities for Role Expansion

Originally, the major focus of the ACNP role was unit-based, collaborative physician practice based or specialty practice based. Although this offered initial opportunities for ACNP practice, research depicts that there are now more ACNPs employed in collaborative and specialty-based practice (Kleinpell, et al., 2005). ACNPs are often employed by a hospital or health care system or hired in collaborative practice arrangements. Currently, hospitals remain the largest employer of ACNPs (Kleinpell & Goolsby, 2006). Specialty-based practice in traditional inpatient hospital areas, such as cardiac surgery, neurology, pulmonary medicine, orthopedics, oncology, infectious disease, endocrinology, transplantation, general surgery, and trauma, remain a large practice base for ACNPs. Additional practice settings include ambulatory clinics, collaborative practices, and nontraditional practice areas such as holistic clinics, sports medicine, and correctional facilities. Collaborative practice models for ACNPs include the establishment of advanced practice roles as hospitalist, intensivist, and surgical first assistant positions. Opportunities for ACNP practice have tremendously expanded since the creation of national board specialty certification in acute care. ACNP certification validates the professional nursing expertise of the role and will be pivotal in the future expansion of this role.

Considerations for ACNP Practice: Challenges to Practice

Along with increasing opportunities for ACNP practice come challenges for practice including credentialing and privileging, ensuring clinical competency, promoting awareness of the role, ensuring practice based on existing scope of practice, education, and reimbursement issues. Petitioning for full credentials and privileges based on education and training and scope of practice, providing education regarding the

Exhibit

1.3 Strategies for Ensuring Clinical Competency in the ACNP Role

Several strategies can be used to ensure clinical competency for NPs working in acute care. These include the following:

- Education and training for acute care skills set
- Credentialing and privileging for acute care skills
- Preceptorship and mentorship with a collaborating physician to verify skill competency
- Formal post-master's education for acute care
- Certification through advanced courses such as the Society of Critical Care Medicine's Fundamentals of Critical Care Support Course
- Attendance at conference sessions focusing on skills, such as the American Academy of Nurse Practitioner's annual conference offering arterial and central line insertion workshops, and work shops on chest tube insertion
- Use of a formal log to verify clinical skills and procedures
- Use of simulation laboratory
- Incorporation of clinical and procedural skill sets within the acute care programs

Adapted from Melander S. et al., (2008). *Journal of the American Academy of Nurse Practitioners, 20,* 63–68.

role of the ACNP, and awareness of worth in terms of billable revenue will lead to continued role recognition and role acceptance (Hravnak, et al., 2008; Magdic, et al., 2005). Several mechanisms exist to ensure clinical competency for NPs working in acute care including continued education and training for acute care skill sets, specialty certification, credentialing, and privileging for acute care skills (Exhibit 1.3).

In addition to the strategies outlined by Melander et al. (2007), the importance of mentorship cannot be underestimated in the refinement and evolution of the ACNP role. The ACNPs, who adopted the initial roles and established the need for ongoing education and training, scrutiny of policy and legislative changes enabling additional scope of practice, were trailblazers. They serve as role models and provide mentorship and preceptorship opportunities for future generations of ACNPs.

ACNPs are positively impacting outcomes for patient care in many clinical settings. An ongoing challenge for ACNPs is to demonstrate their direct contributions to patient care, patient and family education, nursing staff education and competence, as well as on traditional outcome measures such as costs of care. The value of the ACNP role has been demonstrated in several studies assessing outcomes of ACNP practice (Burns & Earven, 2002; Hoffman, et al., 2005; Gawlinski, et al., 2001; Russell, et al., 2002; Rudy, et al., 1998; Sole, et al., 2001; Cooper, et al., 2002; Meyer and Miers, 2005, Garcias et al., 2003). ACNPs are noted to contribute to excellence in collaborative care, promote evidence-based practice, and impact patient care outcomes. Acute care nursing experts directly impact patient care through the provision of high quality, cost-effective care, improved patient satisfaction, reduced length of stay in acute care units, lower mortality rates, decreased nosocomial infection rates, decreased rates of skin breakdown, and reduced readmission rates.

Summary

The ACNP role is an ideal extension for the advanced practice nurse expert in acute and critical care specializations. Currently, nurses who have completed a master's level of education and specific advanced knowledge and skills, outlined by the ACNP scope of practice, serve complex patients in health care settings. In the future, it is anticipated that ACNP programs will adapt to doctoral levels for entry into practice. The Doctorate of Nursing Practice (DNP) concept was developed in response to the American Association of Colleges of Nursing's ([AACN], 2005) vision of advanced practice nursing entry-level practice at the doctorate level. Practice opportunities for the growing specialty area of ACNP practice will continue to increase because of the complex health care needs for patients with acute and chronic disease states. The ACNP role represents an exciting career trajectory to advance nursing practice in acute and critical care.

References

American Academy of Nurse Practitioners. (2006). *Scope of practice for nurse practitioners*. Washington, DC: Author.
American Academy of Nurse Practitioners. (2006). *State regulatory and prescriptiveauthority*. Washington, DC: Author.

American Association of Colleges of Nursing AACN. (2005). *The essentials of doctoral education for advanced practice nursing.* Washington, DC: Author.

American Association of Critical Care Nurses. (2006). *Scope and standards of practice for the acute care nurse practitioner.* Aliso Viejo, CA: Author.

Barkley T. W., & Myers C. M. (2001). *Practice guidelines for acute care nurse practitioners.* Philadelphia: WB Saunders.

Becker, D., Kaplow, R., Muenzen, P. M., & Hartigan, C. (2006). Activities performed by acute and critical-care advanced practice nurses: American Association of Critical Care Nurses Study of Practice. *American Journal of Critical Care, 15,* 130–148.

Burns, S. M., & Earven, S. (2002). Improving outcomes for mechanically ventilated medical intensive care unit patients using advanced practice nurses: A 6-year experience. *Critical Care Nursing Clinics of North America, 14,* 231–243.

Cooper, M. A., Lindsay G. M., Kinn S., & Swann I. J. (2002). Evaluating emergency nurse practitioner services: a randomized controlled trial. *Journal of Advanced Nursing, 40,* 721–730.

Daly, B. F. (1997). *The acute care nurse practitioner.* New York: Springer Publishing.

Gawlinski A., & Hamwi, D. (Eds.) (1999). *Acute care nurse practitioner clinical curriculum and certification review.* Philadelphia: WB Saunders.

Gawlinski, A., McCloy, K., & Jesurum, J. (2001). Measuring outcomes in cardiovascular APN practice. In R. Kleinpell (Ed.). *Outcome assessment in advanced practice nursing* (pp. 131–188). New York: Springer.

Goolsby, M. J. (2005). 2004 AANP National Nurse Practitioner Sample Survey. *Journal of the American Academy of Nurse Practitioners, 17,* 337–341.

Garcias V. H., Sicoutris C. P., Meredith D. M., Haut E., et al. (2003). Critical care nurse practitioners improve compliance with clinical practice guidelines in the surgical intensive care unit. *Critical Care Medicine 31,* 12:A93.

Hoffman, L., Tasota, F., Zullo, T. G., Scharfenberg, C., & Donahoe, M. P. (2005). A controlled trial of nurse practitioner-managed care in a sub acute medical intensive care unit. In review.

Howie-Esquivel, J., & Fontaine, D. K. (2006). The evolving role of the acute care nurse practitioner in critical care. *Current Opinion in Critical Care, 12,* 609–613.

Hravnak, M., & Kleinpell R. M. (2005). The acute care nurse practitioner. In A. B. Hamric, J. A. Spross, & C. M. Hanson. *Advanced practice nursing: An integrative approach.* St. Louis: Elsevier, In Press.

Keane, A., & Richmond, T. (1993). Tertiary nurse practitioners. *Image Journal of Nursing Scholarship, 25*(4), 281–284.

Keeling, A.W., & Bigbee, J.L. (2005). The history of advanced practice nursing in the United States. In A. B. Hamric, J. A. Spross, & C. M. Hanson. *Advanced practice nursing: An integrative approach.* New York: Elsevier Saunders.

Klein, T. A. (2005). Scope of practice and the nurse practitioner: Regulation, competency, expansion, and evolution. Retrieved July 01, 2005 from http://www.medscape.com/viewprogram/4188_pnt

Kleinpell, R. M. (2005). Acute care nurse practitioner practice: Results of a 5-year longitudinal study. *American Journal of Critical Care, 14,* 211–219.

Kleinpell, R. M., & Goolsby, M. J. (2006). 2004 American Academy of Nurse Practitioner National Nurse Practitioner Sample Survey: Focus on acute care. *Journal of the American Academy of Nurse Practitioners, 18*, 393–394.

Kleinpell, R. M., & Hravnak, M. M. (2005). Strategies for success in the acute care nurse practitioner role. *Critical Care Nursing Clinics of North America, 17*, 177–181.

Kleinpell, R. M., Hravnak, M., King, J., & Miller, K. (2008). Post-masters certification programs for nurse practitioners: Population specialty role preparation. *Journal of the American Academy of Nurse Practitioners, 20*, 63–68.

Kleinpell, R. M., Hravnak, M., Werner, K. E., & Guzman, A. (2006). Skills taught in acute care NP programs: A national survey. *The Nurse Practitioner, 31*, 7–13.

Kleinpell, R. M., Perez, D.F., & McLaughlin, R. (2005). Educational options for acute care nurse practitioner practice. *Journal of the American Academy of Nurse Practitioners, 17*, 460–471

Logan P. (Ed.). (1999). *Principles of Practice for the Acute Care Nurse Practitioner* Stamford: Appleton & Lange.

Magdic, K. S., Hravnak, M., & McCartney, S. (2005). Credentialing for nurse practitioners: An update. *AACN Clinical Issues, 16*(1), 16–22.

Melander S. Kleinpell R. McLaughlin R. (2007) Ensuring clinical competency for NPs in acute care. Nurse Practitioner. 32(4):19–20.

Meyer, S. C., & Miers L. J. (2005) Effect of cardiovascular surgeon and acute care nurse practitioner collaboration on postoperative outcomes. *AACN Clinical Issues,*16, p.149–158

National Organization of Nurse Practitioner Faculties. (2005). *A preceptor manual for NP programs, faculty, preceptors, and students.* Washington DC: Author.

National Panel for Acute Care Nurse Practitioner Competencies. (2004). *Acute aare nurse practitioner competencies.* Washington, DC: National Organization of Nurse Practitioner Faculties.

Phillips, S. J. (2007). A comprehensive look at the legislative issues affecting advanced practice nursing. *The Nurse Practitioner, 35,* p.14–42.

Russell, D., VorderBruegge, M., & Burns, S. M. (2002). Effect of an outcomes-managed approach to care of neuroscience patients by acute care nurse practitioners. *American Journal of Critical Care, 11*, 353–364.

Rudy, E. B., Davidson, L. J., Daly, B., Clochesy, J. M., Sereika, S., Baldisseri, M., et al. (1998). Care activities and outcomes of patients cared for by acute care nurse practitioners, physician assistants, and resident physicians: A comparison. *American Journal of Critical Care. 7*, 267–281.

Sole, M. L., Hunkar-Huie, A. M, Schiller, J. S., & Cheatham, M. L. (2001). Comprehensive trauma patient care by nonphysician providers. *AACN Clinical Issues, 12*, 438–446.

Steel, J. E. (1997). Development of the acute care nurse practitioner role: Questions, opinions, consensus. In B. J. Daly (Ed.), *The acute care nurse practitioner.* New York: Springer.

Todd, B. (2002). *Acute Care Nurse Practitioner Certification Examination: Review Questions and Strategies.* Philadelphia: FA Davis.

Todd, B. A. (2005). *Acute Care Nurse Practitioner Secrets.* St Louis: Elsevier Mosby.

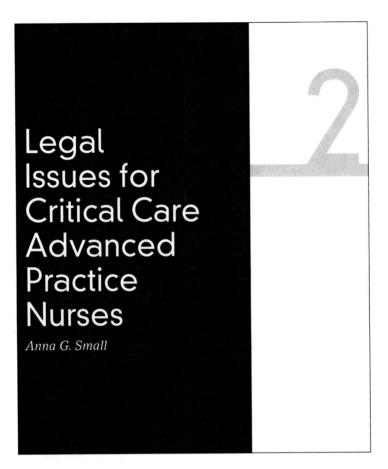

Legal Issues for Critical Care Advanced Practice Nurses

Anna G. Small

Introduction

The decision to become an acute/critical care nurse practitioner (ACNP) is associated with several values including the significant responsibility that comes with the certification and the potential interesting cases, invasive procedures, compassionate care, and their cumulative effect on the patient and his or her family. There is also a legal and ethical side of advanced practice in critical care nursing, and it is our responsibility as practitioners to stay abreast of, and knowledgeable about, such laws and ethical considerations. As such, this chapter will review basic legal issues related to nursing and ACNP practice. Because the specifics may vary from state to state, a nurse practitioner may need to research the regulations within the state of intended practice to become knowledgeable about ACNP regulations. State boards of nursing and state nursing associations are essential resources for initiating such research; their Web sites often have extensive information regarding the issues at hand.

The Nurse Practice Act

Every state has a Nurse Practice Act (NPA). The NPA is part of the laws or statutes of the state and provides an outline of nurses' legal rights and responsibilities. The NPA typically outlines the way in which nurses are licensed and regulated by the specific state, defines various terms related to nursing, and establishes the state's Board of Nursing (BON). NPAs further outline the scope of practice and licensure requirements for the nurses at all levels of practice. The NPA identifies standard actions for licensed nurses, describes violations, states disciplinary actions and penalties, and sets standards for educational programs. Many states include additional regulatory issues in the NPA.

Although NPAs are often written in dry legal prose, it is essential that ACNPs are aware of NPA regulations. Without astute awareness, unintentional violations of the law can occur. Because ignorance of the law is no excuse, accountability for violations of the law will be enforced even if the ACNP acted in good faith. Upon acceptance of an ACNP license in a state, the ACNP agrees to abide by the NPA in that state and is accountable to the law, and is required to know of the law. NPAs as part of the laws of the states are included in the code or the statutes of the state and are available online, generally from a link on the state's BON Web site. Most BONs have staff available to answer questions regarding the legal requirements of their individual states.

The National Council of State Boards of Nursing has developed a Model Nursing Practice Act and Rules. Although these have not been universally accepted in every state, portions of these models are recognizable in each state's NPA. The NPA is the law of the state, but the state legislatures would be overwhelmed with work if they had to enact laws on every issue concerning nursing. To address these issues, the legislature delegates rule-making authority to the executive branch agencies, typically the Department of Health.

Usually through the BON, the Department of Health promulgates rules that are relevant to the practice of nursing. In seven states, the rules that govern practice of nurses are promulgated with input from both the Board of Medicine and the BON (American Academy of Nurse Practitioners [AANP], 2008). These rules reflect the same topics covered by the NPA but fill in some of the details missing in the actual laws. The BON may not exceed its legislative authority by promulgating rules that exceed the scope of the law or the grant of authority from the legislature.

An example of the rule-making process is when the legislature enacts a law that requires nurses to have 25 hours of continuing education credit every 2-year licensure period. The legislature will then delegate the task to the BON to define the details regarding which topics are most significant to nurses. The BON might then promulgate rules that would require that nurses take 2 hours of education on recognizing domestic violence and 2 hours on prevention of medical errors with the remaining hours on a topic of the nurse's choice. The legislature would specify in the law that the BON is to establish rules that specify the continuing education requirements for nurses, which includes education in domestic violence and prevention of medical errors as the BON deems appropriate.

Licensure Issues

All nurses are regulated and licensed by their states. Typically, each state has a Department of Health, which licenses nurses. Generally, there is a BON that acts under the auspices of the Department of Health. The BON licenses licensed practice nurses, registered nurses, advanced practice nurses, and sometimes nursing assistants.

The BON staff work for the state agency that houses it. It is important to note that BON employees may or may not be nurses but are responsible for the daily running of the BON including the processing of applications for licensure. Because the BON is responsible for licensing different types of nurses, it develops and accepts applications for licensure and is responsible for verifying the information on a nurse's application and attaining required background checks. BON employees also may be responsible for certifying continuing education providers and for auditing nurses to verify that they are keeping up with their continuing education requirements. In this respect, the BON may have some authority to establish fees for license types and then is responsible for collecting such fees at the time of application. Requirements for licensure and the specific guidelines on the NPA and BON are found on each state's Web site. Completing license renewal in a timely manner is essential. Practicing nursing without a license can subject the health care provider to disciplinary actions by the BON as well as to possible criminal actions. Compliance with continuing education requirements and maintenance of the proof of completion are responsibilities of each nurse and must be met in accordance to the BON requirements. One of the most common disciplinary issues is failure on the part of the licensee to maintain his or her continuing education requirements.

Case Study

Jane Doe, an acute care nurse practitioner, works hard at a hospital by managing the care for multiple patients. When she gets her renewal notice from the state's Board of Nursing, she puts it in her to-do pile on her desk. Unfortunately, Jane is very busy and forgets to renew her license on time. About 2 weeks after her date of renewal, her hospital asks her for a copy of her new license. Jane suddenly remembers that she forgot all about renewing her license! She rushes to the BON Web site and renews online. However, for the past 2 weeks, she has been seeing patients without a current license. Her employer is upset and tells Jane that she is going to be reported to the BON for disciplinary action for practicing without a current license. The employer wants Jane to pay back all the money it would have billed Medicare for her services during the past 2 weeks. The employer states it has consulted its attorney and it cannot bill for her services unless she is in compliance with all state laws. Because she was out of compliance with her renewal, she was out of compliance with state law. Jane is faced with bills from her employer for over $10,000, possible loss of her employment, and possible disciplinary action from the state's BON.

Scope of Practice

As an ACNP, it is critical to understand the nurse practitioner's scope of practice. There are two definitions of scope of practice that should be similar, if not exactly the same. There is the legal scope of practice and the scope of practice based on education, training, and experience. Remember as well that the scope of practice may vary tremendously from state to state. For example, some advanced practice nurses attain what is deemed "independent" practice. This is more common in the western states where advanced practice nurses (APN) have played an important role in large geographical regions that house an inadequate number of physician providers (Christian, Catherine, & O' Neil, 2007). Arizona and Alaska are two prime examples here. Other states have more restricted practices. Florida APN must sustain a relationship with a supervising physician and file a protocol every 2 years with the BON, which reviews the protocol and publishes it online (The Florida Senate, 2004). At the time of this publication, Florida is one of three remaining states that do not permit APN to prescribe controlled substances.

The scope of practice for an advanced practice nurse encompasses the scope of the registered nurse and is generally defined in the state's NPA. The Model Nursing Practice Act of 2004 defines the scope of practice of the registered nurse as follows:

> *Practice as a registered nurse means the full scope of nursing, with or without compensation or personal profit, that incorporates caring for all clients in all settings; is guided by the scope of practice authorized in this section, through nursing standards established or recognized by the board and includes, but is not limited to:*
>
> A. *Providing comprehensive nursing assessment of the health status of clients.*
> B. *Collaborating with health care team to develop an integrated client-centered health care plan.*
> C. *Developing a strategy of nursing care to be integrated within the client-centered health care plan that establishes nursing diagnoses; setting goals to meet identified*

health care needs; determining nursing interventions; and implementing nursing care through the execution of independent nursing strategies and regimens requested, ordered or prescribed by authorized health care providers.

D. Delegating and assigning nursing interventions to implement the plan of care.

E. Providing for the maintenance of safe and effective nursing care rendered directly or indirectly.

F. Promoting a safe and therapeutic environment.

G. Advocating for clients by attaining and maintaining what is in the best interest of clients.

H. Evaluating responses to interventions and the effectiveness of the plan of care.

I. Communicating and collaborating with other health care providers in the management of health care and the implementation of the total health care regimen within and across care settings.

J. Acquiring and applying critical new knowledge and technologies to the practice domain.

K. Managing, supervising and evaluating the practice of nursing.

L. Teaching the theory and practice of nursing.

M. Participating in development of policies, procedures and systems to support the client.

N. Other acts that require education and training as delineated by the board commensurate with the registered nurse's continuing education, demonstrated competencies and experience. Each nurse is accountable for complying with the requirements of this act and for the quality of nursing care rendered; and for recognizing limits of knowledge, experience and planning of situations beyond the nurse's expertise (National Council of State Boards of Nursing [NCSBN], 2008).

While the Model Nursing Practice Act's definition is quite lengthy and detailed, many of the individual states have more abbreviated definitions. For example, Florida defines the practice of professional nursing as follows:

"Practice of professional nursing" means the performance of those acts requiring substantial specialized knowledge, judgment, and nursing skill based upon applied principles *of psychological, biological, physical, and social sciences, which shall include, but not be limited to:*

1. *The observation, assessment, nursing diagnosis, planning, intervention, and evaluation of care; health teaching and counseling of the ill, injured, or infirm; and the promotion of wellness, maintenance of health, and prevention of illness of others.*
2. *The administration of medications and treatments as prescribed or authorized by a duly licensed practitioner authorized by the laws of this state to prescribe such medications and treatments.*
3. *The supervision and teaching of other personnel in the theory and performance of any of the above acts (Florida Statutes s. 464.003(2008)).*

There are advantages and disadvantages to having a more abbreviated definition. With Florida's definition, there might be different interpretations for a nurse who has practiced on the borders of accepted practice and faces disciplinary action. Consequently, if a nurse is informed of the definition, like the one in the Model Nursing Practice Act, then the nurse has a strong reference guide to know whether he or she is about to cross the line of the defined scope of practice.

For its part, Alaska's more abbreviated definition defines the practice of professional nursing as follows:

"Practice of professional nursing" means the performance for compensation or personal profit of acts of professional service that requires substantial specialized knowledge, judgment, and skill based on the principles of biological, physiological, behavioral, and sociological sciences in assessing and responding to the health needs of individuals, families, or communities through services that include:

A. *Assessment of problems, counseling, and teaching*
B. *Clients to maintain health or prevent illness; and in the care of the ill, injured, or infirm;*
C. *Administration, supervision, delegation, and evaluation of nursing practice;*
D. *Teaching others the skills of nursing;*
E. *Execution of a medical regimen as prescribed by a person authorized by the state to practice medicine;*

    F. *Performance of other acts that require education and training that are recognized by the nursing profession as properly performed by registered nurses;*

    G. *Performance of acts of medical diagnosis and the prescription of medical therapeutic or corrective measures under regulations adopted by the board; (AS 08.68.410(9)).*

Alaska's abbreviated definition also has the potential for different interpretations, whereas, the Model Nursing Practice Act provides more detail and clearly defines the scope of practice.

An ACNP's scope of practice is significantly broader and is complicated with additional duties, rights, and responsibilities. Confusing matters further, there are different types of ACNPs and the legal definition of their scope of practice can vary greatly from state to state. In some states, all ACNPs are regulated by the same section of the Nurse Practice Act and have similar rights and responsibilities. In other states, certified nurse midwives, certified registered nurse anesthetists, and clinical nurse specialists may have a legal definition and scope that is unique to their practice. In the Model Nursing Practice Act , all four types of ACNPs are defined together as follows:

Advanced practice registered nursing by nurse practitioners, nurse anesthetists, nurse midwives, or clinical nurse specialists is based on knowledge and skills acquired in basic nursing education; licensure as a registered nurse; graduation from or completion of a graduate level advanced practice registered nurse (APRN) program accredited by a national accrediting body and current certification by a national certifying body acceptable to the board in the specified APRN role and specialty.

Practice as an APRN means a scope of nursing in a category approved by the board, with or without compensation or personal profit, and includes the registered nurse scope of practice. The scope of an APRN includes, but is not limited to, performing acts of advanced assessment, diagnosing, prescribing, selecting, administering and dispensing therapeutic measures, including over-the-counter drugs, legend drugs and controlled substances, within the APRN's role and specialty appropriate education and certification.

The APRN scope of practice supersedes the registered nurse scope of practice.

APRN are expected to practice within standards established or recognized by the board. Each APRN is accountable to clients, the nursing profession and the board for complying with the requirements of this Act and the quality of advanced nursing care rendered; for recognizing limits of knowledge and experience, planning for the management of situations beyond the APRN's expertise; and for consulting with or referring clients to other health care providers as appropriate (NCSBN, 2008).

According to the definition, the Model Nursing Practice Act delegates authority to the BON to define more specific guidelines with the words, "Advanced practice registered nurses are expected to practice within standards established or recognized by the board." The Model Nursing Administrative Rules provided within the Model Nursing Practice Act do not provide more specific guidelines, but some of the individual states do provide specific guidelines in statute or rule and it is the responsibility of the ACNP to know these specifics.

Collaborative Practice Agreements

In many states ACNPs must have collaborative practice agreements (CPA). These agreements are public records and document a collaborative or supervisory relationship with a physician. These documents may also be called protocols, standardized procedures, patient care guidelines, and standing orders (Likis, 2003). Although CPAs can service an important purpose in clinical practice, the legal requirement of CPAs in Nurse Practice Acts has also been seen by critics as restricting ACNPs.

Ideally, a collaborative practice agreement can define who nurses treat, who they see, and under what circumstances they can provide care (McCabe & Burman, 2006). However, in today's world of high technology and decreasing access to care, the lines between specialties become blurred. The question then becomes an ethical one: "Should we take care of something not traditionally within our scope of practice because there is no other way for the client to get the care they need?" (McCabe & Burman).

In addition to its ethical character, this situation also raises legal issues particularly in the area of medical malpractice and licensure discipline. Data from Nursing Service Organization (NSO) in 2004 indicated that 6% of their claims were related to scope of practice issues in the advanced practice setting (McCabe & Burman, 2006). Plaintiff lawyers seek collaborative practice agreements to determine ultimate responsibility when things go wrong (Atkinson, 2007). Because of the supervisory nature relationships involved in a "collaborative" practice agreement, plaintiffs' attorneys will investigate to determine the liability of the ACNP, the "supervising" or "sponsoring" physician, and the nurse's employer (NCSBN, 2008).

When the scope of practice is rigidly defined in the NPA, deviations are more likely to occur. Any deviation from the existing definition could have serious ramifications for continued licensure. Practicing outside the scope of practice may result in a citation, licensure suspension, or even revocation. Before a CPA is written, however, it is critical that the NPA is examined in detail. The legally required elements should be clearly identified in the document. There are many samples or form protocols available from the BON, prospective employer, or professional organizations.

The CPA generally must contain information regarding contact information, practice address, the contract information for the collaborating physician, the nature of the practice including the conditions that may be treated, the medication and treatments prescribed or performed the duties of the physician, and the occasions during which the physician must directly supervise the ACNP. All parties to the protocol must sign the agreement. ACNPs who are employed by physicians or physician groups will typically have their protocol agreements signed by their employers. ACNPs who seek independent practice will hire a physician to enter into a collaborative practice agreement. Physicians' compensation will vary dependently on time, need for coverage, and consultation. In addition, most physicians feel that they may be accepting additional liability for the ACNP's actions when they enter into a collaborative agreement and may expect additional compensation for assuming this potential liability. The following exhibits are important in this regard (Exhibits 2.1 through 2.4).

2.1 Sample Collaborative Agreement I

I. Requiring Authority:
   A. Nurse Practice Act, cite your state here
   B. Your State's Administrative Code, applicable provisions

II. Parties to Protocol:
   A. Nancy R. Nurse, APRN Lic. # 123456
      123 Main Street
      Somewhere, USA 99999

   B. Ian M. Doctor, MD, MX 999999, DEA 999999
      Practice Name
      456 Center Street
      Somewhere, USA 99999

III. Nature of Practice:
   This collaborative agreement is to establish and maintain a practice model in which the nurse practitioner will provide health care services under the general supervision (collaboration) of Dr. Ian M. Doctor. This practice shall encompass family practice and shall focus on health screening and supervision, wellness and health education and counseling, and the treatment of common health problems. (Use appropriate description for your specialty and activities) Practice Location(s):

   List all practice locations here.

IV. Description of the duties and management areas for which the APRN is responsible.
   A. Duties of the APRN:
      The nurse practitioner is responsible for providing health services to clients of the (name of clinic or agency). The nurse practitioners will provide health promotion, screening, safety instructions, and management of acute episodic illness and stable chronic diseases. Referrals will be made, as needed, to other health care providers.

   B. The conditions for which the APRN may initiate treatment include, but are not limited to:
      Otitis media and externa
      Conjunctivitis
      Upper respiratory tract infections
      Sinusitis

(continued)

Exhibit

2.1 Sample Collaborative Agreement I *(continued)*

C. Treatments that may be initiated by the ARNP, depending on the patient condition and judgment of the ARNP:
1. Suture of simple and complex lacerations not requiring ligament or tendon repair.
2. Incision and drainage of abscesses.
3. Removal of ingrown toenail.

D. Drug therapies that the ARNP may prescribe, initiate, monitor, alter, or order:

Any prescription medication which is within the scope of training and knowledge base of the nurse practitioner.

-or-

Antibiotics

Antihypertensives

etc.

V. Duties of the Physician:

The physician shall provide general supervision for routine health care and management of common health problems, and provide consultation and/or accept referrals for complex health problems. The physician shall be available by telephone or by other communication device when not physically available on the premises. If the physician is not available, his associate, John R. Doctor, MD, MX 999999 (or other description of designated doctor(s) or groups), will serve as backup for consultation, collaboration and/or referral purposes.

VI. Specific Conditions and Requirements for Direct Evaluation:

With respect to specific conditions and procedures that require direct evaluation, collaboration, and/or consultation by the physician, the following will serve as a reference guide:

Clinical Guidelines in Family Practice, X Edition, by Constance R. Uphold, ARNP, PhD, and Mary Virginia Graham, ARNP, PhD (or other reference text or practitioner created reference guide)

-or-

Consultation will occur:

■ Whenever situations arise that go beyond the intent of the protocols or the competence, scope of practice, or experience of the nurse practitioner.

▓ Whenever the patient's condition fails to respond to the management plan within an appropriate time frame, based on the provider's clinical judgment.

▓ For any uncommon, unfamiliar, or unstable patient condition.

▓ For any patient condition which does not fit the commonly accepted diagnostic pattern for a disease/condition.

▓ For any unexplained physical examination or historical finding or abnormal diagnostic finding.

▓ Whenever a patient requests.

▓ For all emergency situations after initial stabilizing care has been initiated.

VII. All parties to this agreement share equally in the responsibility for reviewing treatment protocols as needed and no less than annually.

_____ / _____ License # RN9999999
Nancy R. Nurse, APRN/ Date

_____ / _____ License #ME 999999
Ian M. Doctor, MD/ Date DEA # 999999
(Longworth, 2008; Florida Board of Nursing, 2008)

Interestingly, the Model Nursing Practice Act only refers to a CPA in the context of controlled substance prescribing. However, comprehensive, written, collaborative practice agreements are required in 21 states (Christian et al., 2007).

Disciplinary Process

Many ACNPs find that some aspects of practice are regulated by the state's Board of Medicine. However, the state's BON is charged in all states with regulating the practice of nursing. The BON will investigate complaints against licensees and will contact the licensee to seek the licensee's version

Exhibit

2.2 Sample Collaborative Agreement II (Acute Care Surgical Intensive Care Unit [SICU] Protocols)

TO: Agency for Health Care Administration
Board of Nursing/Compliance Department
4052 Bald Cypress Way Bin C02
Tallahassee, Florida 32399-3252

FROM: Jane Brown, PhD, ACNP, BC, CCNS

DATE: March 10, 2009
SUBJECT: Annual Update of Protocols

Enclosed is a copy of the protocol / joint practice agreement as Pursuant to Florida Board of Nursing Rules Chapter 59S-4.

TO: Board of Medicine
Agency for Health Care Administration
1940 North Monroe Street
Suite 60
Tallahassee, Florida 32399-0770
           ATTN: MARM HARRIS

FROM: Dr. F. Franks, M.D., FACS
Chief of Trauma / Surgical Critical Care
University of Miami / Jackson Health System

Dr. J. Johns, MD
Medical Director Anesthesia Critical Care Medicine
University of Miami / Jackson Health System

DATE: March 10, 2009
SUBJECT: UPDATE of Joint Practice Agreement with an Advanced Practice Registered Nurse (Mary Wyckoff, PhD, MSN, ACNP, BC, FNP-BC, CCNS, CCRN, NNP)

As pursuant F.S. 458.348, this is to notify the Board of Medicine that a formal joint agreement has been established between the physicians and the above named nurse practitioner (APRN) of the Department of Trauma/Surgical/Anesthesia Critical Care Services at the University of Miami/Jackson Health System.
An updated copy of the agreement is enclosed.

JOINT PRACTICE AGREEMENT

I.   REQUIRING AUTHORITY

Nurse Practice Act, Florida Statute, Chapter 464
Florida Board of Nursing Rules, Chapter 59S-4,
Administrative Policies
Pertaining to Advanced Practice Registered Nurse,
Florida Administrative Code.

II. ADVANCED PRACTICE REGISTERED NURSE CERTIFICATION

Jane Brown, PhD, ACNP, BC, CCNS,
NNP is Board Certified in Acute Care and Family Practice
and License # _____, as issued by the Florida Board
of Nursing (copy attached).

III. GENERAL AREA OF PRACTICE

Jane Brown, PhD, ACNP, BC, CCNS
NNP may manage the health care for those clients for
which he/she has been educated.

IV. SPECIFIC MANAGEMENT AREAS

A.   The APRN may prescribe, initiate, or alter medication
     regimens of any FDA approved drugs or OTC
     preparations, oral, topical, intravenous, intramuscular,
     subcutaneous and as a continuous drip.
B.   Controlled substances may be initiated by the APRN
     within the practicing facility under the appropriate federal
     and state guidelines.
C.   Other measures may be initiated or performed within the
     boundaries of the APRN's education, depending upon the
     client's condition and judgement of the APRN.

V.   SUPERVISION

General supervision will be provided through consultation with
the physicians as needed via on site and/or telephone
communication.

(continued)

Exhibit

Sample Collaborative Agreement II (Acute Care Surgical Intensive Care Unit [SICU] Protocols) *(continued)*

2.2

VI. PARTIES INVOLVED

A joint practice agreement has been established between the following APRN, Jane Brown, PhD, ACNP, BC, CCNS and the physicians of the Trauma / Surgical / Anesthesia Critical Care Services Departments at the University of Miami / Jackson Health System.

All of the above functions stated in sections III and IV may be performed under general supervision

---

Mary Wyckoff, PhD, MSN, ACNP, BC, FNP-BC,CCNS,CCRN
Chief of Trauma/Surgical
Critical Care Services
License #
March 10, 2009

Francis Franks, FACS, MDACNP, BC,
Trauma/Surgical/Anesthesia
Critical Care Services
License #

March 10, 2009

Jonathan Johns, MD
Medical Director/Anesthesia Critical
Care Medicine
License # ME
March 10, 2009

of events. At this point in time, the ACNP should seek advice from an attorney. The attorney will be able to focus on the legal arguments in the disciplinary case from a legally directed perspective. A nurse who faces disciplinary action may have acted in a manner unbecoming to a professional nurse, or acted in a manner that exceeded the scope of practice. Disciplinary action may be the result of something as simple as failing to update contact information with BON or failing to participate to the required continuing education.

Exhibit

2.3   Privileges and Activities List

PRIVILEGES AND ACTIVITIES LIST

Name: Jane Brown, PhD, ACNP, BC, CCNS
        Acute Care Nurse Practitioner
        Advanced Practice Registered Nurse
        Division of Trauma/Surgical/Anesthesia Critical Care Services

Category of practice: Board Certified Acute Care Nurse Practitioner
                        Certified Critical Care Nurse Specialist

Privileges & Activities:

1. Obtain health histories.

2. Perform physical examinations.

3. Order and interpret laboratory and diagnostic studies.

4. Order restraints as indicated.

5. Monitor and manage patients with chronic diseases.

6. Monitor and manage patients with acute injury and illness.

7. Monitor and manage patients preoperatively and postoperatively.

8. Monitor and manage patients pretransplant and posttransplant.

9. Make referrals to consult services as indicated.

10. Prescribe, initiate, monitor, and alter medications and treatments.

11. Provide counseling and teaching.

12. Under the general supervision and at the discretion of a Florida licensed physician (the Chief of Service or his/her designee), the APRN may perform select procedures for which he/she has been educated.

13. Under the general supervision of the Chief of Service and his/her designee, the APRN may perform medical acts of diagnosis and develop a treatment plan for such diagnosis, based upon the history, physical examination, and diagnostic findings.

(continued)

Exhibit

2.3   Privileges and Activities List *(continued)*

14. The APRN must practice under the general supervision of the Chief of Service or his/her designee.

15. General supervision will be provided through consultation with the physicians of the Division of Trauma / Surgical / Anesthesia Critical Care Services as needed via on-site and/or telephone communication.

_____ ACNP, BC
Jane Brown, PhD, ACNP, BC, CCNS
Acute Care Nurse Practitioner
Trauma/Surgical/Anesthesia Critical
Care Svcs
License # RN / APRN
March 10, 2009

_____ MD
Francis Franks, MD, FACS
Chief of Trauma/Surgical
Critical Care Svcs
University of Miami/Jackson
Memorial Hospital
License # ME
March 10, 2009

_____, MD
Jonathan Johns, MD
Medical Director/Anesthesia
Critical Care Medicine
ME
March 10, 2009
Trauma/Surgical/Anesthesia
Critical Care Services

Nurses who are confronted with state disciplinary action must comprehend the serious legal and regulatory nature of the Board of Nursing. The BON is made up primarily of nurses, and it would be a logical, but misguided, assumption on the part of a nurse to believe that the BON will be overly sympathetic to an admission of guilt. The nurses who comprise the BON are fallible; however, they are charged with maintaining the standard of the profession and do not lightly dismiss conduct unbecoming to the profession.

Exhibit

2.4   Nurse Practitioner Job Description

NURSE PRACTITIONER JOB DESCRIPTION
Jane Brown, PhD, ACNP, BC, CCNS

The Advanced Practice Registered Nurse (APRN) for the Trauma/Surgical/
Anesthesia Critical Care Services at the University of Miami/Jackson Health
System will assume the following responsibilities:

1. Admission history and physical exams, admission orders for in-house.

2. Discharge orders and dictation of discharge summaries for those patients
   discharged by the APRN.

3. Monitor and management of preoperative and postoperative patients in
   the critical care setting, including, patients with acute injury, illness, and
   transplant.

4. Obtain referrals to consulting services as indicated.

5. Prescribe, initiate, monitor, and alter medications and treatments.

6. Provide ongoing ventilator management.

7. Provide counseling and teaching.

8. Monitor and provide appropriate nutrition.

9. Order and interpret radiographic studies.

10. Privileges and activities as outlined in the Privileges and Activities List and
    Joint Practice Agreement and nurse practitioner protocols.

11. Perform procedures as designated by the Chief of the Department of Trauma
    Surgical Critical Care and Medical Director Anesthesia Critical Care or his/her
    designee. These include but are not limited to advanced cardiac life support,
    electrical cardioversion, open chest intracardiac defibrillation, placement of
    central line, pulmonary catheter, arterial line, peripherally inserted central
    catheter, chest tube, dialysis catheter, feeding tubes placement, intubation,
    tracheostomy and bronchoscopy, insertion of percutaneous drains, and
    removal of drainage tubes, facilitate extracorporeal membrane oxygenation,
    insertion, removal, and management of intraortic balloon pumps, removal
    epicardial wires, management of ventricular assist devices.

(continued)

2.4 Nurse Practitioner Job Description (continued)

12. Participate in writing orders as recognized during rounds.

NOTE: The above responsibilities are shared with the interns / residents of Trauma / Surgical / Anesthesia Critical Care Services Team and are not solely the responsibility of the nurse Practitioner.

Approved by:

_____, MD

Francis Frank, M.D., FACS
Chief of Trauma/Surgical Critical Care Svcs
University of Miami/Jackson
Memorial Hosp.
License # ME
March 10, 2009

_____, MSN, RN

Rachel Ray, MSN, RN
Director of Nursing
Critical Care Nursing Director
Jackson Memorial Hospital
March 10, 2009

_____, MD

Jonathan Johns, MD
Medical Director/Anesthesia Medicine
Trauma /Surgical/Anesthesia
Critical Care Svcs
March 10, 2009

_____, PhD, ACNP, BC

Jane Brown, PhD, ACNP, BC, CCNS
Advanced Registered Nurse
Critical Care
Practitioner ME
License # RN/APRN
March 10, 2009

When the BON completes the investigation and decides that further action should be taken, judicial action will be pursed against the licensee. The BON has the power to seek revocation or suspension of a nurse's license. Less significant penalties can include citations, fines, extra continuing education hours, and public admonishments.

Some states have laws that require certain events be reported to the BON. Nurses may end up facing possible disciplinary action when they are involved with an adverse incident at work

Case Study

Nancy Klein is an acute care nurse practitioner who practices in a state that requires her to have a collaborative practice agreement with a supervising physician. In accordance with her protocol, she administers conscious sedation to intensive care unit (ICU) patients who are undergoing procedures by her supervising physician. One day, Nancy is in the ICU and is asked by a consulting podiatrist to administer conscious sedation for a procedure. Nancy has never worked with the podiatrist before and feels some hesitance. She calls a lawyer she has consulted before and asks if she may administer the sedation for the podiatrist. The lawyer tells her that she may only administer the sedation if the administration of conscious sedation for podiatrists is in her protocol. As it is not, Nancy declines to administer the sedation in this case.

or when they are involved in a medical malpractice case. Additionally, some institutions will have policies regarding when to report an employee or medical staff to the BON.

When faced with possible disciplinary action, the ACNP should consider consulting an attorney. Many types of professional liability insurances cover licensure defense and disciplinary matters, therefore consulting an attorney does not have to be a significant out-of-pocket expense. However, even if one neglects to obtain insurance coverage for disciplinary matters, it is almost certainly worth the expense to consult a lawyer. Do not panic or react rashly when faced with the prospect of disciplinary action, but follow the advice of legal counsel. There are several nurses who are also attorneys and these nurse–attorneys can address your legal issues while having the additional knowledge and insight of the nursing perspective. Additional information regarding nurse attorneys can be obtained through the Web site of The American Association of Nurse Attorneys.

Medical Malpractice

There is significant angst among health care providers regarding medical malpractice claims. There are many examples of physicians and ACNPs who are practicing defensive medicine in order to avoid lawsuits but it is unclear if this has had any effect on reducing claims. In addition, there is considerable concern regarding the cost of medical malpractice insurance or professional liability insurance. Although ACNP insurance is generally less expensive than physician counterparts, it is still quite expensive and may be difficult to obtain. Investigating through professional organizations may be helpful.

In a claim for medical malpractice, a plaintiff must show (a) the existence of the duty of the health care provider to the plaintiff, (b) a breach of that duty, and (c) resultant damages. Many states have instituted tort reform, which has made it more difficult for plaintiffs to file medical malpractice lawsuits. In addition, there are short periods during which a case may be filed, limits or caps on damages amounts, and presuit screening requirements. In order to understand the liability situation for medical malpractice, the ACNP must comprehend the duty of a plaintiff to have to prove the case against a nurse. This is highlighted in the following case study.

Case Study

Mr. J is admitted to the ICU after having a fall at home resulting in a fractured hip. He is a 92-year-old white man with a history of hypertension and non–insulin-dependent diabetes. Mr. J receives surgery prior to his admission to your unit. He is receiving pain medication and is reluctant to get out of bed. Over the course of the next few days, Mr. J's pain level is difficult to control and he declines to eat full meals or participate in physical therapy. Mr. J develops some skin breakdown in his sacral area and a wound care consult is ordered, including a specialty air mattress and a speech therapist consult. Mr. J continues to improve and is ready for discharge to rehabilitation on postoperative day 10. Eighteen months later, as the ACNP who provided care for Mr. J, you are served with a notice to initiate litigation against you for failing to meet the standard of care for Mr. J because his wound has worsened in rehab and has progressed to a stage IV pressure ulcer. Mr. J ultimately developed *Escherichia coli* sepsis and died before his 93rd birthday. The family alleges that the ACNP has failed to diagnose Mr. J's malnutrition.

The family will have to prove that the ACNP had a duty of care to Mr. J and it was the responsibility of the ACNP to diagnose his problems, including malnutrition. If the ACNP named was his care provider, proving duty is not difficult. As an ACNP and a health care provider, you have a duty to provide care to your patients in a nonnegligent manner.

The family would be responsible to show that the ACNP has breached this duty (Florida Statutes s. 766.102 (2008) "Medical Malpractice Act"). In a medical malpractice case, this is shown by proving that the health care provider has breached the standard of care. The standard of care is defined as "that level of care, skill, and treatment which, in light of all relevant surrounding circumstances, is recognized as acceptable and appropriate by reasonably prudent similar health care providers" (Florida Statutes s. 766.102 (2008) "Medical Malpractice Act"). In this case, the family would have to show that this is the standard of care to conduct testing for malnutrition (i.e., an albumin, prealbumin levels [monitoring] completed and a dietician consult completed).

The third element of a medical malpractice case is to show that Mr. J was damaged by the breach of the standard of care (Florida Statutes s. 766.102 (2008) "Medical Malpractice Act"). When Mr. J died, he was damaged, but the family will have to prove causation. In other words, the family will have to prove that his death was secondary to damages caused to Mr. J by the breach in the standard of care.

Without proof of the three elements of a medical malpractice claim, there is no case against the ACNP. At the very first hint of a medical malpractice claim, the ACNP should notify their insurance carrier. The carrier will identify an attorney as appropriate. Competent and careful health care providers should not live in fear of a malpractice suit but should acknowledge the existence of the litigious climate in contemporary health care. The prudent ACNP should be prepared and seek advice from professional legal council when appropriate.

End-of-Life Issues

ACNPs are confronted daily with patients and families coping with end-of-life issues. Regardless of how people reach the final stages of their lives, emotions run high and families are forced to make decisions that they would prefer not to make.

There are ethical and legal issues surrounding end-of-life care. Increasing medical technologies provide treatments and interventions for diseases and conditions that were once considered fatal. Bioethicists describe the sense of entitlement Americans have toward health care and their typical expectation for curative measures. Despite a limited expectation for recovery, futile care is expected and many times mandated as a "right." The role of the ACNP includes guiding patients and families through difficult decisions that occur with end-of-life care. There are many cases cited in the literature regarding dignity in death, hope of miracles and cures, and care that has become futile.

Case Study

Karen Ann Quinlan was an unfortunate young woman who inadvertently became a major figure in the right to die movement. She was a 22-year-old woman who stopped breathing after an evening out with friends. The report indicated that alcohol and prescription narcotics led to irreparable brain damage caused by prolonged anoxia and left her in a persistent vegetative state that requires ongoing ventilatory support. After some months of waiting for improvement, Karen Ann's parents recognized the futility of the care and requested that the hospital remove their daughter from the ventilator. The hospital declined and the parents sought judicial intervention (In re Quinlan, 1976).

The Quinlans sought the court's permission to terminate life support for their daughter (In re Quinlan, 1976). Prior to the Quinlan case, the general philosophy was that physicians should make end-of-life decisions for their patients and spare the families these difficult decisions. Although the philosophy could be argued to be part of that traditional "doctor-knows-best" theory, it was also meant to spare families the mental and emotional agony that end-of-life decisions can cause.

In addition to Karen's doctors and the hospital, the Attorney General of New Jersey intervened in the case arguing that the state has a compelling interest in the preservation of life (In re Quinlan, 1976). The Quinlans argued that Karen

Ann would not have wanted to continue life in a persistent vegetative state when there was no hope for a cure or even improvement (Wijdicks, 2002). However, the court chose not to consider this argument because it was felt there was no credible evidence that Karen Ann had ever expressed such an opinion. The court instead examined the Quinlans' right to privacy and their right to make their own personal, ethical, moral, and religious decision about treatment for Karen Ann (In re Quinlan, 1976). Although there is no explicit right to privacy in the United States Constitution, courts have consistently described a personal right of privacy and have held that certain areas of life are too private to justify state intervention (Eisenstadt v. Baird, 1972).

The New Jersey Supreme Court ultimately upheld that decisions made with regard to end-of-life care, at least in Karen Ann's case, are private ones that families may make without state interference. Karen Ann Quinlan's respiratory support was removed after the court's decision. She continued to live for another decade until she died of pneumonia in 1985 (Karen Ann Quinlan, Wikipedia, 2008). Karen Ann's family's tragedy has been attributed with the development of ethics committees in hospitals and with the proliferation of advanced directives.

Case Study

Nancy Cruzan was another young woman who made national headlines when she was left in a persistent vegetative state after an automobile accident (Ashley, 2005). Nancy's family sought the right to discontinue artificial hydration and nutrition in order to allow their daughter to die. Like Karen Ann's family, Nancy's family argued that Nancy would not have wanted to live in her present condition (*Cruzan, by her parents and co-guardians v. Missouri Department of Health,* 1990).

The Missouri Supreme Court and then the United States Supreme Court upheld that there was insufficient evidence that Nancy had expressed such an opinion prior to her accident and declined to allow the family to remove artificial nutrition and hydration. However, the court did recognize the right of a competent person to decline treatment including artificial nutrition and hydration if done in advance (*Cruzan, by her parents and co-guardians v. Missouri Department of Health*, 1990).

Following the decision by the court, congress enacted the Patient Self-Determination Act of 1990 (Ashley, 1990). The act requires hospitals to give inpatients information on advanced directives at the time of admission and to inform patients of their rights to refuse treatment.

Case Study

Terri Schiavo repeatedly made national headlines during an intense family battle regarding whether to withhold nutrition and hydration in order to allow Terri to die in 1990. Terri collapsed one evening in her home and suffered permanent brain damage caused by severe anoxia. Terri's husband, Michael, and her parents, the Schindlers, were initially highly motivated to seek treatment for Terri. But by 1998, a disagreement arose regarding the use or futility of treatment for Terri. Michael Schiavo and the Schindlers parted ways and Michael filed a petition in Pinellas County Circuit Court to remove Terri's feeding tube so as to allow her to die. The Schindlers maintained that Terri would not have wanted to die and a lengthy and acrimonious 7-year court battled ensued.

The Schiavo case resulted in national and international headlines and resulted in over 14 reported court opinions. Ultimately, the Schindlers' appeals were unsuccessful and the laws enacted by congress and the Florida legislature were held unconstitutional. Terri Schiavo died on March 31, 2005 after having hydration and nutrition withheld for 13 days (Terri Schiavo, Wikipedia, 2008).

During the Schiavo–Schindler legal battle, Terri Schiavo became a household name and an exemplar for the necessity of advanced directives. Emotions ran high and numerous religious, right-to-life, right-to-die, dignity in death, elders rights, disabilities rights, and other public interest groups intervened and spoke out on their feeling and beliefs concerning what was right for Terri. Florida Governor Jeb Bush, the Florida Legislature, and the United State Congress intervened as well. Ultimately, one must wonder how Terri would have felt about her life in the public eye for the last 7 years of her life. As ACNPs, probably the most important lesson learned from Terri Schiavo is the importance of advanced directives.

Each type of advanced directive serves a distinct purpose, and as an ACNP, basic understanding of advanced documentation is critical especially the living will and health care proxy. Ideally, these documents are thoughtfully considered by patients, discussed with family or significant others and will be prepared by an attorney well in advance of the time they are needed.

A living will is a type of advanced directive. This document describes when the treatments should be given or in what circumstances it should be withheld. This document may be as specific or as broad as the author intends. A person may specify his or her desire to enact, withhold, or withdraw treatment, not to initiate heroic measures, or even nutrition and hydration. Although each state may have separate legal requirements regarding the specific language that must be in a living will, what follows is a good example and complies with the law of Illinois (Living Will, n.d.) (Exhibit 2.5). However, each individual must be sure to comply with the legal requirements in their state, or the living will could be declared void by a court of law.

A legally correct living will must be signed and witnessed in some manner. The specific manner will be in accordance with appropriate state law: generally a correctly executed living will requires two witnesses. A health care proxy or health care power of attorney is another legal document that gives decision-making power to someone other than the patient. A person who is of sound mind may appoint a health care proxy to make health care decisions in the event that they become unable to do so. Presumably, the individual will have had some type of conversation with the health care proxy and the proxy will have an understanding of their desires and wishes. A legal document appointing a health care proxy can be similar to a living will, as in Exhibit 2.6, which complies with New York state law (New York State, n.d.). The significant difference is that a health care proxy is enacted when

Exhibit

2.5 Living Will Sample

LIVING WILL OF JANE DOE

This declaration is made this _____ day of _____(month, year).

I, _____, being of sound mind, willfully and voluntarily make known my desires that my moment of death shall not be artificially postponed.

If at any time I should have an incurable and irreversible injury, disease, or illness judged to be a terminal condition by my attending physician who has personally examined me and has determined that my death is imminent except for death-delaying procedures, I direct that such procedures which would only prolong the dying process be withheld or withdrawn, and that I be permitted to die naturally with only the administration of medication, sustenance, or the performance of any medical procedure deemed necessary by my attending physician to provide me with comfort care.

In the absence of my ability to give directions regarding the use of such death delaying procedures, it is my intention that this declaration shall be honored by my family and physician as the final expression of my legal right to refuse medical or surgical treatment and accept the consequences from such refusal.

Signed _____

City, County and State of Residence _____

The declarant is personally known to me and I believe him or her to be of sound mind. I saw the declarant sign the declaration in my presence (or the declarant acknowledged in my presence that he or she had signed the declaration) and I signed the declaration as a witness in the presence of the declarant. I did not sign the declarant's signature above for or at the direction of the declarant. At the date of this instrument, I am not entitled to any portion of the estate of the declarant according to the laws of intestate succession or, to the best of my knowledge and belief, under any will of declarant or other instrument taking effect at declarant's death, or directly financially responsible for declarant's medical care.

Witness _____ Date _____ Witness _____ Date _____

the patient can not make their own decisions and appoints a specific person to make health care decisions.

A document appointing a health care proxy must also comply with the requirements of the law of the state in which it is meant to be effective. Similar to a living will, this document will likely need to be witnessed by two witnesses. Generally, witnesses do not sign in any attempt to attest to the contents of the document but only to the authenticity of the signature of the patient.

Exhibit

2.6 Health Care Proxy Form

New York State Health Care Proxy Form

1. I, _____ hereby appoint
_____

(name, home address and telephone number)

as my health care agent to make any and all health care decisions for me, except to the extent that I state otherwise. This proxy shall take effect when and if I become unable to make my own health care decisions.

2. Optional instructions: I direct my agent to make health care decisions in accord with my wishes and limitations as stated below, or as he or she otherwise knows. (Attach additional pages if necessary.)

_____

_____

_____

(Unless your agent knows your wishes about artificial nutrition and hydration (feeding tubes), your agent will not be allowed to make decisions about artificial nutrition and hydration.

See instructions on reverse for samples of language you could use.)

(continued)

Exhibit

2.6   Health Care Proxy Form *(continued)*

3. Name of substitute or fill-in agent if the person I appoint above is unable, unwilling, or unavailable to act as my health care agent.

_____

(name, home address, and telephone number)

_____

4. Unless I revoke it, this proxy shall remain in effect indefinitely, or until the date or conditions stated below. This proxy shall expire (specific date or conditions, if desired):

_____

5. Signature _____

   Address _____

   Date _____

Statement by Witnesses (must be 18 or older)

I declare that the person who signed this document is personally known to me and appears to be of sound mind and acting of his or her own free will. He or she signed (or asked another to sign for him or her) this document in my presence.

Witness 1 _____

Address _____

Witness 2 _____

Address _____

Most states' Department of Health Web sites will contain the information needed to make sure that the living wills and health care proxy forms that are in use are legally sound. Hospitals have these forms available and it is likely that hospital attorneys have assisted in the development of the forms.

Case Study

A young woman, Amy, is involved in an automobile accident and has devastating injuries. She is hospitalized on life support and cared for by a team including an acute care nurse practitioner, Lisa Smith. Lisa asks the family if the young woman has a living will or a health care proxy and the family tells her she does not. Amy's parents feel that she would not have wanted to live on life support and wonder if there is hope for meaningful recovery. Amy's brother feels that everything should be done for her that is medically possible. The family, already experiencing a high level of stress, begins to argue. Lisa watches in dismay as the family's interactions deteriorate. She knows that had Amy had a living will or had appointed a health care proxy, many of the decisions involving Amy's care would be in line with Amy's wishes. As it stands now, the family will have to negotiate these difficult decisions amongst themselves or their family's tragedy may end up in the court system.

Conclusion

The role of the ACNP is complex and multidimensional. There are primary legal elements required to attain and maintain licensure, guide practice, and direct clinical practice agreements. In an effort to provide optimal care to patients, families, and society, ACNPs must comprehend and demonstrate a working knowledge of contemporary legal and ethical issues. Consultation with legal professionals should be viewed as a proactive strategy in establishing and maintain advanced clinical practice.

References

Ashley, R. C. (1990) Legal Counsel. Patient Self-Determination Act, Pub L No. 101–508 § 4206, 4751 (OBRA), 42 USC 1395 cc(a) et seq (1990). Cruzan, by her parents and co-guardians v . . . Critical Care Nurse, 25 (3): 60. Retrieved March, 2008, from ccn.aacnjournals.org/cgi/content/full/25/3/60

Ashley, R. C. (2005). Why are advanced directives legally important. *Critical Care Nurse, 25*(4), 56–57. Retrieved February 10, 2008, from http://ccn.aacnjournals.org/cgi/content/full/25/4/56

Atkinson, L. (2007). Who's in Charge. *Trial,* May.

American Academy of Nurse Practitioners. (n.d.). Map of Nurse Practitioner

Regulatory Authority. Retrieved March 22, 2008, from http://www.aanp.org

Christian, S., Catherine, D., & O'Neil, E. (2007). Chart Overview of Nurse Practitioner Scopes of Practice in the United States [Brochure]. Oakland, CA: UCSF Center for the Health Professions.

Cruzan, by her parents and co-guardians v. Missouri Department of Health, Supreme Court of the United States, 497 U.S. 261. (1990). [Electronic version]. Retrieved March 2008, from www.law.umkc .edu/faculty/projects/ftrials/conlaw/cruzan.html

Eisenstadt v. Baird, 405 US 438. (1972). Eisenstadt v. Baird. No. 70-17. [Electronic version] Retrieved March, 2008, from supreme.justia .com/us/405/438/case.html

Florida Administrative Weekly (2003) 29(39) Fla. Stat 464.003(3)(a) (2008). Retrieved March 2008, from http://www.leg.state.fl.us/STATUTES/

Florida Board of Nursing. (n.d.). ARNP Protocol. Retrieved April 22, 2008, from http://www.doh.state.fl.us/mqa/nursing/ProtocolSample.htm

In re Quinlan, 70 N.J. 10, 355 A.2d 647 (1976). [Electronic version] Retrieved March 2008, from law.jrank.org/pages/9617/Quinlan-in-Re.html

Likis, F. E. (2003). A novel model for collaborative practice guidelines. *Nurse Practitioner, 28*(7), 54–55.

Living will. (n.d.). Retrieved March, 2008, from Illinois Department of Public Health Web site: http://www.idph.state.il.us/public/books/Livin.PDF

Longworth, J. C. (n.d.). Sample Collaborative Practice Agreement. Retrieved February 25, 2008, from http://www.nonpf.com/fpcollab agreesample.htm

McCabe, S., & Burman, M. (2006). A Tale of Two APNs: Addressing Blurred Practice Boundaries in APN Practice. *Perspectives in Psychiatric Care, 42*(1), 3–12.

Model Nursing Practice Act (2004). Retrieved March, 2008, from National Council of State Boards of Nursing Web site: www.ncsbn.org

New York State Health Care Proxy Form. (n.d.) Retrieved March, 2008 from http://www.oag.state.ny.us/health/proxy_form.pdf

Terri Schiavo. (n.d.). Retrieved April 7, 2008, from Wikipedia Web site: http://en.wikipedia.org/wiki/Terri_Schiavo

The American Association of Nurse Attorneys. (n.d.). Retrieved March, 2008, from www.taana.org

The Florida Senate (Fla. Stat. § 456.0391). (2004). Review of data on physician availability and patient access to physician services [Electronic version]. Retrieved, March 22, 2008 from http://www .flsenate.gov/data/Publications/2004/Senate/reports/interim_reports/ pdf/2004-164hc.pdf

Wijdicks, E. F. (2002). Brain death worldwide: Accepted fact but no global consensus in diagnostic criteria. *Neurology, 58,* 20–25.

766.102 Florida Statutes - Definition of the Standard of Care [Electronic version]. Retrieved March, 2008, from www.floridamalpractice.com/ stat766.102.htm

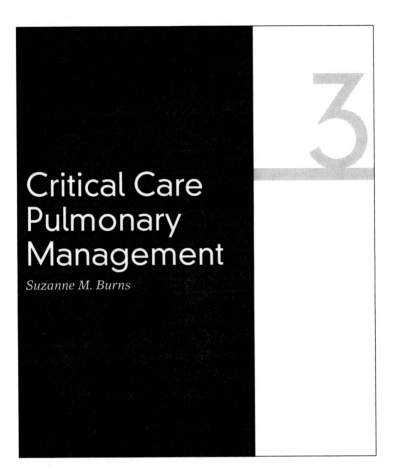

Critical Care Pulmonary Management

Suzanne M. Burns

Introduction

An essential component of critical care is the management of acute respiratory failure. Respiratory failure can result from a pulmonary or nonpulmonary insult and often requires the application of mechanical ventilation. This chapter focuses on the ventilatory management of patients with critical illness from intubation to weaning. To ensure that the application of mechanical ventilation is appropriately applied, a discussion of the pathophysiology of selected restrictive and obstructive conditions is included.

Restrictive and Obstructive Conditions

Restrictive Pathology

Restrictive conditions are those that result in decreased lung expansion. The conditions may be caused by thoracic chest wall abnormalities, such as a fibrothorax, or lung and/or pleural conditions. Restrictive conditions common to critical care are acute respiratory distress syndrome (ARDS), pneumonia, atelectasis, pulmonary edema, pleural effusions, and pneumothorax. Other less common conditions include bronchiolitis obliterans organizing pneumonia (BOOP) and neuromuscular conditions, such as myasthenia gravis, that result in a relative decrease in lung expansion secondary to weakness. Regardless of the condition, the pathology is often similar and is helpful to understand so that application of mechanical ventilation is appropriate. Table 3.1 (pages 52 through 55) lists selected obstructive and restrictive conditions.

When restrictive conditions exist, the result is a decrease in lung expansion and, subsequently, lung volume. Functional residual capacity (FRC) is reduced and compliance is decreased. Laplace's law describes how spherical air-filled objects, such as the alveoli, behave under these conditions. With a reduction in volume, the pressures acting on the sphere are increased and directed inward with the result being closure or collapse of the sphere. In contrast, with restoration of volume, the work associated with distending the sphere decreases. With restrictive diseases like ARDS, FRC is greatly reduced and the pressure, and subsequently the work of breathing required to open the alveoli, is high. Alveolar collapse results in the shunting of blood; oxygenation suffers and is refractory to provision of applied oxygen. Thus recruitment of the alveoli is necessary, and prevention of derecruitment is required. Whereas recruitment is an inspiratory maneuver (and will be described in detail later in this chapter), derecruitment is generally managed with the provision of applied positive end-expiratory pressure (PEEP).

Obstructive Pathology

Obstructive conditions are those in which there is limitation to airflow. Airway resistance results in a decrease in the flow of gases down the airways. To maintain flow, the pressure must be increased, which results in an increase in the work of breathing. Emphysema/chronic bronchitis and asthma are examples. For the purposes of this chapter, emphysema and chronic bronchitis are considered together and will be referred to as chronic obstructive pulmonary disease (COPD). Asthma will be discussed separately.

In COPD, the loss of alveolar surface area results in a decrease in the elastic properties of the lung and a resultant increase in FRC. The patient works at a mechanical disadvantage because the diaphragm is displaced downward and the chest is distended, requiring additional effort during exhalation to assure emptying. Exhalation is active, and early airway closure is common and contributes to airflow limitation and further hyperinflation. The net result is the increased work of breathing. Mucous plugging and bronchospasm may also exist and exacerbate airflow limitation.

With asthma, the major determinant of airflow limitation is airway resistance secondary to bronchospasm and, to some degree, mucous plugging. Bronchospasm makes exhalation difficult and results in hyperinflation of the lungs, especially with mechanical ventilation. This dynamic hyperinflation, or auto-PEEP (when on the ventilator), may result in pneumothorax and subsequent hypotension, and should be avoided.

Mechanical Ventilation: Modes and Methods

Criteria for intubation and initiation of mechanical ventilation generally fall into the following categories: apnea (and/or need for anesthesia with surgery), severe hypoxemia (PaO_2 ≤ 50 mmHg on room air), progressive or impending respiratory failure (serial arterial blood gases indicating worsening status with clinical signs and symptoms of fatigue), and acute respiratory failure (uncompensated respiratory acidosis and hypoxemia on room air). Once the patient is intubated, it is necessary to select a mechanical ventilator mode and associated parameters. Understanding the pathology of the condition necessitating mechanical ventilation is essential if the lung is to be protected while meeting hemodynamic and acid–base management goals.

Microprocessor technology has increased the versatility of traditional modes and has resulted in a wide variety of new

3.1 Examples of Selected Restrictive and Obstructive Pulmonary Conditions That Require Mechanical Ventilation

Condition	Category	Pathophysiology	Management	Comments
Acute Respiratory Distress Syndrome (ARDS)	Restrictive	Noncardiogenic pulmonary edema. pulmonary capillary leak. bilateral diffuse infiltrates, PaO_2/FiO_2 ratio < 200. Etiology is indirect or direct injury. High mortality.	*Treat etiology:* infection, trauma. hypotension. etc. *Supportive:* oxygenation. ventilation. cardiac output. *Optimize lung recovery and prevent lung injury:* avoid O_2 toxicity ($FiO_2 <$ .5–.6). tidal volumes: 6 ml/kg. (plateau pressures < 30). Maintain lung recruitment with PEEP. consider prone positioning.	Hypercarbia and associated acidosis may be the outcome of using lung protective strategies such as low lung volume ventilation and is referred to as permissive hypercarbia. PEEP at higher levels (14–16 cm H_2O range) may be necessary to recruit the lung.
Pneumonia	Restrictive	*Community Acquired:* Common organisms include *Streptococcus pneumoniae. Haemophilus Influenzae. Moraxella catarrhalis,* viruses, and atypicals (*Legionella. Mycoplasma etc.*)	Treatment of all pneumonias is dependent on diagnostic category: start with empiric coverage first and adjust with recovery of organism or treatment failure.	If the patient is immune compromised, bronchoscopy is done early to recover organism.

	Hospital Acquired: (within 3–5 days of being in the hospital, recent hospitalization, nursing home, etc.). These pneumonias are often the result of an aspiration and resistant bacteria such as methicillin-resistant *Staphylococcus aureus* (MRSA), *Pseudomonas, Enterobacter, and Serratia* are often responsible. *Ventilator Associated Pneumonia (VAP):* after 3–5 days of mechanical ventilation.	VAP is preventable and measures should be put in place upon intubation (elevate head of bed >30 degrees, etc.)
Bronchiolitis Obliterans Organizing Pneumonia or Cryptogenic Organizing Pneumonitis (BOOP/COP)	Restrictive	BOOP is seen with connective tissue disorders, solid organ transplantation, and infections such as *Legionella.* It is called idiopathic BOOP or cryptogenic organizing pneumonia (COP) when its etiology is undetermined. Commonly, the patient presents with a community acquired pneumonia that fails to respond to antibiotics. The course is usually subacute, developing over 2 weeks to 6 months of the initial event. Biopsy findings may show a widespread inflammatory response with terminal and respiratory bronchiole involvement as well as the alveolar ducts.	The majority of patients respond to corticosteroids. Treatment is usually required for at least 6 months. Cytotoxic therapy is considered early if failure to respond to steroids is seen.

(continued)

3.1

Examples of Selected Restrictive and Obstructive Pulmonary Conditions That Require Mechanical Ventilation *(continued)*

Condition	Category	Pathophysiology	Management	Comments
Idiopathic Pulmonary Fibrosis (IPF)	Restrictive	It is an uncommon inflammatory/fibrotic interstitial lung disorder of unknown etiology.	Corticosteroids are the mainstay of treatment, although their role is now being questioned. Cyclophosphamide can be used as a second immunosuppressive agent. Single-lung transplant is the definitive therapy	The disease was originally described by Hamman and Rich as a fulminant form of pneumonitis.
COPD (emphysema /bronchitis)	Obstructive	*Chronic Bronchitis:* Chronic or recurrent excess mucus production in bronchial tree. Occurs 3 months in a year for 2 consecutive years. Common to have repeated respiratory infections (RSV: respiratory syncytial virus, strep pneumonia, H-flu) *Emphysema:* Abnormal permanent enlargement of airspaces distal to terminal bronchiole, accompanied by destruction of the walls. Centrilobular proximal, most common. Panlobular (panacinar), entire acinus involved. Lower lobes more involved with alpha 1-antitrypsin deficiency	Relieve reversible airway obstruction, cough control, and sputum production. Eliminate/prevent airway infections. Increase exercise tolerance and control complications (cardiovascular and hypoxemia)	Generally, emphysema and bronchitis are considered together because they often have similar pathology.

| Acute Severe Asthma (ASA) | Obstructive | Severe acute bronchoconstriction that is intense, unrelenting, and unresponsive to usual therapy. Pathology includes airway inflammation, bronchoconstriction, and mucus production. | *Bronchodilators*: beta 2-agonists (1st line), anticholinergics (2nd but often given in combination with beta agonists), steroids (always a first line drug). Oxygen. Hydration. Antibiotics if infection suspected. | Methylxanthine and magnesium have been used but rarely. |

sophisticated mode options. However, despite many available mode options, there is little scientific evidence supporting the selection of any one mode over another. Instead, the clinician must carefully apply the options to selected conditions to assure good outcomes. To that end, a discussion of volume and pressure modes follows. Table 3.2 (pages 56 through 58) describes traditional and common mode parameters found on most ventilators. Table 3.3 (pages 58 through 61) describes the parameters required for selected volume and pressure modes.

3.2 Traditional Ventilator Parameters

Parameter	Settings	Comments
Fraction of Inspired Oxygen (FiO_2)	Variable from .21–1.00	High levels of FiO_2 (>50%) are considered toxic. Positive end-expiratory pressure (PEEP) is added to recruit lung and decrease shunt and ventilation/perfusion mismatch.
Tidal Volume (Vt)	8–12 ml/kg. With acute lung injury or ARDS use 6 ml/kg	Remember the combination of Vt, f, and Ti contribute to hyperinflation in obstructive conditions.
Respiratory Rate/ frequency (f)	Rate is initially set between 10–20. Once the Vt is determined, the rate is adjusted to attain desired $PaCO_2$ level.	"Normal" $PaCO_2$ is not a goal for all mechanical ventilation. In ARDS, lung protection using small Vts will result in anticipated hypercarbia and acidosis. This is referred to as "permissive hypercarbia".
Inspiratory time (Ti)	Average adult Ti = .7–1.0 seconds	Ti is determined by the flow rate of the gas. The higher the flow, the shorter the Ti (for any given Vt). Increasing flow increases pressure. Very high fs result in very short Tis; the flow pattern becomes very turbulent, and gas distribution is poor.

Parameter	Settings	Comments
	I/E ratio is usually 1:2 or 1:3	Generally, obstructive conditions require longer expiratory times to prevent auto-PEEP. In contrast, restrictive conditions do not require long expiratory times.
Sensitivity (Pressure and/or flow triggering)	*Pressure sensing:* generally set between −1 to −2 cm H_2O. The greater the negative pressure, the harder the patient work to get a breath.	Flow triggering (if set correctly) results in less patient work than does pressure sensing.
	The smaller the flow sensitivity number (e.g., 500 ml/min), the more sensitive the ventilator. The higher the setting (e.g., 1–2L/min), the less sensitive. Set at the minimal level above auto-triggering.	Generally, flow sensing will default to pressure sensing if not set correctly (i.e., the flow trigger is too large)
Positive End-Expiratory Pressure (PEEP)	PEEP of 5 cm H_2O is considered "physiologic." Weaning below this level is rarely necessary. Higher levels are required to "recruit the lung".	Maintains positive pressure at end exhalation. "Recruits" alveoli & holds them open. Restores functional residual capacity (FRC).
	When exhalation is inadequate, auto-PEEP (occult or hidden PEEP) is the result. Auto-PEEP may be an anticipated result of some ventilator modes such as PC/IRV, or an undesirable result of inadequate ventilator settings.	Factors that contribute to auto-PEEP include expiratory resistance, low elastic recoil, high MV, short expiratory time, mucus hypersecretion, increased wall thickness and airway closure or collapse. Mechanical factors like water in the circuit may also result in auto-PEEP.

(continued)

3.2 Traditional Ventilator Parameters (continued)

Parameter	Settings	Comments
Continuous Positive Airway Pressure (CPAP)	Pressure is maintained continuously above baseline (i.e., "0"). CPAP is a spontaneous breathing mode. As with PEEP, it is used to restore FRC. Other uses are as a spontaneous breathing method for weaning and for noninvasive ventilation as in obstructive sleep apnea (serves as a pneumatic splint to keep the upper airway open during sleep).	

3.3 Volume and Pressure Modes and Corresponding Ventilator Parameters

Mode Name	Main Parameters	Comments
Assist Control (A/C)	V_t f_x T_i Sensitivity FiO_2 PEEP	Generally considered a support mode. Must switch to another mode or method for weaning.
Synchronized Intermittent Mandatory Ventilation (SIMV)	V_t RR T_i Sensitivity FiO_2 PEEP	Originally used as a "weaning mode"; however, work of breathing is high at low IMV rates. Often used in conjunction with PSV.

Mode Name	Main Parameters	Comments
Pressure Support Ventilation (PSV)	PS level Sensitivity FiO_2 PEEP	Pressure is often arbitrarily selected (e.g., 10–20 cm H_2O) then adjusted up or down to attain the desired tidal volume. Some use the plateau pressure if transitioning from volume ventilation as a starting point.
Pressure Control Ventilation (PCV)	IPL *fx* *Ti* Sensitivity FiO_2 PEEP	Varients of PCV include *Volume Assured Pressure Options* and some other modes such as *Airway Pressure Release Ventilation* and *BiLevel Ventilation*. They are listed below.
Pressure Controlled-Inverse Ratio Ventilation	As for PCV, an inverse I/E ratio is attained by lengthening the *Ti*. Inverse ratios include 1:1, 2:1, 3:1, and 4:1.	Some ventilators allow for the I/E ratio to be selected.
Airway Pressure Release Ventilation	Pressure high (P_{HIGH}) - the high CPAP level Pressure low (P_{LOW}) which is generally 0–5 cm H_2O Time high (T_{HIGH}) Time low (T_{LOW}) FiO_2	Generally, the CPAP level is adjusted to assure adequate oxygenation, whereas the *fx* of the releases are increased or decreased to meet ventilation goals. *Vt* is variable dependent on the CPAP level, compliance and resistance of the patient, and patient spontaneous effort.
Volume Assured Pressure Modes (1–5 below)	These modes provide pressure breaths with a volume guarantee.	These modes are ventilator specific. Although the simi larities are greater than the differences, they are called different names. Often, the names suggest that the mode is a volume mode yet a decelerating flow pattern (associated with pressure ventilation) is always provided.
1. Volume Support (VS)	*Vt.* Sensitivity FiO_2 PEEP	The pressure level is automatically adjusted to attain the desired *Vt*. If control of pressure is desired, it must be carefully monitored.

(continued)

3.3 Volume and Pressure Modes and Corresponding Ventilator (continued)

Mode Name	Main Parameters	Comments
2. Pressure-Regulated Control (PRVC)	fx and Ti set in addition to those set for VS	As with VS, the difference is that this is a control mode. Spontaneous breaths however may also occur.
3. Volume Support (VS)	Vt Sensitivity FiO_2 PEEP	This mode is one option in a category called "Volume Ventilation Plus." This is the spontaneous breathing option in this category and is similar to VS above.
4. Volume Control Plus (VC+)	fx and Ti are set in addition to those set for VS	This mode is also a mode option listed in the category called "Volume Ventilation Plus". To access this mode, the user selects the SIMV or assist control (both control modes) then selects VC+. For some clinicians, this is confusing as it appears that the patient is on two different modes versus VC+.
Bilevel Positive Airway Pressure (Bilevel or BiPAP)	$PEEP_H$ $PEEP_L$ fx and Ti	If additional support is desired for patient-initiated breathing, Psupp may be selected as well. Attention to Vt is important, because the patient can augment Vt significantly with supported spontaneous breaths.
Adaptive Support Ventilation (ASV)	Body weight %MinVol (minute volume) High pressure limit	Once basic settings are selected, ASV is started and %MinVol is adjusted if indicated. Spontaneous breathing is automatically encouraged, and when the inspiratory pressure (Pinsp) is consistently $= 0$ and fx control (rate) $= 0$, extubation may be considered.

Mode Name	Main Parameters	Comments
Proportional Assist Ventilation (PAV)	Proportional Pressure Support- PPS$_{TM}$ (Drager Medical, Canada): PEEP, FiO$_2$, % volume assist, and flow assist Proportional Assist Plus ([PAV+] Puritan Bennett, now Covidien) PEEP, FiO$_2$, % Support	Depending on the ventilator, the amount of "assist" that is provided is determined by the clinician, and different parameters are selected to do so. Default % support numbers are recommended, but the clinician must determine the timing of reductions of the same.
Automatic Tube Compensation (ATC)	Endotracheal tube internal diameter % compensation	This is not a mode but rather a pressure option to offset the work associated with tube resistance. It can be combined with other modes or can be used alone as in a CPAP weaning trial.

Adapted with permission from Burns SM. Pressure Modes of Mechanical Ventilation: The good, bad and the ugly. *Advanced Critical Care*. 2008; 19: 399–411.
Key: *Vt*: tidal volume; PS: pressure support; FiO$_2$: fraction of inspired oxygen; PEEP: positive end-expiratory pressure; IPL: inspiratory pressure level; *fx*: respiratory frequency; *Ti*: inspiratory time; PEEP$_H$: high PEEP; PEEP$_L$: low PEEP; Psup: pressure support in bilevel mode; MinVol: minute volume.

Volume Versus Pressure Modes

Volume ventilators are still in use but are increasingly being supplanted by pressure modes. One reason for the current popularity of pressure modes is the characteristic decelerating flow pattern of pressure breath delivery that is associated with improved gas distribution (Figure 3.1).

With volume ventilation, a predetermined volume is delivered with each breath regardless of changes in compliance or resistance (Figure 3.2). Pressure increases or decreases accordingly on a breath to breath basis. In contrast, when pressure modes were first introduced, pressure was selected by the clinician and it remained stable, whereas volume varied with changing compliance and resistance. Unlike the earlier pressure mode options, newer pressure modes no longer sacrifice volume for pressure. Current ventilators allow for guaranteed volumes while delivering the pressure breath with the characteristic decelerating flow pattern.

3.1

Decelerating Flow Pattern With Pressure Ventilation

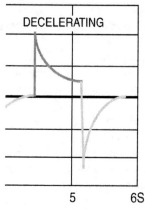

Reprinted by permission from Nellcor Puritan Bennett LLC. Boulder, Colorado, part of Covidien.

3.2

Square Flow Pattern With Volume Ventilation (A-B)

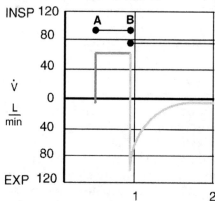

Reprinted by permission from Nellcor Puritan Bennett LLC. Boulder, Colorado, part of Covidien.

Although it is not within the scope of this chapter to describe every mode available on ventilators manufactured today, categories of ventilator modes are described for the reader's reference. The Acute Care Nurse Practitioner (ACNP) is encouraged to access specific manufacturer ventilator operating user manuals for specific details related to the modes and how to adjust ventilators to assure proper mode operation.

Volume Modes

Control Mandatory Ventilation (CMV). CMV is the term used when the goal is to prevent patient–ventilator interaction. This is usually accomplished with the aid of sedation and sometimes neuromuscular blockade. (Figure 3.3).

Assist/Control Ventilation (A/C) A/C delivers volume breaths at a predetermined rate and inspiratory time. Between the control breaths, the patient can initiate a respiration and upon doing so receives a volume breath as configured for

3.3

Pressure Waveform: Control Mandatory Ventilation

(A: No spontaneous effort noted, all breaths are control breaths.)

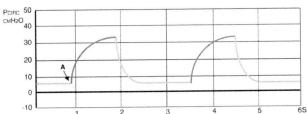

Reprinted by permission from Nellcor Puritan Bennett LLC, Boulder, Colorado, part of Covidien.

3.4

Pressure Waveform: Assist Control Ventilation

The arrow points to a negative deflection representing a patient-initiated breath. Once the patient initiates the breath, a volume as set for the control breaths is delivered.

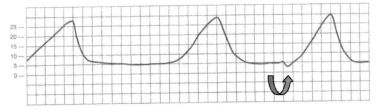

3.5

Pressure Waveform: Synchronized Mandatory Ventilation

Note: The first arrow is pointing to a mandatory volume breath. The second arrow is pointing to one of the patient-initiated breaths.

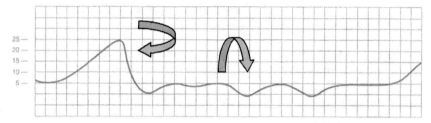

the control breaths (Figure 3.4). This mode is useful when the goal is to provide full ventilatory support. The patient must be transitioned to another mode when able to be weaned from mechanical ventilation.

Synchronized Intermittent Mandatory Ventilation (SIMV). With SIMV, the ventilator synchronizes the delivery of volume breaths at a predetermined rate and inspiratory time. The patient may breathe spontaneously between mandatory breaths at his/her own respiratory rate and tidal volume. (Figure 3.5).

Early studies on the use of SIMV suggest that the work of breathing associated with spontaneous breathing at low SIMV rates is excessive. Thus, pressure support ventilation (PSV) is often used to support the patient-initiated breaths. Although this combination of pressure-supported and volume-supported breaths is common, weaning times may be prolonged with the combination mode. This will be discussed later in the section on weaning.

The manner in which the traditional volume modes operate related to patient–ventilator interaction is important to remember. Some of the new ventilator pressure mode options require the user to select a mode setting that is called SIMV or A/C, so that pressure breath delivery is configured similarly. For example, a pressure mode may be selected, but how the breaths are delivered may depend on the selection of either an A/C or SIMV setting. If A/C is selected, the control pressure breaths will be delivered at the predetermined rate and inspiratory time, and when the patient initiates a breath, a control pressure breath is delivered. With the selection of SIMV, the spontaneous breaths will be patient controlled (e.g., inspiratory time, volume, and rate).

Pressure Modes

Pressure Support Ventilation (PSV). PSV is a spontaneous breathing mode. With PSV, the clinician selects the pressure level, but the patient determines the rate (f), tidal volume (Vt), and inspiratory time (Ti). Spontaneous inspiration is augmented with the PSV level. (Figure 3.6). High levels of PSV provide almost full ventilatory support, whereas the gradual reduction in the pressure level allows for a progressive increase in workload (MacIntyre, 1997).

Pressure Control Ventilation (PCV) and Pressure Control Inverse Ratio Ventilation (PC/IRV). PCV was first introduced as a mode used in patients with ARDS. The idea was to control airway pressure while providing a decelerating flow pattern. At the time, it was not known if peak airway pressure or plateau pressure was responsible for lung injury. Inverse ratio ventilation (IRV) was used to lengthen inspiration in an attempt to keep the lung open for longer periods of time (Tharrat, Allen, & Albertson, 1988). Given the restrictive nature of ARDS, the prolonged inspiratory to expiratory (I/E) ratio could be adjusted from 1:1 to 4:1 to assure improved oxygenation. (Figure 3.7). These modes require that the clinician designate a pressure level, rate, and inspiratory time.

A common problem encountered with the use of traditional PC/IRV is the inability of the patient to receive adequate gas flow

3.6

Pressure Waveform: Pressure Support (square pressure waveform)

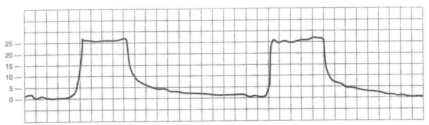

3.7

Pressure Waveform: Pressure Controlled/Inverse Ratio Ventilation

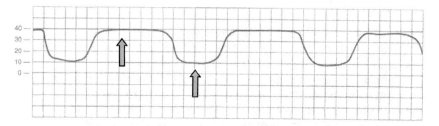

with spontaneous effort. Thus, sedatives and paralytic agents have been required to assure patient–ventilator synchrony. Although traditional PC/IRV is rarely used today (newer technology allows for improved flow to the patient upon demand), the concept of preventing derecruitment of alveoli with a prolonged inspiratory time is incorporated into more sophisticated modes such as airway pressure release ventilation.

Airway Pressure Release Ventilation (APRV) and Biphasic Ventilation. APRV is a spontaneous breathing mode that requires the selection of a relatively high level (15–20 cm H_2O) of continuous positive airway pressure (CPAP) and short timed-frequency releases (1–1.5 sec) to a baseline pressure. This mode is designed for use in patients with ARDS who require a high level of pressure to recruit alveoli (Cane, Peruzzi, & Shapiro, 1991). The short releases prevent derecruitment and aide in the elimination of CO_2. The extremely short airway pressure releases are the hallmark of APRV and set it apart from PCV and biphasic ventilation (Putensen et al., 2001). (Figure 3.8)

Biphasic ventilation may be considered a form of PCV and/or PC/IRV, depending on the inspiratory to expiratory ratio. Similar to the two modes, an inspiratory pressure level and PEEP level are selected in addition to *Ti* and *f*. In contrast to traditional PC or PC/IRV, biphasic ventilation allows for patient breathing during all portions of the respiratory cycle. Spontaneous breathing may be assisted with PS if additional support is desired. Parameters for the inspiratory pressure and PEEP levels are referred to as *high PEEP* and *low PEEP or high pressure and low pressure.* (Figure 3.9)

3.8

Airway Pressure Release Ventilation

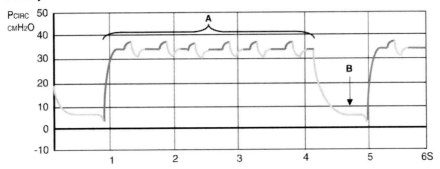

Reprinted by permission from Nellcor Puritan Bennett LLC, Boulder, Colorado, part of Covidien.

Both APRV and biphasic modes appear to be safe and effective and may have the additional advantage of not requiring the use of muscle relaxants or heavy sedatives to assure patient–ventilator synchrony (Rathgeber et al., 1997). The microprocessor technology in these modes allows for rapid delivery of flow throughout the cycles for the support of spontaneous patient breathing.

Volume-Assured Pressure Modes. This category includes several ventilator mode options that provide a pressure breath

3.9

Biphasic or Bilevel Ventilation

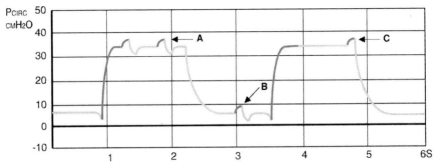

Reprinted by permission from Nellcor Puritan Bennett LLC, Boulder, Colorado, part of Covidien.

(with a decelerating pressure waveform) combined with a volume guarantee. Despite the mode names, which often have *volume* in the title, these modes are designed to deliver pressure breaths. Some examples of volume assured pressure modes are volume support (VS), pressure-regulated volume control (PRVC), and volume control plus (VC+) (Puritan Bennett product information, 2008; Maquet product information, 2008).

VS is a spontaneous breathing mode, whereas PRVC is not. With each mode, the ventilator automatically adjusts the pressure level (in 3 cm H_2O increments) on a breath-to-breath basis to attain the clinician-desired volume (Figure 3.10). Similar to PRVC, VC+ is the mandatory option of a volume guaranteed pressure mode. Both PRVC and VC+ are considered *control* modes and require that respiratory frequency (*fx*) and inspiratory time (*Ti*) are selected for the control breaths.

Adaptive Support Ventilation (ASV) (Hamilton medical product information 2008). This mode is referred to by the manufacturer as *intelligent ventilation*. The mode is designed to assess lung mechanics on a breath-to-breath basis (controlled loop ventilation) for spontaneous and control settings. It automatically adjusts mandatory *fx* and *Ti* to attain the optimal *Vt* (as determined by the ventilator calculations). The ventilator is designed to adapt workload so that elastic and resistive loads are minimized. It automatically promotes spontaneous breathing in all modes, and parameter adjustments are few. Settings include body weight, % min volume, and a high

3.10

Volume Support Ventilation

Note that the pressure level is increased on a breath-to-breath basis to maintain the volume, and that all breaths are patient initiated. Pressure-regulated volume control is similar, but the rate is set.

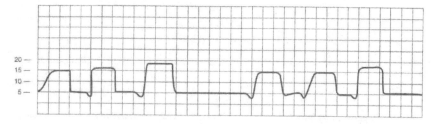

pressure limit. The ventilator has built-in lung protective algorithms that activate automatically. They include strategies to minimize auto-PEEP, prevent apnea, tachypnea, excessive dead space, and excessively large breaths.

Proportional Assist Ventilation (PAV) (Draeger product information, 2008; Puritan Bennett product information, 2008). PAV was designed to assist breath-to-breath ventilation in proportion to the resistance and elasticity of the system. To that end, current PAV modes take measurements throughout the inspiratory cycle and then automatically adjust the pressure, flow, and volume proportionally. Different names for the modes are provided by specific manufacturers and parameters that require varying adjustments. Essential parameters in which to apply this mode include the percent of volume assist and flow assist.

Automatic Tube Compensation (ATC). ATC is available in many of the microprocessor ventilators and is designed to overcome the work of breathing induced by artificial airways. Although it is not a mode of ventilation per se, it does adjust pressure (proportional to tube resistance) required to provide a variable fast inspiratory flow during spontaneous breathing. The clinician must enter the internal diameter of the artificial airway and the proportion of compensation for the ventilator to accurately compensate for tube resistance.

What Modes are Best?

Although the new modes of ventilation are attractive because of their sophistication, versatility, and potential applications, little data exists that demonstrates their superiority. Instead, application, understanding, and familiarity with the modes are the key to good outcomes. Variation in practice breeds mistakes and should be decreased when possible. When clinicians do not understand the modes, the potential for inaccurate and inefficient management exists. This is true throughout the continuum of ventilation (from the acute stage to the weaning stage). Thus, it is essential that the ACNP understand the modes, so that they are appropriately applied.

Perhaps the greatest challenge with regard to mechanical ventilation is the management of the most complex patients. ARDS and acute severe asthma (ASA) are two extreme examples of restrictive and obstructive pathology. A discussion of the ventilatory management of these conditions follows.

Ventilatory Management of ARDS and ASA

Background

As noted in Table 3.1, ARDS is often referred to as non-cardiac pulmonary edema. The precipitating event may be nonpulmonary, as in the case of sepsis, or pulmonary, as in the case of aspiration pneumonia. Regardless of the etiology, the result is a pulmonary capillary leak. Pathologic changes include ventilation abnormalities, decreased lung compliance (and atelectasis), shunting, and refractory hypoxemia. Work of breathing is very high, and high pressures are required to open the lung (Dreyfuss & Saumon,1993). Most patients with ARDS require mechanical ventilation as a supportive measure, while treatment of the underlying condition that precipitated the ARDS is accomplished. Mortality continues to be as high as 50% (TenHoor, Mannino, & Moss, 2001).

Over 20 years ago, investigators studying the ARDS lung in animal models began to recognize the relationship of high distending pressures to lung injury. They noted that with the use of large traditional volumes (at that time between 12 and 20 ml/kg) and pressures >35 cm H_2O, animals that were ventilated for >72 hours suffered alveolar fractures and edema. The lung injury was referred to as *volutrauma* (Dreyfuss, Bassset, Soler & Saumon, 1985; Dreyfuss, Soler, Bassett, & Saumon, 1988; Dreyfuss & Saumon, 1998, Fu, Z. et al., 1992).

Subsequent studies clarified other potential mechanisms of injury in the noncompliant ARDS lung. Computed tomography (CT) scans taken of the ARDS lung demonstrated that the disease distribution was not homogeneous, meaning that the pressure delivered to the lung was preferentially being delivered to "open" areas (Gattinoni et al., 1986). This syndrome was referred to as *baby lung*, and it was noted that these areas were especially prone to injury from the distending forces of a big breath.

An additional study noted that when the lung is not fully recruited, the forces needed to open the stiff alveoli are large and with repetitive tidal opening; the associated stress resulted in injury. It was suggested that recruitment with PEEP was necessary to keep the lung open and prevent this "repetitive opening injury."

Amato et al., (1995) subsequently noted in a randomized controlled trial that higher PEEP levels were associated with improved mortality and other outcomes in patients with ARDS. Using inflection pressures to determine the optimal PEEP level to recruit the lung, they noted that levels of 14–16 cm H_2O were often necessary to achieve lung recruitment (Amato et al., 1995; Amato et al., 1998).

Tidal volume (*Vt*) and the related pressures to attain *Vt* were also the focus of randomized controlled trials (RCT). Hickling, Henderson, and Jackson (1990) noted that patients ventilated with low volume ventilation had lower mortality than those ventilated with traditional lung volumes. In a multisite study sponsored by the National Heart, Blood, and Lung Institute of the National Institutes of Health, 800 patients meeting the criteria for ARDS (i.e., PaO_2 /FiO_2 < 300, noncardiac, bilateral infiltrates) were assigned to low-volume ventilation or traditional volume ventilation (6 vs. 12 ml/kg, respectively). FiO_2 and PEEP were assigned in an algorithmic approach (The ARDS Clinical Trials Network, 2000). The results of the study noted 25% lower mortality in those ventilated at the lower lung volumes. Although the results were dramatic, it was difficult to determine what part PEEP (and/or auto-PEEP) contributed to the improved outcomes. In a subanalysis of the data, it was also noted that the plateau pressure associated with the low and traditional tidal volume ventilation strategies were ~26 and 35, respectively (The ARDS Clinical Trials Network, 2000). These plateau pressures were substantially less than those noted to be injurious in animal models. See Exhibit 3.1 for the definition and measurement of plateau pressure.

The evidence related to mechanical ventilation of patients with ARDS suggests that application of selected protective lung strategies is essential. They include the use of low tidal volume ventilation (6 ml/kg), lung recruitment with PEEP, and the prevention of derecruitment (The Acute Respiratory Distress Syndrome Network, 2003)

Application of Protective Lung Strategies in ARDS.

- *Low lung volume ventilation.* Volume modes of ventilation are useful to assure that tidal volumes of 6 ml/kg (lean body weight) are consistently delivered. To maintain a pH that is within an acceptable range, *fx* is generally high (20–30). If this protective strategy results in hypercarbia and acidosis, it may be necessary to sedate and paralyze the patient to depress respiratory drive.

Exhibit

3.1 Measurements of Compliance and Resistance

Compliance (or how easy it is to distend the lungs and chest wall) is measured with a plateau pressure.
Resistance (how easy it is to move gases down the airways) is measured by noting the difference between peak airway pressure and plateau pressure.

Plateau pressure (also known as distending pressure, static pressure, and alveolar pressure) is the pressure required to hold the lungs and chest wall open. It is referred to as a "static" measurement because it is measured at the end of a full inspiration during a breath hold (no air flow). The resultant pressure is generally 10–15 cm H_2O less than the *peak airway pressure*. This occurs because the pressure required to assure the flow of gas down the airways contributes to the peak airway pressure (which is the result of both airways resistance and lung/chest wall compliance). During the end-inspiratory hold maneuver, this flow is eliminated. With decreased compliance, the plateau pressure will increase. In obstructive conditions such as asthma, resistance to airflow is high and pressure must increase to maintain flow. Resistance is measured by performing a plateau pressure maneuver and is the difference between peak airway pressure and plateau pressure. Increased resistance will result in an increase in peak airway pressure and, with severe hyperinflation, an increased plateau pressure as well.

Measurement of plateau pressure:
1. Switch to volume mode of ventilation for measurement.
2. At the end of inspiration, activate the end-inspiratory hold button.
3. Hold briefly while observing the peak airway pressure.
4. The peak pressure will drop, and the resulting pressure is the plateau pressure.
5. This maneuver is difficult to do in a spontaneous breathing patient and may require sedation (and sometimes neuromuscular blockade) to accomplish accurately.

Permissive hypercarbia is relatively well tolerated in many patients, but it is contraindicated in those with elevated intracranial pressure and in some with cardiac conditions (Hickling et al., 1990). When pressure modes are used, constant attention to the delivered volumes is necessary. Furthermore, it is important to remember that the plateau pressure necessary to prevent lung injury is unknown. Based on the ARDS network study, the required plateau pressure may be within a 26–30 cm H_2O range; however, plateau pressure is reflective of chest wall as well as lung, thus making it difficult to determine what the pressure goal should be.

■ *Lung recruitment* is generally accomplished with PEEP. Unfortunately, it is clinically very difficult to determine what critical opening pressure is required to uniformly recruit the ARDS lung. Some have used maneuvers such as the "40/40 or 60/60 maneuvers" for lung recruitment (Foti et al., 2000; Fujino et al., 2001). These consist of using critical opening pressures (PEEP) of 40 or 60 cm H_2O for 40–60 seconds. The techniques are difficult to accomplish and carry the additional risk of barotrauma. Instead, many use high levels of PEEP (e.g., 14–16 cm H_2O) and monitor the effect on PaO_2. Unfortunately, improved oxygenation may result from recruitment or may be the result of redistribution of blood flow to aerated areas of the lung. Definitive methods of assessing lung recruitment are few and include serial CT scans with changes in PEEP (very unrealistic cost and labor intensive). Another method is to monitor plateau pressure with increases in PEEP. With this technique, plateau pressure should remain stable or decrease with increases in PEEP. In contrast, an increase in plateau pressure with the addition of PEEP may be reflective of overdistention. Prone positioning may also be used to "recruit lung" (Tobin & Kelly, 1999, Albert, Lesa, Sanderson, Robertson, & Hlastala, 1987) although definitive data demonstrating positive effects on mortality secondary to prone positioning are lacking (Gattinoni et al., 2001; Mancebo et al., 2006). However, subanalyses in the existing studies do suggest that the technique may result in improved outcomes in those with the most severe ARDS (PaO_2/FiO_2 ratios of <100) (Gattinoni et al., 2001; Mancebo et al., 2006). Further studies are necessary to clarify the use of prone positioning, especially as related to duration, frequency, and timing of the technique. Regardless of the method used to assure recruitment, it is important to remember that derecruitment occurs quickly, such as when the ventilator circuit is broken, and is to be avoided.

Acute Severe Asthma (ASA)

Background. The hallmark pathologies in asthma include airway inflammation, bronchospasm, and mucus production. With ASA, therapy consists of aggressive pharmacologic management and mechanical ventilation when necessary. Pharmacologic management includes treatment of inflammation with steroids, bronchodilators (specifically β-2 agonists and anticholinergics), and fluid resuscitation. Despite definitive pharmacologic therapies, many of these patients require admission to a critical care unit and support with mechanical ventilation. Unfortunately, ventilating patients with ASA is difficult and must be carefully achieved if lung injury and death are to be avoided. Mortality associated with ventilation of the ASA patient is generally low but is noted to be as high as 22% in some patients (Mansel, Stogner, Petrini, & Norman, 1990). Morbidity associated with the mechanical ventilation of patients with asthma includes dynamic hyperinflation and auto-PEEP, hypotension (the effect of intrathoracic pressure on venous return), and barotrauma (Pepe & Marini, 1982; Mansel et al., 1990).

Dynamic hyperinflation refers to the overdistension of the lung related to bronchospasm and is common with ASA. Exhalation is incomplete as a result of airway narrowing and noncommunicating airways (from bronchospasm or mucus plugging). The diaphragm is displaced into a disadvantageous downward position in the chest. This mechanical disadvantage results in a substantial increase in the work of breathing. With mechanical ventilation, inadequate exhalation time results in hyperinflation and is called auto-PEEP. Factors contributing to auto-PEEP include expiratory resistance, low elastic recoil, high minute ventilation, high rates, short expiratory times, mucus hypersecretion, increased wall thickness, and airway closure or collapse. Mechanical factors, such as water in circuits, also can result in auto-PEEP. Thus, interventions are aimed at preventing and/or reducing auto-PEEP.

Application of Protective Lung Strategies for ASA

■ Prevent hyperinflation and auto-PEEP by decreasing the rate, shortening the inspiratory time, and decreasing the volume. In severe cases, sedation and even neuromuscular blockade will be necessary to accomplish these interventions because they will result in hypercarbia and acidosis (and increased respiratory drive). The goal is to prevent morbidity and mortality associated with auto-PEEP. Measurement of resistance and plateau pressure may be done to track progress and assess adequacy of interventions. Refer to Exhibit 3.1 on page 72.

▨ Assume hyperinflation and auto-PEEP in patients with ASA. Measure auto-PEEP. The absence of auto-PEEP does not necessarily mean it is not present. Instead, it simply may not be measurable. Noncommunicating airways secondary to early airway closure during exhalation, mucus, and/or severe bronchoconstriction may prevent measurement (Leatherman & Ravenscraft, 1996). Occasionally, applied PEEP will help by preventing closure of the airways during exhalation and will allow for better emptying (refer to Exhibit 3.2).

Exhibit

3.2 Measurements of Auto-PEEP

Auto-PEEP or occult PEEP is a result of inadequate exhalation time from any cause.

Measurement:
1. At the end of a full expiration (right before inspiration), activate the end-expiratory hold button.
2. Observe the baseline pressure (set PEEP level or zero). As gases in the system equilibrate, the baseline pressure will rise to a higher pressure if auto-PEEP is present.
3. Auto-PEEP is the difference between the higher pressure and the baseline pressure.
4. In some cases, noncommunicating airways secondary to early airway closure during exhalation, mucus plugging and bronchospasm preclude accurate measurement of auto-PEEP. Applied PEEP may help by preventing premature airway closure. To assess, a plateau pressure is checked following application of PEEP. If no increase in plateau pressure occurs (or if it decreases), the addition of PEEP is resulting in more complete exhalation. If, however, the plateau pressure increases with the addition of PEEP, it is contributing to alveolar overdistension and should be decreased.

▓ If hypotension is noted with mechanical ventilation of the patient with ASA, consider a brief cessation of mechanical ventilation. This may be lifesaving as the hypotension may be the result of extreme levels of auto-PEEP. This is often noted with vigorous or over-zealous mechanical ventilation of these patients.

Summary: Ventilatory Management of ARDS and Asthma

Ventilating the sickest patients requires an understanding of the pathophysiology of the conditions and knowledge of existing evidence related to the appropriate application of management strategies. In the case of ARDS (a restrictive disorder) and ASA (an obstructive disorder), lung protection is essential to assure good outcomes, yet the methods to do so differ greatly. Although many other obstructive and restrictive conditions may require mechanical ventilation, different concepts related to ventilation of these individual conditions, exemplified with the discussions of ARDS and ASA, may be applied.

Weaning From Mechanical Ventilation

The process of weaning from mechanical ventilation has evolved greatly over the last 10 years. Prior to studies that employed protocols for weaning trials, weaning was accomplished with a wide variety of modes and methods; variability in practice was the norm. We know that protocols for weaning trials work because they decrease practice variability. Randomized controlled trials indicated that the combination of weaning trial screens (to determine when to start a trial); protocols for how to accomplish the weaning trial (mode, method, and when to stop); and multidisciplinary approaches to weaning resulted in improved outcomes (Esteban et al., for the Spanish Lung Failure Collaborative Group, 1995; Ely et al., 1996; Marelich et al., 2000; Kollef et al., 1997; Burns et al., 1998; Burns et al., 2003; Smyrnios et al., 2002).

Weaning is not just about ventilator management. As noted in two systematic reviews, prior to weaning, attention to the myriad of pulmonary and nonpulmonary factors that affect weaning should be corrected (Cook, Meade, Guyatt, Griffith, &

Booker, 1999; MacIntyre, Cook et al., 2001). In addition, research in the area of sedation management and other care elements, such as glucose control, suggest that ventilator duration, ICU and hospital length of stay, including mortality data, may also be positively affected with the use of standardized management algorithms and protocols (Brook et al., 1999; Kress, Pohlman, O'Connor, & Hall, 2000; Van den Berghe, et al., 2001).

A discussion of sedation management, assessment of readiness to wean, and the design and use of weaning protocols follows. In addition, a brief discussion related to the timing of tracheostomy is included.

Weaning Assessments

Although it is understood that the underlying condition or disease resulting in the need for mechanical ventilation must be improved prior to weaning, rarely is that enough to assure weaning success, especially in those requiring mechanical ventilation for longer than 3 days. These patients suffer from iatrogenic insults that further compromise their recovery. Ventilator-associated pneumonia (VAP), gastro-intestinal bleeding, urinary tract infection (UTI), pneumo-thorax, immobility, and venous thromboembolism (VTE) are just a few subsequent sequelae that can emerge over time (Cook. et al., 1996; Geerts et al., 2001; Chastre & Fagon, 2002). Thus, management of the ventilator patient actually begins with intubation and must include interventions to eliminate impediments to weaning and prevent complications with appropriate prophylaxis and treatments.

One very important factor to assess is the need for seda-tion in the ventilated patient with critical illness. Sedation, especially infusions of sedatives, although necessary in some cases, may adversely affect the ventilated patient. Brook, et al., (1999) and Kress, et al., (2000) found that standardized sedation management methods, such as daily sedative inter-ruptions, sedation vacation, and algorithmic approaches, respectively resulted in better outcomes, such as ventilator duration and length of stay (LOS) (Brook et al., 1999; Kress et al., 2000). Additional work by Kress et al., demonstrated that daily sedation infusion interruptions decreased long-term psychological stress and resulted in fewer iatrogenic complications in patients compared with the outcomes of those who did not experience daily sedative interruptions

(Kress et al., 2003; Schweickert, Gehlbach, Pohlman, Hall, & Kress, 2004).

Perhaps most intriguing, is the link between sedation and delirium (Dubois, Bergeron, Dumont, Dial, & Skrobik, 2001). Benzodiazepines are an independent risk factor for delirium (Pandharipande et al., 2006) And some individuals who experienced delirium developed an unanticipated long-term cognitive dysfunction (Ely et al., 2001; Ely et al., 2004). Thus, the ACNP should consider stopping sedatives as early as feasible in the course of a patient's stay. As noted in Table 3.4 below, sedation protocols and methods to systematically decrease sedation are linked with improved outcomes.

Although head–to-toe assessments are part of routine ACNP care management, there are many key elements, such as sedation, that represent impediments to weaning, and these should be addressed systematically. "Checklists" prevent omissions and errors that may delay care or even result in untoward events (Gawande, 2008). Thus, the use of a checklist to assure "weaning readiness" is helpful to the team and keeps care planning on target. One such checklist is the *Burns Wean Assessment Program* (BWAP) (Exhibit 3.3). The use of this checklist, in combination with a systematic comprehensive care management model, is associated with improved weaning times, ICU and hospital LOS, and subsequent mortality (Burns, S., Burns J., & Truwit, 1994; Burns et al., 1998; Burns et al., 2003).

3.4	Effect of Sedation Management Protocols on Selected Outcomes by Author			
Author (type of protocol)	Vent Duration	ICU-LOS	Hosp-LOS	Mortality
Kress et al[10] (sedation protocol)	Yes*	Yes*	No	No
Brook et al[9] (sedation protocol)	Yes*	Yes*	Yes*	No

*Statistically significant.

Exhibit

3.3 Burns Wean Assessment Program (BWAP) (©1990)

GENERAL ASSESSMENT

YES	NO	NOT ASSESSED	
___	___	___	1. Hemodynamically stable? (Pulse rate, cardiac output)
___	___	___	2. Free from factors that increase or decrease metabolic rate (seizures, temperature, sepsis, bacteremia, hypo/hyper thyroid)?
___	___	___	3. Hematocrit >25% (or baseline)?
___	___	___	4. Systemically hydrated? (weight at or near baseline, balanced intake and output)?
___	___	___	5. Nourished? (albumin >2.5, parenteral/enteral feedings maximized) If albumin is low and anasarca or third spacing is present, score for hydration should be "no."
___	___	___	6. Electrolytes within normal limits? (including Ca^{++}, Mg^+, PO_4). *Correct Ca^{++} for albumin level.
___	___	___	7. Pain controlled? (subjective determination)
___	___	___	8. Adequate sleep/rest? (subjective determination)
___	___	___	9. Appropriate level of anxiety and nervousness? (subjective determination)
___	___	___	10. Absence of bowel problems (diarrhea, constipation, ileus)?
___	___	___	11. Improved general body strength/endurance? (i.e., out of bed in chair, progressive activity program)?
___	___	___	12. Chest x-ray improving or returned to baseline?

(continued)

Exhibit

3.3   Burns Wean Assessment Program (BWAP) (©1990) *(continued)*

RESPIRATORY ASSESSMENT

YES	NO	NOT ASSESSED	

Gas Flow and Work of Breathing

___   ___   ___   13. Eupneic respiratory rate and pattern (spontaneous RR <25, without dyspnea, absence of accessory muscle use).
*This is assessed <u>off</u> the ventilator while measuring #20–23.RR = ___

___   ___   ___   14. Absence of adventitious breath sounds? (rhonchi, rales, wheezing)

___   ___   ___   15. Secretions thin and minimal?

___   ___   ___   16. Absence of neuromuscular disease/deformity?

___   ___   ___   17. Absence of abdominal distention/obesity/ascites?

___   ___   ___   18. Oral ETT > #7.5 or trach > #6.0 (I.D.)

Airway Clearance

___   ___   ___   19. Cough and swallow reflexes adequate?

Strength

___   ___   ___   20. NIP <−20 (negative inspiratory pressure)
<u>NIP</u> = ___

___   ___   ___   21. PEP >+30 (positive expiratory pressure)
<u>PEP</u> = ___

Endurance

___   ___   ___   22. STV >5 ml/kg (spontaneous tidal volume)?
Spont VT = ___   <u>STV/BW in kg</u> =

___   ___   ___   23. VC > 10–15 ml/kg (vital capacity)?
<u>VC</u> =

ABGs

___   ___   ___   24. pH 7.30–7.45

___   ___   ___   25. $PaCO_2$~40 mm/hg (or baseline) with M.V. <10 L/min
*This is evaluated while on ventilator.
<u>$PaCO_2$</u> = ___   MV =

___   ___   ___   26. PaO_2 >60 on FiO_2 <40%

Weaning Screens

Weaning screens were first introduced by Esteban et al., (1995) in a research protocol seeking to determine the best weaning method (Esteban et al., Spanish Lung Failure Collaborative Group, 1995). This RCT first "screened" ventilated patients using a short list of criteria that represented stability using such clinical measures such as FiO_2 and PEEP levels and the need for vasopressors and other clinical criteria. Patients meeting the screening criteria were assigned to a 2-hour spontaneous breathing trial (SBT). If signs of intolerance emerged during the trial interval, mechanical ventilation was resumed, and the patient was randomized to one of three protocol-driven weaning methods. Those that tolerated the 2-hour trial were extubated. Of the extubated cohort, 20% required reintubation.

Intrigued with this study, Ely et al., (1996) sought to determine the safety and efficacy of SBTs in coronary and medical intensive care patients. Using a weaning screen similar to that used by Esteban et al., (1995), patients who passed the screen were randomly assigned to a SBT or traditional weaning (as determined by the team on a daily basis). The study results demonstrated that ventilator duration was significantly improved in those assigned to the intervention and that the reintubation rate was only 4%. The conclusion indicated that use of a protocol-driven SBT in patients who passed a simple weaning screen was both safe and effective.

The weaning screen, in contrast to a full assessment of potential impediments to weaning, is a tool used to provide a rapid snapshot of the patient's stability. The screen is not comprehensive, but rather is designed to assure that an aggressive weaning trial may be safely attempted while preventing delays. With the implementation of the weaning screen, the next step is to attempt a spontaneous breathing trial. The choice of ventilator mode is somewhat arbitrary and, to some degree, determined by clinician preference. Regardless, the most common methods for SBTs include CPAP at a low level (e.g., 5 cm H_2O) or T-piece trials. Many also use PSV at a low level. Decisions related to protocol development and selection of mode follow.

Protocol Development: Modes, Methods, etc.

Studies suggest that a weaning trial method using SBTs of CPAP or T-piece for 2 hours or less are effective and safe (Esteban, et al., Spanish Lung Failure Collaborative Group, 1995; Ely et al.,

1996). Some prefer to use PSV for trials in those who are weak or who have cardiac problems that preclude the more stressful CPAP or T-piece trials. It is likely that any of these methods will work well provided that they do not result in delayed progression of weaning trials and assure prompt return to the ventilator when the patient demonstrates intolerance.

One exception to selection of modes for weaning may be the combined use of SIMV and PSV. In a survey seeking to determine methods of weaning and subsequent ventilator duration, the combination of SIMV plus PSV was associated with significantly longer ventilator times than other methods (Esteban, Alia, Ibanez, Benito, & Tobin, 1994). Although it continues to be unclear why such a result occurred, it is possible that the main problem with using these modes in combination is that doing so increases the complexity of the plan. The process of weaning SIMV and/or PSV is more complicated than if simply placed on an SBT of CPAP for example. In busy critical care units, multiple changes in mode parameters are difficult to accomplish in a timely fashion and lead to variation in practice. The less complicated the better.

The most effective protocols are easy to apply and clearly understood by caregivers. Essential elements of the protocol include mode, method, signs of intolerance (and what to do if they emerge), and duration of the trial. Finally, how to rest the patient between trials and at night are important to delineate. Exhibit 3.4 is an example of a weaning trial protocol that incorporates all these elements.

Timing of Tracheostomy

Clinicians and scientists have long debated the merits of early versus delayed tracheostomy placement. Retrospective and observational studies suggest that early tracheostomy is associated with lower costs, shorter duration of ventilation, ICU LOS, and hospital LOS (Brook, Sherman, Malen, & Kollef, 2000; Freeman, Borecki, Coopersmith & Buchman, 2005). In addition, one study noted that patients with tracheostomies required less sedation, spend less time heavily sedated, and achieve more autonomy earlier in the course of the hospitalization (Nieszkowska et al., 2005).

Recently in a prospective, randomized study of patients who were projected to require mechanical ventilation for >14 days, medical patients with critical illness were assigned

Exhibit

3.4 Example of Weaning Trial Protocol: CPAP

Weaning Trial Screen:

1. Hemodynamic stability (no dysrhythmias, HR ≤120, absence of pressors—low dose dopamine and dobutamine are exceptions)
2. FiO_2 ≤50%
3. PEEP ≤8 cm H_2O
4. Patient comfortable and able to interact

CPAP Protocol:

1. One trial for 1 hour on CPAP of no more than 8 cm H_2O.
2. With any signs of intolerance, the trial is discontinued and the patient is returned to a resting mode until the next trial.
3. When trial is completed without signs of intolerance, the team is approached and extubation potential is discussed.
4. Full respiratory muscle rest is provided between trials and at night.

Intolerance is defined as any of the following:

1. RR ≥35 for 5 mins.
2. O_2 sat ≤90% or a decrease of 4%
3. HR ≥140 and/or a 20% sustained change of HR in either direction
4. Systolic BP ≥180, ≤90 mm Hg
5. Excessive anxiety or agitation
6. Diaphoresis

Rest:

1. PSV max: PSV max is that pressure level required to attain a RR of 20 or less and a Vt of 8–12 ml/kg. Respiratory pattern should be synchronous and there should be no accessory muscle use.
2. Other modes: With volume modes of ventilation (i.e. A/C or IMV), respiratory muscle rest is not assured unless there is cessation of respiratory muscle activity. Therefore, rest is considered that level of support required to prevent patient initiated breaths. When IMV is used, PSV may be added for protection (i.e. as a "safety"). Regardless, the goal is cessation of spontaneous effort

to early percutaneous dilatational tracheotomy (within 48 hours of intubation) or to delayed tracheotomy (Rumbak et al., 2004). Mortality, incidence of pneumonia, and accidental extubations were all statistically significant and showed improvement in the early tracheostomy group compared with the controls. Although the reason why early tracheostomy resulted in better outcomes is not known, it is possible that the lower requirement for sedation was responsible. In addition, the presence of tracheostomy provides an element of safety that is not possible with an endotracheal tube; reintubation following an unsuccessful trial is not necessary. Thus, earlier and potentially more aggressive trials with a tracheostomy are possible.

In patients with tracheostomies who require excessively prolonged stays on the ventilator (i.e., weeks or months), spontaneous breathing trials can be progressed gradually. A plan incorporating daytime trials, with nighttime rest on the ventilator works well until they can tolerate a full 12 hours. At that point, extension of the trial into the nighttime hours is reasonable.

Summary

Managing complex patients with respiratory failure requires attention to a myriad of factors that affect outcomes from the acute to the weaning stages of mechanical ventilation. An understanding of the pathophysiology of conditions resulting in respiratory failure, modes of ventilation and their appropriate applications, and how best to wean patients is essential. The application of evidence-based methods and systematic, comprehensive approaches goes a long way in assuring good outcomes. Continuity and consistency clearly showed decreasing variations, which is an important step in the weaning process.

References

Albert, R. K., Lesa, D., Sanderson, M., Robertson H. T., & Hlastala, M. P. (1987). The prone position improves arterial oxygenation and reduces shunt in oleic-acid- induced acute lung injury. *American Review of Respiratory Disease*, 628–633.

Amato, M. B. P., Barbas, C. S., Medeiros, D. M., Shettino, G de., Lorenzi-Filho, G., Kairalla, R.A., et al. (1995). Beneficial effects of the "open lung approach" with low distending pressures in acute respiratory distress syndrome. A prospective randomized study on mechanical ventilation. *American Journal of Respiratory and Critical Care Medicine, 152,* 1835–1846.

Amato, M. B., Barbas, C. S., Medeiros, D. M., Magaldi, R. B., Schettino, G. P., Lorenzi-Filho G, et al. (1998). Effect of protective ventilation strategies on mortality in the acute respiratory distress syndrome. *New England Journal of Medicine, 338,* 347–354

Brook, A. D., Ahrens, T. S., Schaff, R., Prentice, D., Sherman, G., Shannon, W., et al. (1999). Effect of a nursing-implemented sedation protocol on the duration of mechanical ventilation. *Critical Care Medicine, 27,* 2609–2615.

Brook, A. D., Sherman, G., Malen, J., & Kollef, M. H. (2000). Early versus late tracheostomy in patients who require prolonged mechanical ventilation. *American Journal of Critical Care, 9,* 352–359.

Burns, S. M., Burns, J. E., & Truwit, J. D. (1994). Comparison of five clinical weaning indices. *Journal of Critical Care, 3,* 332–352

Burns, S. M., Earven, D., Fisher, C., Lewis, R., Merrel, P., Schubart, J. R., et al. (2003).Implementation of an institutional program to improve clinical and financial outcomes of patients requiring mechanical ventilation: One year outcomes and lessons learned. *Critical Care Medicine, 31,* 2752–2763.

Burns, S. M., Marshall, M., Burns, J. E., Ryan, B., Wilmoth, D., Carpenter, R., et al. (1998). Design, testing, and results of an outcomes-managed approach to patients requiring prolonged ventilation. *Journal of Critical Care, 7,* 45–57.

Cane, R. D., Peruzzi, W. T., & Shapiro, B. A. (1991). Airway pressure release ventilation in severe acute respiratory failure. *Chest, 100,* 460–463.

Chastre, J., & Fagon, J. (2002). State of the art: ventilator–associated pneumonia. *American Journal of Respiratory Critical Care Medicine, 165,* 867–903.

Cook, D., Meade, M., Guyatt, G., Griffith, L., & Booker, L. (1999). *Evidence report on criteria for weaning from mechanical ventilation.* Contract No. 290-97-0017. Agency for Health Care Policy and Research, 6010 Executive Blvd., Suite 300, Rockville, MD, 20852. USA.

Cook, D. J., Reeve, B. K., Guyatt, G. H., Heyland, D. K., Griffith, L. E., Buckingham, L., et al. (1996). Stress ulcer prophylaxis in critically ill patients. Resolving discordant meta-analyses. *Journal of American Medicine Association, 275,* 308–314.

Draeger Critical Care Product information: retrieved January 2, 2008, from http://www.draeger.com/MT/internet/pdf/CareAreas/CriticalCare/cc_evita_atcpps _br_en.pdf

Dreyfuss, D., Basset, G., Soler, P., & Saumon, G. (1985) Intermittent positive-end expiratory pressure hyperventilation with high inflation pressures produces pulmonary microvascular injury in rats. *American Review of Respiratory Disease, 132,* 880–884

Dreyfuss, D., & Saumon, G. (1998). Ventilator induced lung injury. *American Review of Respiratory Disease, 157,* 294–323.

Dreyfuss, D., & Saumon, G. (1993). The role of tidal volume, FRC and end-inspiratory volume in the development of pulmonary edema following mechanical ventilation. *American Review of Respiratory Disease, 148,* 1194–1203.

Dreyfuss D., Soler P., Bassett, G., & Saumon, G. (1988). High inflation pressure pulmonary edema. *American Review of Respiratory Disease, 137,* 1159–1164.

Dubois, M. J., Bergeron, N., Dumont, M., Dial, S., & Skrobik, Y. (2001). Delirium in an intensive care unit: a study of risk factors. *Intensive Care Medicine, 27,* 1297–1304.

Ely, E. W., Baker, A. M., Dunagan, D. P., Burke, H. C., Smith, A. C., Kelly, P. T., et al. (1996). Effect on the duration of mechanical ventilation of identifying patients capable of breathing spontaneously. *New England Journal of Medicine, 335,* 1964–1969.

Ely, E. W., Gautam, S., Margolin, R., Francis, J., May, L., Speroff, T., et al. (2001). The impact of delirium in the intensive care unit on hospital length of stay. *Intensive Care Medicine, 27,* 1892–1900.

Ely, E. W., Shintani, A., Truman, B., Speroff, T., Gordon, S. M., Harrell, F. E., Jr., et al. (2004). Delirium as a predictor of mortality in mechanically ventilated patients in the intensive care unit. *Journal of American Medicine Association, 291,* 1753–1762.

Esteban, A., Alia, I., Ibanez, J., Benito, S., & Tobin, M. J. (1994). Modes of mechanical ventilation and weaning a national survey of Spanish hospital. *Chest, 106,* 1188–93.

Esteban, A., Frutos, F., Tobin, M. J., Alía, I., Solsona, J. F., Valverdú, I., et al. (Spanish Lung Failure collaborative Group). (1995). A comparison of four methods of weaning patients from mechanical ventilation. *New England Journal of Medicine, 332,* 345–350.

Foti, G., Cereda, M., Sparacino, M. E., De Marchi, L., Villa, F., & Pesenti, A. (2000). Effects of periodic lung recruitment maneuvers on gas exchange and respiratory mechanics in mechanically ventilated acute respiratory distress syndrome (ARDS) patients. *Intensive Care Medicine, 26,* 501–507.

Freeman, B. D., Borecki, I. B., Coopersmith, C. M., & Buchman, T. G. (2005). Relationship between tracheostomy timing and duration of mechanical ventilation in critically ill patients. *Critical Care Medicine, 33,* 2513–2520.

Fu, Z., Costello, M. L., Tsukimoto, K., Prediletto. R., Elliott, A. R., Mathieu-Costello, O., et al. (1992). High lung volume increases stress failure in pulmonary capillaries. *Journal of Applied Physiology, 73,* 123–133.

Fujino, Y., Goddon, S., Dolhnikoff, M., Hess, D., Amato, M. B., & Kacmarek, R. M. (2001). Repetitive high-pressure recruitment maneuvers required to maximally recruit lung in a sheep model of acute respiratory distress syndrome. *Critical Care Medicine, 29,* 1579–1586.

Gattinoni, L., Presenti, A., Torresin, A., Baglioni, S., Rivolta, M., Rossi, F., et al. (1986) Adult respiratory distress syndrome profiles by computed tomography. *Journal of Thoracic Imaging, 1,* 25–30.

Gattinoni, L., Tognoni, G., Pesenti, A., Taccone P, Mascheroni D, Labarta V., et al. (2001). Effect of prone positioning on the survival of patients with acute respiratory failure. *New England Journal of Medicine, 345,* 568–573.

Gawande, A. (2008). *The Checklist.* retrieved February 22, 2008, from http://www.newyorker.com/reporting/2007/12/10/071210fa_fact_gawande?currentPage=1

Geerts, W. H., Heit, J. A., Clagett, G. P., Pineo, G. F., Colwell, C. W., Anderson, F. A., Jr., et al. (2001). Prevention of venous thromboembolism. *Chest, 119*(1 Suppl), 132S–175S.

Hamilton Medical Product information: retrieved January 2, 2008, from http://www.hamilton-medical.com/GALILEO-ventilators.37.0.html

Hickling, K. G., Henderson, S. J., & Jackson, R. (1990). Low mortality associated with low volume pressure limited ventilation with permissive hypercapnia in severe adult respiratory distress syndrome. *Intensive Care Medicine, 16,* 372–377.

Kollef, M. H., Shapiro, S. D., Silver, St John, R. E., Prentice, D., Sauer, S., et al. (1997). A randomized, controlled trial of protocol-directed versus physician-directed weaning from mechanical ventilation. *Critical Care Medicine, 25,* 567–574.

Kress, J. P., Gehlbach, B., Lacy, M., Pliskin, N., Pohlman, A. S., & Hall, J. B. (2003). The long-term psychological effects of daily sedative interruption on critically ill patients. *American Journal of Respiratory Critical Care Medicine, 168,* 1457–1461.

Kress, J. P., Pohlman, J. S., O'Connor, M. F., & Hall, J. B. (2000). Daily interruption of sedative infusions in critically ill patients undergoing mechanical ventilation. *New England Journal of Medicine, 342,* 1471–1477.

Leatherman, J., & Ravenscraft, S. A. (1996). Low measured auto-positive end expiratory pressure during mechanical ventilation of patients with severe asthma: hidden auto-positive end-expiratory pressure. *Critical Care Medicine, 24,* 541–546.

MacIntyre, N. R. (1997). Ventilatory muscles and mechanical ventilatory support. *Critical Care Medicine, 25,* 1106–1107.

MacIntyre, N. R., Cook, D. J., Ely, E. W., Epstein, S. K., Fink, J. B., Heffner, J. E., et al. (2001). Evidence-based guidelines for weaning and discontinuing ventilatory support: a collective task force facilitated by the American College of Chest Physicians; the American Association for Respiratory Care; and the American College of Critical Care Medicine. *Chest, 120*(6 Suppl), 375S–395S.

Mancebo, J., Fernandez, R., Blanch, L., Rialp, G., Gordo, F., Ferrer, M., et al. (2006). A multicenter trial of prolonged prone ventilation in severe acute respiratory distress syndrome. *American Journal of Respiratory Critical Care Medicine, 173,* 1233–1239.

Mansel, J. K., Stogner, S. W., Petrini, M. F., & Norman, J. R. (1990). Mechanical ventilation in patients with acute severe asthma. *American Journal of Medicine, 89,* 42–48.

Maquet Product information: Retrieved January 2, 2008, from http://www.maquet.com/productPage.aspx?m1=112599774495&m2=112808545902&m3=105584076919&productGroupID=112808545902&productConfigID=10 5584076919&languageID=1&titleCountryID=224

Marelich, G. P., Murin, S., Battistella, F., Inciardi, J., Vierra, T., & Roby, M. (2000). Protocol weaning of mechanical ventilation in medical and surgical patients by respiratory care practitioners and nurses: effect on weaning time and incidence of ventilator associated pneumonia. *Chest, 118,* 459–467.

Nieszkowska, A., Combes, A., Luyt, C., Ksibi, H., Trouillet, J., Gilbert, C., et al. (2005). Impact of tracheotomy on sedative administration, sedation level, and comfort of mechanically ventilated intensive care unit patients. *Critical Care Medicine, 33,* 2527–2533.

Pandharipande, P. P., Shintani, A., Peterson, J., Pun, B. T., Wilkinson, G. R., Dittus, R. S., et al. (2006). Lorazepam is an independent risk factor for transitioning to delirium in intensive care unit patients. *Anesthesiology, 104,* 21–26.

Pepe, P. E., & Marini, J. J. (1982). Occult positive end-expiratory pressure in mechanically ventilated patients with airflow obstruction. *American Review of Respiratory Disease, 126,* 166–170.

Puritan Bennett product information: Retrieved January 2, 2008, from http://www.puritanbennett.com/prod/Product.aspx?S1=VEN&S2=SOF&id=292

Putensen, C., Zech, S., Wrigge, H., Zinserling, J., Stuber, F., Von Spiegel, T., et al. (2001). Long-term effects of spontaneous breathing during ventilatory support in patients with acute lung injury. *American Review of Respiratory Critical Care Medicine, 164,* 43–49

Rathgeber, J., Schorn, B., Falk, V., Kazmaier, S., Speigel, T., & Burchardi, H. (1997). The influence of controlled mandatory ventilation (CMV), intermittent mandatory ventilation (IMV) and biphasic intermittent positive airway pressure (BIPAP) on duration of intubation and consumption of analgesics and sedatives. A prospective analysis in 596 patients following adult cardiac surgery. *European Journal of Anaesthesia, 14,* 576–582

Rumbak, M. J., Newton, M., Truncale, T., Schwartz, S. W., Adams, J. A., & Hazard, P. B. (2004). A prospective, randomized study comparing early percutaneous dilatational tracheotomy to prolonged translaryngeal intubation (delayed tracheotomy) in critically ill medical patients. *Critical Care Medicine, 32,* 1689–1694.

Smyrnios, N. A., Connolly, A., Wilson, M. M., Curley, F. J., French, C. T., Heard, S. O., et al. (2002). Effects of a multifaceted, multidisciplinary, hospital-wide quality improvement program on weaning from mechanical ventilation. *Critical Care Medicine, 30,* 1224–1230.

Schweickert, W. D., Gehlbach, B. K., Pohlman, A. S., Hall, J. B., & Kress, J. P. (2004). Daily interruption of sedative infusions and complications of critical illness in mechanically ventilated patients. *Critical Care Medicine, 32,* 1272–1276.

TenHoor, T., Mannino, D. M., & Moss, M. (2001). Risk factors for ARDS in the United States: analysis of the 1993 National Mortality Followback Study. *Chest, 119,* 1179–1184.

Tharrat, R. S., Allen, R. P., & Albertson, T. E. (1988). Pressure-controlled inverse ratio ventilation in severe adult respiratory failure. *Chest, 94,* 755–762.

The Acute Respiratory Distress Syndrome Network (2000). Ventilation with lower tidal volumes as compared with traditional tidal volumes for acute lung injury and the acute respiratory distress syndrome. *New England Journal of Medicine, 342,* 1301–1307.

The ARDS Clinical Trials Network; National Heart, Lung and Blood Institute: National Institutes of Health. (2003). Effects of recruitment maneuvers in patients with acute lung injury and acute respiratory distress syndrome ventilated with high positive end-expiratory pressure. *Critical Care Medicine, 31,* 2592–2597

Tobin, A., & Kelly, W. (1999). Prone ventilation-it's time. *Anaesthesia Intensive Care, 27,* 194–201.

Van den Berghe, G., Wouters, P., Weekers, F., Verwaest, C., Bruyninckx, F., et al. (2001). Intensive Insulin Therapy in Critically Ill Patients. *New England Journal of Medicine, 354,* 1359–1367.

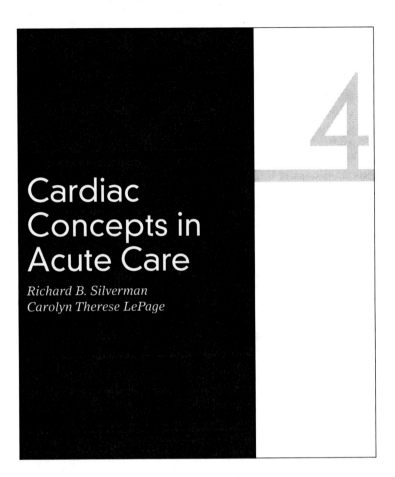

Cardiac Concepts in Acute Care

Richard B. Silverman
Carolyn Therese LePage

Introduction

In 1999, the American Heart Association (AHA) set a strategic
goal of reducing the death rates from coronary heart disease
and stroke and reducing 25% of the risk factors for these diseases by 2010 (AHA, 2008). The most current data reflects that
in 2005, the United States had achieved this initial goal (CDC,
2008). The reduction equates to approximately 160,000 lives
saved in 2005 compared to the 1999 baseline data. The AHA
cites this progress in the reduction of death rates as a landmark
achievement.

These accomplishments have been achieved as a result of
tremendous efforts from many partners in practice, research,
health care, government, business, and communities. Despite

this encouraging data, heart disease remains number one and stroke remains number three as the leading causes of death in the United States (CDC, 2008). There are goals that have not been achieved, such as reductions in the risk factors that lead to heart disease and stroke, as well as eliminating the striking disparities in care for women and minority populations. Continuous attention by health care providers is essential to address both acute and primary care issues required to reduce death and disability among the population in the United States.

The AHA regularly publishes scientific statements, guidelines, performance measures, and clinical data standards. Their purpose is to increase knowledge and awareness of health care professionals regarding effective, state-of-the art science related to the causes, prevention, detection, and management of cardiovascular diseases (AHA, 2008). AHA scientific statements represent the consensus of the leading experts in cardiovascular disease and stroke and are subjected to blind peer review prior to approval by the highest scientific body of the AHA (AHA, 2008).

In 2000, the AHA launched the "Get with the Guidelines" program to help hospitals treat patients with evidence-based strategies to optimize patient outcomes for heart disease and stroke. These guidelines have affected more than one million people to date. Consistent with the national focus on health care quality, the American College of Cardiology (ACC) and the AHA have developed a multifaceted strategy to facilitate the process of improving clinical care. One aspect of this effort is the creation of clinical practice guidelines that carefully synthesize available evidence to guide better patient care. Such guidelines are written to suggest diagnostic or therapeutic interventions that apply to patients in most circumstances, but clinical judgment is required to adapt these guidelines to the care of individual patients. The guidelines are based on available evidence, providing varying degrees of recommendation.

Clinical guidelines, as defined by the Institute of Medicine's definition, are "systematically developed statements to assist practitioner and patient decisions about appropriate health care for specific clinical circumstances." The AHA often develops practice guidelines in conjunction with the ACC, but may also independently institute practice guidelines or develop a partnership with other organizations as appropriate. All current guidelines adhere to the levels of evidence and classes of recommendation as established by the ACC/AHA Guidelines Task Force (AHA, 2008).

Another element of the ACC/AHA effort is to improve the quality of cardiovascular care by the development of performance measures. Multidisciplinary committees address both retrospective and prospective data with explicit documented clinical criteria (AHA, 2008). Furthermore, the data elements required for the performance measures are linked to existing ACC/AHA clinical data standards to encourage uniform measurements of cardiovascular care. By facilitating measurements of cardiovascular health care quality, ACC/AHA performance measurement sets may serve as vehicles to accelerate appropriate translation of scientific evidence into clinical practice. These documents are intended to provide practitioners with tools to measure the quality of care and identify opportunities for improvement.

Ongoing scientific research has led to improvements in medications and technology. The development of evidence-based practice guidelines has helped health care providers know what is effective both for the treatment and prevention of cardiovascular disease. Some of the advances are complex and others are quite simple, though important. More than 94% of heart attack patients are now receiving aspirin on admission, compared to 76.4% at baseline (AHA, 2007). Patients with cerebral vascular accidents (CVA) arriving at a facility within 2 hours of onset of symptoms now receive thrombolysis >63% of the time versus 23.5% at baseline (AHA, 2007).

Evidence-based data has shifted the paradigm of cardiac care in United States. "Time is muscle" was a common mantra among health care teams in the 1990s. The importance of access to care and timely presentation to the hospital are central to saving lives. Rapid response of emergency teams and interventions, such as angioplasty, which facilitates blood flow through blocked coronary arteries, or thrombolysis may be performed when primary angioplasty is not available or appropriate. These prompt interventions are making a critical difference in morbidity and mortality.

Community commitment to establish primary stroke centers and competent acute care specialists who provide rapid and improved care for stroke victims has all made positive impacts. Improving the quality of care through the dissemination of evidence-based clinical guidelines can help patients benefit from research, facilitating longer lives, and reducing their risk of a second heart attack, stroke, or long-term secondary sequelae (AHA, 2008).

Acute care nurse practitioners (ACNPs) are confronted with many challenges in caring for the cardiovascular needs of patients with primary and secondary cardiovascular disease processes. Common cardiovascular diagnoses include acute coronary syndromes or coronary artery disease, hypertension, heart failure, valvular disease, peripheral vascular disease, pulmonary hypertension, cardiac rhythm disturbances, pericarditis, tamponade, cardiomyopathy, aneurysms, and endocarditis. Although it is beyond the scope of this chapter to provide expert cardiology knowledge, the chapter will review aspects of care that promote optimal outcomes of these areas for the ACNP.

Key Concepts in Cardiology

Electrophysiology

The potential resting membrane of the myocardium is about -90 mV with the inside being negatively charged comparative to the outside, which is relatively positive. The diffusion of ions across the membrane, their concentration gradients, and cyclic permeability are the basis for depolarization, action potential, and return to a resting state. The concentration gradient is produced by the work of the sodium–potassium adenosine 5′-triphosphate (ATP) pump by which sodium is pumped out of the cell and potassium into the cell.

By producing concentration equilibrium, this creates an electrical potential and as ions flux, this causes the interior to be less negative and thus there is a cycle of depolarization. There are two basic cardiac action potentials, *fast* and *slow*.

Electrical Conduction System

The cardiac electrical impulses arise in the sinus node, which is approximately 10–20 mm long near the junction of the superior vena cava (SVC) and the right atrium (RA). The specialized muscle tract conducts the impulses to the atrioventricular (AV) node, which is located under the right atrial endocardium at the level of the septal leaf of the tricuspid. This is the only normal conduction pathway between the atria and the ventricles. After stimulation of the AV node and a brief delay, the impulse is carried down the bundle of His posterior along the interventricular septum, giving rise to the right and left bundle branches. The left side divides again into the anterior and posterior fascicles. Both bundle branches continue to divide into Purkinje fibers and finally conduct to the ventricular myocardium.

Understanding the ECG

The electrocardiogram (ECG) is essential for interpretation and monitoring of the cardiac patient. The standard 12-lead pattern involves 10 electrodes placed in a specific pattern; one on each limb and six across the chest known as the *V leads*. Together, these leads record the electrical difference of two leads at a time. The standard leads I, II, III and the augmented leads aVR, aVL, and aVF predominately record the potentials from the frontal plane, whereas the V leads (1–6) record across the horizontal plane. Together they reflect the magnitude and direction of the electrical signals. The augmented leads are unipolar in that they record the potential difference between one limb and an indifferent composite electrode.

In general, the standard lead II is best for seeing the P wave and thus looking for arrhythmia. The V5 chest lead is the most sensitive for diagnosing myocardial ischemia. Together, these two leads should be monitored continuously in the acute care setting. Although complete interpretation of ECG is beyond the scope of this chapter, there are some myocardial abnormalities that can have serious consequences if not detected and may negatively affect overall patient outcomes. As a result, the ACNP must be confident in advanced ECG interpretation and integrate essentials with patient's clinical symptoms and cardiac risk factors.

Once establishing the overall heart rate, the clinician proceeds in evaluating cardiac conduction. The P wave must be identified, the presence or absence of the wave, and if present, whether it is positive or negative in deflection (except in V1 where they are usually biphasic). The duration of the P wave should be <0.12 seconds and the height <0.25 mV. Large P waves may be present in right atrial hypertrophy. The absence of a discernable P wave will point to an atrial arrhythmia.

The PR interval is a reflection of intracardiac conduction and should be 0.10–0.22 seconds. A prolonged PR interval is seen in first- and second-degree heart block. The

QRS morphology begins with the small Q wave deflection. These can be seen normally in all the leads except for the chest leads. When Q waves appear in the chest leads, they are indicative of a transmural myocardial infarction. The next component of the QRS is the R wave, which typically increases incrementally in size from V1–V4. The absence of this phenomenon is referred to as *poor R-wave progression* and may indicate prior infarction. The QRS complex should have duration of 0.07–0.10 seconds. Abnormally long QRS could indicate abnormal intracardiac conduction. The amplitude of the QRS ranges considerably; the larger amplitude may reflect physical fitness or conversely ventricular hypertrophy. A small QRS is suggestive of emphysema, pericardial effusion, or obesity.

The QRS axis is the net direction of electrical flow of the heart. The normal vector is −30° to +90°. When the leads' vector is −30° to −90°, this is left axis deviation and may be caused by left anterior hemiblock, inferior myocardial infarction, chronic obstructive pulmonary disease (COPD), and left ventricular (LV) hypertrophy. When the vectors are in the range of +90° to 180°, it is referred to as right axis deviation and the causes include left posterior hemiblock, right ventricular (RV) hypertrophy, and myocardial infarction.

The T wave representing ventricular repolarization is normally positive in leads aVR and V1. If these T waves are inverted, this is a sign of ischemia and perhaps infarction. A flattened T wave is indicative of hypokalemia and a peaked T wave would indicate hyperkalemia.

The next and perhaps most important component of the ECG is the ST segment. While there may be slight upslope or downslope, the truly elevated ST segment may indicate myocardial infarction or pericarditis. Depending on the pattern of the ST segments and their elevation, this information may be used to help diagnose which part of the heart is infarcting. The ST-segment elevation across a range of leads is common in postoperative patients and ST-segment depression is usually associated with myocardial ischemia, but may also be secondary to strain, digoxin, or hypokalemia.

The positive deflection following the T wave is an abnormal entity known as the U wave, which may represent hypokalemia, but may also be present in hypercalcemia, thyrotoxicosis, and exposure to digoxin, epinephrine, and class 1A and III antiarrhythmics, as noted in Exhibit 4.1.

Exhibit

4.1 Antiarrhythmic Drugs (AHA, 2007)

Class I — Sodium-channel blockers
Disopyramide (Norpace)
Flecainide (Tambocor)
Lidocaine (Xylocaine)
Mexiletine (Mexitel)
Moricizine (Ethmozine)
Procainamide (Procan, Procanabid, Pronestyl)
Propafenone (Rythmol)
Quinidine (Cardioquin, Quinaglute Dura-Tabs, Quinidex Extentabs, Quinora)
Tocainide (Tonocard)

Class II — Beta-blockers
Acebutolol (Sectral)
Atenolol (Tenormin)
Betaxolol (Kerlone)
Bisoprolol (Zebeta)
Carvedilol (Coreg)
Esmolol (Brevibloc)
Metoprolol (Toprol-XL, Lopressor)
Nadolol (Corgard)
Propranolol (Inderal)
Sotalol (Betapace, Betapace AF, Sorine)
Timolol (Blocadren)

Class III — Potassium-channel blockers
Amiodarone (Cordarone, Pacerone)
Azimilide (Stedicor)
Bepridil (Vascor)
Dofetilide (Tikosyn)
Ibutilide (Corvert)
Tedisamil (Pulsium)

Class IV — Calcium-channel blockers
Diltiazem (Cardizem, Tiazac, Cartia XT, Dilacor XR, Diltia XT)
Verapamil (Calan, Covera-HS, Isoptin SR, Verelan)

Miscellaneous
Adenosine (Adenocard, Adenoscan)
Digoxin (Lanoxin, Digitek)

An inverted U wave may further represent myocardial ischemia or LV volume overload. The U wave represents the repolarization of the papillary muscles or Purkinje fibers. Lastly, the
QT interval can vary significantly with heart rate and should
be corrected for this variation (QTc). Although most ECG programs will calculate this information, the manual formula is
the division of the QT by the square root of the RR interval. The
upper measure of normal is 0.44 seconds, if longer; this reflects
a potential prolongation, delay, or repolarization. This can be
congenital or acquired secondary to some medications and
can predispose the patient to a potentially deadly dysrhythmia
known as torsades de pointes ventricular tachycardia.

General Treatment of Arrhythmias

The approach to the patient with arrhythmias is individual,
but should be centered on history, physical examination, ECG,
vital signs, and stability. In general, the patient who presents
with severe symptoms requires aggressive evaluation and
treatment. Syncope adds a level of confusion and mandates
a comprehensive evaluation to rule out cardiac versus neurological origins. Family history, especially consistent with
sudden death or arrhythmias, warrants a higher degree of
concern. The physical examination should be focused on
presentation of cardiac disease, but the absence does not
ensure that an arrhythmia is benign. In contrast, the identification of cardiac or respiratory findings in the presence of
palpitations or syncope is a worrisome sign.

In approaching arrhythmias, the initial consideration must
be rate. In the presence of fast arrhythmias, the next step is
to determine if it is narrow or wide, regular or irregular, and
most importantly, the hemodynamic stability of the patient. A
slower arrhythmia may be physiologic or pathologic, the latter
needing consideration of a permanent pacemaker. Medication
history is paramount to determine if the rate is iatrogenic. See
Exhibit 4.2 for common etiologies.

Ventricular Arrhythmias

A premature ventricular complex is noted by the early occurrence of a QRS complex that is distinctively different and lasts
greater than 120 ms. A large T wave results from opposition

Exhibit

4.2 Common Etiologies of Ventricular Arrhythmias

- Ischemia
- Metabolic abnormalities
- Acidosis
- Hypoxia
- Hyperkalemia
- Hypokalemia
- Hypomagnesium
- Cardiomyopathy
- Valvular disorders
- Stimulants: cocaine, alcohol, caffeine
- Medications: digoxin, theophylline, antipsychotics, antidepressants, antiarrhythmics with proarrhythmic potential (i.e., flecainade, quinidine)

polarity to the QRS complex. A compensatory pause typically follows the premature beat. Ventricular bigeminy is used to denote alternating normal sinus beats and premature ventricular complexes (PVC). Three or more successive PVCs are defined as ventricular tachycardia. Premature ectopic beats, arising from the ventricle, increase with age and may be aggravated by exposure to precipitating stimuli. Studies have demonstrated an increased risk for life-threatening arrhythmias in individuals with 10 or more ectopic beats per hour or the presence of three to five consecutive impulses on Holter monitoring (Hebbar & Hueston, 2002). Evidence supports structural heart disease, and diminished LV functions are the key factors in determining treatment options and prognosis.

Ventricular tachycardia is defined by chaotic ventricular ectopy at a rate >100 beats per minute (bpm). The ECG reveals wide-complex tachycardia in the absence of conducted P waves (Table 4.1). Wolff–Parkinson–White (WPW), bundle branch block (BBB), aberrant conduction, and supraventricular tachycardia (SVT) can appear similar to ventricular tachycardia. Because of the potentially catastrophic outcomes associated with untreated ventricular tachycardia, all wide-complex tachycardia should be assumed to be ventricular tachycardia until proved otherwise. Practitioners must note that patients with ventricular tachycardia may be asymptomatic.

The AHA guidelines for the treatment of ventricular tachycardia in mildly symptomatic patients, advise the initial use of amiodarone. Patients with stable ventricular tachycardia may also benefit from amiodarone until there is a conversion to sinus rhythm or a less harmful rhythm is evident. Lidocaine is a less suitable alternative. Hemodynamically unstable patients require electrical cardioversion according to current ACLS guidelines.

The implantable cardioverter-defibrillator (ICD) is considered the golden standard for patients with life-threatening ventricular tachycardia or fibrillation (Gregoratos, Abrams, Epstein et al., 2002). Multiple studies have shown the ICD to be superior to antiarrhythmic drug therapy in patients with a history of life-threatening ventricular tachyarrhythmias (VT) and ventricular fibrillation (VF) (Kuck, Cappato, Siebels, & Rüppel, 2000, Moss et al., 2002). ICDs are typically prescribed as initial therapy, poststabilization, for sustained VT in association with structural heart disease or for those who present secondary to a resuscitated cardiac arrest (Strickberger et al., 2003; Moss et al., 2002). Exceptions include patients with idiopathic VT because the prognosis is excellent, VF caused by rapid rates during preexcited atrial fibrillation (AF), and in patients with specific dysrhythmias such as WPW. The initial therapy should be catheter ablation, once the patient is stabilized, for VT or VF, when this occurs early in an acute transmural infarction. Patients in whom a transient or reversible cause for the arrhythmia is detected are excluded from ICD implantation.

The treatment options for those with polymorphic VT or VF, secondary to acute ischemia, in the absence of an acute transmural infarction are more vague. Although in the past, these patients were frequently treated with revascularization only, the current trend appears to be ICD implantation following revascularization (Goldenberg, Moss, et al., 2005). In addition to ICD use as secondary prophylaxis after ventricular arrhythmia, multiple studies support ICD use as primary prophylaxis in ischemic and nonischemic cardiomyopathy.

The impact of the Multicenter Automatic Defibrillator Implantation Trial II (MADIT) and Multicenter Unsustained Tachycardia Trial (MUSTT) studies support patients with a

prior infarct, ejection fraction <40%, and spontaneous nonsustained VT should receive ICD implantation if the arrhythmia
is inducible (Moss et al., 2002; Klein, & Reek, 2000). Heart failure patients with ischemic or nonischemic cardiomyopathy,
ejection fraction <35% or less, and New York Heart Association
(NYHA) functional class II or III are also considered appropriate candidates for ICD (Goldenberg, Moss, et al., 2005).
Patients who experience syncope of undetermined origin with
hemodynamically significant inducible VT or VF during electrophysiology studies (EPS) or when drug therapy is ineffective or not an option should also be considered for ICD.

Given the poor sensitivity and specificity of EPS in patients
with nonischemic cardiomyopathy, patients with unexplained
syncope in the setting of nonischemic cardiomyopathy are
frequently treated empirically with ICD implantation. High-
risk patients with prolonged QT syndrome, hypertrophic cardiomyopathy, arrhythmogenic RV cardiomyopathy, Brugada
syndrome, which is a genetic disease with high risk of sudden
death, and short QT syndrome are candidates for prophylactic ICD implantation, although what constitutes high risk in
these patient populations remains controversial. Currently,
high-risk features include syncope and a family history of
unexplained sudden cardiac death.

Atrial Arrhythmias

Atrial fibrillation is perhaps the most common ECG arrhythmia found in the intensive care unit (ICU) and postoperative setting. Although considered a disease of aging with
fibrosis of the atrium, the irritated heart from surgery or
electrolyte imbalance lends itself to frequent bouts postoperatively. Atrial fibrillation is a result of multiple reentrant
circuits randomly colliding, dissipating, and reactivating in
the absence of a clear-cut P wave on the ECG. These multiple
depolarizations cause rapid atrial contractions with a highly
variable and irregular ventricular response. Although generally not life threatening once controlled, the disorganized
atrial to ventricular contractions and "loss of atrial kick" or
complete emptying of the atrium and thus reduced ventricular filling results in modest to severe hypotension dependant
on the interventions.

The AHA 2008 refined atrial fibrillation and atrial flutter guidelines to establish simplicity and clinical relevance.

4.1 ECG Classification of Ventricular Arrhythmias

Nonsustained Ventricular Tachycardia (VT)	Three or more beats in duration, terminating spontaneously in <30 seconds
	VT is a cardiac arrhythmia of three or more consecutive complexes in duration emanating from the ventricles at a rate of >100 bpm (cycle length <600 ms).
	Monomorphic – nonsustained VT with a single morphology
	Polymorphic – nonsustained VT with a changing morphology at cycle length between 600 and 180 ms
Sustained VT	VT >30 seconds and/or requiring termination due to hemodynamic compromise in <30 seconds
	Monomorphic – sustained VT with a single QRS morphology
	Polymorphic – sustained VT with a changing morphology at cycle length between 600 and 180 ms
Bundle branch reentrant tachycardia	VT due to reentry involving the His–Purkinje system, usually with LBBB morphology; usually occurs in the presence of cardiomyopathy
Bidirectional VT	VT with a beat to beat alternans in the QRS frontal plane axis, often in the presence of digoxin toxicity
Torsades de pointes	VT associated with a long QT or QTc and ECG changes reflective of twisting of QRS peak complexes around the isoelectric line during the arrhythmia:
	"Typical" initiated following short-long-short coupling intervals
	Short coupled variant initiated by normal-short coupling
Ventricular Flutter	A regular (cycle length variability 30 ms or less) ventricular arrhythmia approximately 300 bpm (cycle length 200 ms) with a monomorphic appearance; no isoelectric interval between successive QRS complexes
Ventricular Fibrillation	Rapid usually >300 bpm/200 ms (cycle length <180 ms), grossly irregular ventricular rhythm with marked variability in QRS cycle length, morphology and amplitude

Adapted from AHA Guidelines (2006).

Initially, the provider must identify whether the episode of AF is a first episode and whether or not it is symptomatic, and be aware that there may be ambiguity regarding the duration of the episode and the possibility of previously undetected episodes. Recurrent AF is defined as two or more episodes. When AF resolves spontaneously, it is identified as paroxysmal; once sustained, AF is classified as persistent. Persistent AF may be either the initial presentation of the arrhythmia or resultant of recurrent episodes of paroxysmal AF.

The classic description of AF is that the rhythm is irregularly irregular. On the ECG, it is generally impossible to make out a discernable P wave. One caveat when looking for AF is the possibility of AF with complete heart block. The ventricular rhythm may appear equal, but there would still be no preceding P wave.

Reversible AF may be a consequence of acute myocardial infarction, acute pulmonary disease, cardiac surgery, pericarditis, hyperthyroidism, pulmonary embolism, pneumonia, pulmonary edema, or other acute illness. This form of transient AF is considered separately because AF is less likely to recur once the precipitating condition has resolved (ACC/AHA, 2008). In these settings, AF is not the primary problem, and treatment of the underlying disorder concurrently with management of the episode of AF usually results in termination of the arrhythmia without recurrence.

AF may appear as atrial flutter or atrial tachycardia. Atrial flutter is characterized by a sawtooth pattern of regular atrial activation called flutter (f) waves on the ECG, more typically noted in leads II, III, aVF, and V1. The rate ranges from 240–320 beats/min, with f waves inverted in leads II, III, and aVF and upright in lead V1. Upright f waves in II, III, and aVF represent the reversed direction of activation in the right atrium. Atrial flutter may degenerate into AF, and AF may convert to atrial flutter. Although atrial flutter is more commonly identified, misdiagnosis may occur when coarse fibrillatory atrial activity is evident in more than one ECG lead.

Atrial flutter is actually a microreentrant pattern confined to the atrium as there is an anatomic physiologic block to conduction. Usually, there is a ventricular response rate of 1:2 or 1:3. The f waves of atrial depolarization are sent to continually disrupt the ECG and thus produce the classic sawtooth pattern. The morphology of the atrial f waves tends to appear similar or consistent. Usually, these patients are hemodynamically stable. Terminating the atrial flutter is directed at the rate and rhythm with rate being the prime consideration; antiarrhythmic therapy is often ineffective because it only serves to slow conduction. Examining electrolytes and correcting any abnormalities may be of assistance but, if the atrial flutter is persistent and symptomatic, then anticoagulation, defibrillation, or EP ablation may be needed.

Risk stratification for embolic events is as critical for patients with atrial flutter using the same criteria as for AF. The AHA included atrial flutter as an arrhythmia appropriate for performance measures on the basis of several considerations. Most significant is the potential for patients with atrial flutter to be at higher risk for thromboembolism. The current guidelines indicate as a Class I recommendation that it is prudent to stratify patients on the basis of thromboembolic risk and to consider anticoagulation for atrial flutter in a fashion similar to that for patients with AF (ACC/AHA, 2008).

Anticoagulation is essential in patients who have known risk factors for CVA associated with AF (see Exhibit 4.3). Initial treatment with IV heparin is suggested for high-risk patients if the duration of AF is >12 hours and hemodynamic stability is evident. Chronic anticoagulation with warfarin to target the INR between 2 and 3 is recommended in patients with persistent or paroxysmal AF, age consideration should be evaluated based on the potential of secondary injury from anticoagulation. Termination of atrial fibrillation may be necessary because of hemodynamic instability or clinical presentation. Confirmation of anticoagulation status should be documented prior to electrical conversion except in emergent scenarios. After 48 hours of atrial fibrillation, all patients should be anticoagulated because of the increased risk of atrial clot formation. Once the patient is anticoagulated, another attempt at cardioversion may be attempted after approximately 3 weeks. Should the patient require cardioversion prior to this time, an echocardiogram is mandatory to rule out a preformed atrial clot, which could be dislodged by cardioversion.

Exhibit

4.3 Risk Factors for CVA in the Presence of Atrial Fibrillation

History of prior Cerebralvascular Attack or Transient Ischemic Attack	Diabetes Mellitus
>75 years of age	Mitral stenosis
Hypertension	Congestive Heart Failure

Supraventricular Arrhythmias

Premature atrial beats may be normal, abnormal, or nonconducted and typically are followed by a noncompensatory pause.
The important factor is to differentiate aberrantly conducted
premature atrial complexes (PAC) from premature ventricular complexes (PVC). PACs may be unifocal or multifocal. The
apical rate is typically slower, the P wave morphology varies,
and PR interval is slightly shorter than in sinus rhythm.

A multifocal atrial rhythm is an irregularly irregular rhythm
caused by the arbitrary release of multiple ectopic stimuli. This
is defined as a heart rate ≤ 100 beats/min. This arrhythmia most
typically occurs in patients with existing pulmonary disease or
in situations when the patient is hypoxic, acidotic, or experiencing theophylline toxicity. P-wave morphology is distinctive in
each beat and there are three or more dissimilar P waves. The
presence of P waves distinguishes wandering atrial pacemaker
from atrial fibrillation. Multifocal atrial tachycardia is a chaotic
rhythm. By definition, the heart rate is >100 beats/min. The
characteristics are the same as those of wandering atrial pacemaker except for rate. Treatment is focused at improvement of
the underlying respiratory diagnosis.

Atrial Tachycardia

Atrial tachycardia is a result of rapid response from a single
focus. The resultant heart rate is >150 beats/min. The underlying mechanisms include increased atrial automaticity and

intra-atrial reentry. Atrial tachycardia may be caused by atrial irritation such as pericarditis, drugs, alcohol, and toxic gas inhalation. Symptoms include palpitations, shortness of breath, and chest discomfort. The P waves are distinctive from normal sinus P waves because they precede QRS complexes but may be hidden within the preceding T wave. Treatment may include pharmacologic agents or may be terminated by direct-current cardioversion. Drugs used in the treatment of atrial tachycardia include antiarrhythmic drugs in class Ia, Ic, and III (See Exhibit 4.1). Patients who fail to respond to noninvasive measures may require radiofrequency ablation.

Junctional tachycardia is caused by abnormal conduction in the AV node or adjacent tissue and is common after heart surgery, acute inferior MI, myocarditis, or digitalis toxicity. The cardiac monitor reveals regular QRS complexes without P waves or with retrograde P waves (inverted in the inferior leads) that occur preceding or following the QRS complex. The rhythm is differentiated from paroxysmal SVT by the reduced heart rate.

Acute onset of SVT typically requires targeted intervention. The underlying pathology should be quickly identified and, if possible, be addressed (increased atrial pressures, irritating central lines, or electrolyte disturbances). When patients are hemodynamically unstable, then synchronous electrical cardioversion is indicated. The patient that is hemodynamically stable has other options such as vagal maneuvers and medical interventions. There remains some disagreement between those that feel sinus rhythm should be the ultimate goal and those that feel that simple ventricular rate control will suffice.

Adenosine may be an option for SVT of unknown etiology. This short-acting medication causes transient heart block in the AV node, which breaks the SVT and is administered by rapid IV bolus, then by a large saline bolus to ensure prompt administration. Should the initial dosage be ineffective, two subsequent doses are given at 5-minute intervals. Temporary (2–3 second) moments of cardiac standstill are to be anticipated and adequate patient support is necessary to avoid distress. Other methods of restoring sinus rhythm include antiarrhythmics, particularly the class II and III drugs (see Exhibit 4.1). Beta-blockers decrease the conduction through the AV node and may be used as long-term maintenance.

Calcium channel blockers are negative inotropes that decrease the force of contraction and slow down the conduction of electrical activity by blocking the calcium channel during the plateau phase of the action potential of the heart, causing a negative chronotropic effect.

Accessory pathway reentrant tachycardia involves specific areas that bypass normal cardiac conduction. This may be the result of either premature atrial or ventricular ectopy. The most frequent manifestation is WPW syndrome characterized by both accessory pathway and normal conducting path utilization noted in sinus rhythm. This results in early ventricular depolarization. Subsequently, there is a short PR interval and a notable upstroke to the QRS complex referred to as a *delta wave*. This delta wave prolongs the QRS and may depict a normal appearing complex except for the delta wave and in some instances, a Q wave may be noted.

When persistent narrow complex tachycardia persists, AV node blockers are indicated to prevent the firing of the AV node during the reentry cycle. Adenosine is the first choice and other options include verapamil or diltiazem. AV nodal blockers may also be effective in the presence of wide QRS complex tachycardia. The essential goal is to determine the source of the arrhythmia and to specifically exclude ventricular tachycardia as AV nodal blockers may intensify ventricular tachycardias at which point IV procainamide may be initiated. Synchronized cardioversion with 50 joules may be a more acceptable approach to pharmacologic therapy.

For critical or unrelenting nodal reentrant tachycardia, long-term antiarrhythmics or transvenous catheter radiofrequency ablation is typically prescribed. Ablation is preferable since long-term efficacy is rapidly achieved. In unstable patients or those electing to avoid interventional options, drug prophylaxis may be initiated with digoxin, beta-blockers, non-dihydropyridine calcium channel blockers, or other appropriate antiarrhythmics.

Atrioventricular Block

AV block is a temporary or complete disruption of conduction from the atria to the ventricles. Idiopathic fibrosis or sclerosis of the conduction system is cited as the most common underlying pathology. Interventions are dependent on the degree of block and symptomatology with the treatment choice typically including pacing. AV block may be secondary to medications such as beta-blockers, calcium channel blockers, digoxin; increased vagal tone, valvular disease, congenital heart disease, or other disorders.

First-degree AV block is noted when normal P waves are followed by QRS complexes, but the PR interval takes longer than 0.2 seconds. This is typically asymptomatic and does not necessitate intervention. Proactive investigation may determine if the block is secondary to another heart disorder or is drug induced. Second-degree AV block indicates the presence of typical P wave followed by QRS complexes, but in some instances, the P wave is not followed by a QRS. When this occurs, there are two specific types of known blocks: Mobitz I and Mobitz II.

Mobitz I is a lengthening of the PR interval until the atrial stimuli are not conducted and the QRS complex is missing (Wenckebach phenomenon); AV nodal conduction normalizes then the cycle repeats. Mobitz I arises from the junction of the AV node in most patients with a distinctly narrow QRS complex. When an entire block occurs, a junctional escape rhythm may ensue in an attempt to restore function. Intervention is unnecessary unless the block results in symptomatic bradycardia. The recommendation for treatment is pacemaker insertion.

Mobitz II has a regular PR interval. Beats are randomly dropped with a notable absence of QRS, in a repetitive cycle. Frequent patterns may ensue with every 3rd (3:1 block) or 4th (4:1 block) P wave. Mobitz II is indicative of underlying disease along the bundle branches. Symptoms may range from dizziness, weakness, and syncope, depending on the proportion of nonconducted beats. Treatment of 2nd-degree AV block and structural disease includes permanent pacemaker insertion except in the presence of a reversible cause.

Third-degree or complete heart block is resultant of an absence of electrical communication between the atria and ventricles. The ECG depicts no connection between P waves and QRS complexes. The heart attempts to preserve function through junctional escape or ventricular pacemaker beats. Beats originating above the bifurcation of the bundle of His display narrow QRS complexes and the patient exhibits a heart rate >40 beats/min with minimal symptoms. Escape rhythms arising beneath the bifurcation produce wider QRS complexes, lower and more erratic heart rates, and worsening symptom-atology, including loss of consciousness or heart failure.

When the heart block is secondary to drugs, discontinu-ation of the specific medication may restore normal rhythm, but temporary pacing might be necessary. Complete heart block may be produced by acute inferior MI and the dis-turbance typically denotes significant myocardial necrosis. Immediate transvenous pacemaker insertion is indicated with interim external pacing as necessary. Spontaneous resolution may occur, but further diagnostic evaluation of conduction is indicated.

Cardiac Arrest

In adults, acute cardiac arrest or sudden death results pri-marily from underlying cardiac disease. However, it may be the initial manifestation of the disease. Some additional causes include trauma, pulmonary embolism, hemorrhage, or drug overdose. Global ischemia is the consequence of cardiac standstill with cellular damage and edema ensuing quickly. Rapid response and resuscitation decreases the likelihood of death and disability, but even patients with full supportive measures may experience long-term cerebral dysfunction.

Decreased ATP production following arrest creates a loss of cellular membrane integrity with an efflux of potassium and calcium. Elevations of nitrous oxide cause free radical formation and may activate cellular destruction. Abnormal depolarization sets off neurotransmitters including gluta-mate, which triggers an overload of calcium. Inflammatory mediators surge result in increased thrombosis and worsen-ing of edema. Apoptosis as a result of overwhelming isch-emia causes cell death.

Initial evaluation for potential treatable causes including hypoxia, hypovolemia, pneumothorax, or cardiac tamponade is paramount in acute care. Rapid intervention that utilizes current advanced cardiac life support (ACLS) guidelines is essential. A primary survey of airway, breathing, circulation, and defibrillation is always the primary intervention even in the acute care setting. Precordial thump is not indicated except in the absence of a defibrillator. Prompt direct current cardio-version is the most effective intervention for conversion of VF or VT. The success of defibrillation is correlated to time with a 10% decline in success with each minute of pulselessness.

There is little definitive evidence to support the effectiveness of ACLS drugs in survival of cardiac arrest to hospital discharge. Some may enhance circulatory responses such as the first line drugs, which include epinephrine, vasopressin, atropine, and amiodarone. Other agents may be utilized to address individual patient scenarios including metabolic disturbances or drug overdose. Cessation of resuscitation events is determined by patient stability, pronunciation of death, or failure to establish spontaneous circulation within 30–45 minutes. Patients with hypothermia must be rewarmed to 34°C to make an accurate assessment of death.

Heart Failure

Intrinsically, the LV function is tied to cardiac output. Understanding the LV function and thus dysfunction it is best to review the basics; energy supply and demand of the heart. The primary energy demands are heart rate, wall tension, and contractility. The ventricle is largest during diastole, whereas the greatest pressure occurs during systole. Rate will increase contractility and thus use greater energy. With an increase in any of these factors, oxygen demand must be increased to match demand.

With just a resting heart rate, the myocardium already uses 6–8cc $O_2 \cdot min \cdot 100g$ while skeletal muscle only uses 0.15 cc $O_2 \cdot min \cdot 100g$. Furthermore, the myocardium must extract nearly 80% of the oxygen, whereas skeletal muscle needs only 25%. There is not a large reserve for the heart when it needs to increase energy expenditure. The determinants of myocardial oxygen delivery are coronary artery blood flow, hemoglobin concentration, and arterial oxygen saturation. Coronary blood flow can increase from a resting level of 70–80 $cc \cdot min \cdot 100g$ to 400–600 $cc \cdot min \cdot 100g$ when at maximal demand. With inadequate supply, when supply out strips demand, ventricular dysfunction is common. As an extreme example, when the oxygen supply for the heart is interrupted and unable to meet demand, dyskinesia results and can result in pulseless electrical activity.

Cardiac contractility, ventricular function, and myocardial oxygen demand are determined by (a) preload, (b) afterload, (c) heart rate, (d) rhythm, and (e) the presence of substrates including fatty acids, oxygen, glucose, and viable myocardium. Cardiac output is defined as stroke volume × heart rate and is dependent on venous return, peripheral vascular tone, and neurohumoral factors.

Preload is the pressure stretching, which expands the ventricle after passive filling and contraction of the atrium. Preload corresponds to the amount of end-diastolic stretch of cardiac fiber cells and end-diastolic volume. These are products of ventricular diastolic pressure and myocardial structure. LV end-diastolic pressure is synonymously identified as the amount of preload. The factors that create an increased ventricular filling pressure causing a high preload include elevations in central venous pressure, increased ventricular compliance, underlying conditions such as valvular disease and heart failure, increased atrial contractile force, decreased heart rate, and increased aortic pressure. Preload is decreased by factors including low blood volume, atrial arrhythmias, elevated heart rate, ventricular diastolic failure, and mitral and tricuspid stenosis.

Afterload is the force that resists cardiac contraction upon systole and is also defined as the pressure necessary to eject blood from the chamber and is a consequence of systemic arterial pressure. Under normal circumstance as afterload increases, there is a resultant decrease in cardiac output. The Frank-Starling principle illustrates the effects of preload and cardiac performance. Contractility typically requires interventional methods to be measured, but can be reasonably deduced by the ejection fraction estimation on an echocardiogram.

Cardiac reserve reflects the heart's capacity to perform above resting levels secondary to stressors including emotional or physical conditions. Factors affecting cardiac reserve include tachycardia, systolic and diastolic volume, stroke volume, and the difference between oxygen content in arterial blood and mixed venous or pulmonary artery blood. At rest the arterial blood is estimated at 18 ml O_2/dl of blood, or pulmonary artery blood estimates equate to 14 ml/dl. The oxygen extraction is therefore calculated at 4.0 ml/dl, but as demand rises, it may be increased to 12–14 ml/dl. This effect provides some adaptation for blood flow in the presence of heart failure.

There are several causes of primary ventricular failure. Valvular disease is a prominent cause of ventricular dysfunction. Chronic states like endocarditis or acute ischemia may cause failure. The patient with chronic hypertension will generally have increased left ventricle hypertrophy, which results in mitral insufficiency because of the dilation of the ventricle and mitral ring as well as inadequate alignment of the papillary muscle. This increases demand with primary forward and backward dysfunction causing pulmonary edema. The demand is increased at a time when supply is decreased particularly in the subendocardial areas.

Individuals with heart failure experience inadequate blood flow to meet metabolic needs and subsequent elevation of pressure may result in organ congestion. This state creates dysfunction of systolic or diastolic activity or both. During systolic dysfunction, there is poor ventricular inotropy and ineffective emptying, which results in elevated diastolic volume and lowered ejection fraction. Systolic dysfunction can also result from the loss of contractile muscle cells in the heart following acute myocardial infarction. Intracellular calcium modulation and cAMP production prevent effective utilization and storage of energy with resultant electrophysiological and functional abnormalities.

During diastolic disturbances that affect the function, there is a weakened relaxation of the ventricle with impaired filling and a decreased ventricular end-diastolic volume, increased end-diastolic pressure, or both. Primary features of diastolic dysfunction include, but are not limited to, valvular disease, stiffness, and constrictive pericarditis. The ejection fraction may be within normal limits despite the inadequate LV filling. The effects of poor LV filling are evident in lowered cardiac output measurements and the manifestation of systemic symptoms. As right atrial pressures increase, there is pulmonary congestion. Resistance to filling may be secondary to reduction of myocytes and the deposit of collagen. Diastolic dysfunction may be present in hypertrophic cardiomyopathy, hypertrophic ventricular states, and cardiac disease secondary to amyloidal permeation.

LV dysfunction may produce LV failure. This is manifested by decreased cardiac output and elevations in pulmonary venous pressure. The rapid rise in pulmonary capillary pressure surpasses colloidal osmotic pressure resulting in shunting of fluid from the capillaries to interstitial and alveolar areas with poor pulmonary compliance causing respiratory insufficiency. Marked volume pulmonary edema changes ventilation–perfusion reactions. Pulmonary arterial blood passes through alveoli with negligible ventilator capacity thus limiting systemic arterial oxygenation and producing shortness of breath. Dyspnea may occur before ventilation–perfusion mismatch because of rising pulmonary venous pressure and the heightened burden of breathing. Pleural effusions are evident in persistent or severe or chronic dysfunction of the left ventricle and can exacerbate dyspnea. Small increases in ventilation induce lower $PaCO_2$ and produce respiratory alkalosis. Elevations of $PaCO_2$ are ominous signs of respiratory failure representative of interstitial edema of the alveoli.

RV dysfunction and elevation of systemic venous pressure with resultant edema are the manifestations of right heart failure. The liver is affected and gastrointestinal organs exhibit congestion as evident by the presence of ascites. The severe dysfunction of the right ventricle creates hepatic congestion and impairment, specifically high bilirubin levels, elevated PT, and hepatic enzymes. The overloaded liver is unable to meet the demands of circulating aldosterone, thus increasing and adding to increased volume. Patients may develop anorexia, malabsorption, hypoalbuminemia, chronic blood loss, and in rare cases, ischemia of the mesenteric vessels.

Atrial natriuretic peptide is an amino acid that is produced by cardiac cells in response to atrial distension, angiotensin II, and sympathetic stimulation typically in response to hypervolemic states. Brain-type natriuretic peptide (BNP) is peptide produced in the brain and ventricles. BNP is also produced by excessive volume and mimics physiological actions. BNP and NT-pro-BNP are specific diagnostic indications for heart failure. Neutral endopeptidase (NEP) is a complex chemical that degrades the natriuretic peptides. Therefore, it may block natriuretic peptide and intensifies their effects. Natriuretic peptides serve as counterregulatory processes for the renin–angiotensin–aldosterone system. A recombinant human BNP is approved for use in the acute treatment of decompensated heart failure caused by systolic dysfunction. New classes of drugs that are NEP inhibitors prevent enzymatic response in combination with ACE inhibitors.

Ventricular remodeling is a consequence of prolonged elevations of preload and subsequent cardiac output. There is notable change in ventricular shape, width, and weight over time, and then hypertrophy ensues. Compensatory mechanisms result in markedly decreased diastolic capacity thereby compromising cardiac workload especially during stress. Elevated ventricular stiffness raises oxygen demand and stimulates apoptosis of the myocardium. Valvular regurgitation increases in the presence of chronic elevated end-diastolic volumes.

Sepsis may result in ventricular failure because of by-products of inflammation. The circulation of inflammatory products, IL-1, IL-9, tumor necrosis factor, and cytokines, causes a decrease in cardiac function. As sepsis ensues, the patient experiences a decline in SVR and profound hypotension. In an effort to maintain an acceptable blood pressure, the heart must increase demand, thus outstripping the myocardial reserves.

The renin–angiotensin–aldosterone system is stimulated by decreased perfusion to the kidneys. Increases in sodium, water retention, renal, and peripheral vascular tone are evident. The end result is intense sympathetic activation that is seen in heart failure. Heightened sympathetic activity with increased circulating angiotensin II and vasopressin, contribute to an intensified systemic vascular resistance. Drugs that may reduce these mechanisms include angiotensin-converting enzyme inhibitors. The angiotensin receptor blockade agents may improve stroke volume by decreasing afterload. Arterial and venous dilators, such as hydralazine and sodium nitroprusside are indicated for the acute reduction of afterload in patients with critical illness.

Angiotensin II aggravates failure by stimulating vasoconstriction, including efferent renal vasoconstriction, and by raising circulatory aldosterone. This enhances retention of sodium in the distal kidney and is responsible for myocardial and vascular collagen deposition and fibrosis. Norepinephrine, a by-product of Angiotensin II, increases antidiuretic hormone (ADH) and can trigger apoptosis. Angiotensin II is credited with vascular and myocardial hypertrophy and ultimately attributed to the cycle of failure by remodeling the heart and peripheral vasculature.

There is also evidence that other factors such as nitric oxide and endothelin may play a role in the pathogenesis of heart failure. Some drug treatments for heart failure involve attenuating the neurohumoral changes. Beta-blockers have been shown to provide significant long-term benefit, because they block the excessive sympathetic activation in cardiac muscle. Angiotensin-converting enzyme inhibitors, angiotensin receptor blockers (ARBs), and aldosterone receptor antagonists are commonly used to treat heart failure by inhibiting the actions of the renin–angiotensin–aldosterone system.

Ischemia and necrosis of the primary organs produce cytokine, also known as tumor necrosis factor (TNF)-α, is produced. This catabolic entity causes cachexia, which is common in severe failure. Metabolic changes occurring in end-stage heart failure include elevated free fatty acid consumption and decreased glucose utilization. Systemic and cardiac specific factors can impair cardiac performance and cause failure. Biventricular failure results from disorders that affect the entire heart including viral or congenital states.

The term *high-output heart failure* refers to conditions in which the heart requires elevated cardiac output to maintain functionality. Ultimately, the cardiac muscle cannot meet the demand and failure ensues. Some of the underlying causes of high-output failure include, but are not limited to, severe anemia, hyperthyroidism, Paget disease, and persistent tachycardia. Failure may be noted in forms of cirrhosis, but the edema is typically attributed to underlying hepatic mechanisms.

Treatment

Critical intervention is essential for acute or worsening failure in the presence of acute myocardial infarction, atrial fibrillation, severe hypertension, acute valvular regurgitation, as well as for patients with pulmonary edema, new-onset failure, or individuals who are refractory to outpatient treatment. The primary goal is to diagnose and treat the underlying cause (Exhibit 4.4). Initially, therapy is centered on improving hemodynamic stability, avoiding electrolyte imbalance, improving renal insufficiency, lessening symptoms, and correcting neurohumoral activation. Long-term needs must address hypertension, the progression of coronary heart disease, reduction of MI risk, improving cardiac function, reducing acute care days, and improving quality of life.

Pharmacotherapy in Heart Failure

Drug treatment for heart failure includes diuretics, nitrates, ACE inhibitors, ARBs, and beta-blockers for diastolic HF. Severe diastolic dysfunction predisposes patients to

Exhibit

4.4 Treatment Considerations for Heart Failure

Identify and treat arrhythmias

> Aggressive attempts to convert atrial fibrillation

Treat underlying conditions

> Hyperthyroidism, pulmonary emboli, fever, anemia

Correct electrolyte abnormalities

Consider ICD therapy for appropriate patients

Ultrafiltration (venovenous filtration)

> Patients who fail diuretic therapy with worsening cardiorenal syndrome

Intra-aortic counterpulsation balloon pump

Surgery

> Closure of congenital or acquired intracardiac shunts
> Coronary artery bypass graft
> Valve repair or replacement

Heart transplantation

> Patients younger than the age of 60 who have severe, refractory HF and no other life-threatening conditions.

LVAD

> Bridge to transplantation or recovery

hypotension and reduction of plasma volume; therefore, diuretics and nitrates are prescribed in lower doses. Current research supports data on plasma biomarkers that may predict which patients might respond best to which drug or drug combination.

Diuretics are a staple in the management of symptomatic systolic dysfunction and current or previous volume overload. Loop diuretics including furosemide and bumetanide are commonly prescribed and, in refractory cases, increased dosage of furosemide, ethacrynic acid, bumetanide, or metolazone may have an additive effect. Intravenous infusion of furosemide is effective in the presence of severe edema. Side effects include the following: hypovolemia with hypotension, hyponatremia, hypomagnesemia, and severe hypokalemia. Acute doses of diuretic should be targeted to resolve failure and decreased or discontinued as heart function improves. High doses of diuretics lower CO, impair renal function, and increase mortality. These medications should be used judiciously. Serum electrolytes must be monitored closely especially after increasing dose.

Spironolactone or eplerenone may limit the hypokalemia-associated side effects related to higher-dose loop diuretics. Hyperkalemia may result in combination of ACE inhibitors or ARBs and may aggravate renal dysfunction. These drugs have been noted to benefit patients with chronic RV failure as hepatic congestion increases aldosterone levels.

Patients with systolic dysfunction should be maintained on oral ACE inhibitors unless contraindicated (i.e., by plasma creatinine >2.8 mg/dl, bilateral renal artery stenosis, renal artery stenosis, or past medical history of ACE induced angio-edema). ACE inhibitors facilitate vasodilation, lower LV filling pressures, decrease systemic vascular resistance, and resist ventricular remodeling. ACE inhibitors have been credited with prolonged survival and reduced subsequent admissions for failure especially in individuals with diabetic nephropathy (Strippoli, Craig, Schena, et al., 2006). ACE inhibitors may reduce MI and stroke risk in individuals with coronary heart disease and delay the onset of nephropathy in patients with diabetes. Thus, ACE inhibitors may be used in patients with diastolic dysfunction and any of these disorders.

ACE inhibitors may be responsible for temporary elevations in serum creatinine secondary to vasodilation of the efferent glomerular vessels. Subtle increases in creatinine should not be the rationale for termination of therapy but should alert the provider to titrate the dose carefully, reduce diuretics, and avoid use of NSAIDs. Regular evaluation of renal function and electrolytes should be initiated prior to onset of ACE inhibitors, repeated at least 1 month, and following any deviations in clinical condition or dose adjustment. Dehydration or poor renal function may develop because of acute illness and then, the ACE inhibitor dose may need to be reduced or the drug may need to be temporarily withheld.

ARBs are less likely to cause cough and angioedema than the ACE inhibitor and may be indicated if adverse effects prohibit ACE inhibitor use. MI studies revealed that ACE inhibitors and ARBs are equally effective although their equivalence is less clear in chronic failure. Ongoing studies are underway to explore long-term dosing standards. Similar to ACE inhibitors, ARBs may aggravate renal dysfunction, and the dose may need to be reduced or discontinued in acute scenarios. In the presence of severe or repetitive episodes of heart failure, the provider may add an ARB to the ACE inhibitor, beta-blocker, and diuretic regimen. Combination therapy necessitates ongoing evaluation of blood pressure, plasma electrolytes, and renal function.

Aldosterone production is independent of the renin-angiotensin system and the effects cannot be removed despite maximal dosing of ACE inhibitors and ARBs. Spironolactone and eplerenone decrease mortality, including from sudden death, in patients with low ejection fraction severe or acute episodes, or following acute MI. Potassium supplementation should be terminated and monitored frequently.

Beta-blockers are an important addition to ACE inhibitors for chronic systolic dysfunction in most patients. These agents are most effective if initiated in the absence of pulmonary congestion. Research supports the role of beta-blockers for improved ejection fraction and decreased morbidity and mortality in patients with chronic systolic dysfunction (AHQR, 2003). Beta-blockers are efficacious for diastolic dysfunction because of heart rate reduction, prolonging diastolic filling time, and may possibly improve ventricular relaxation. During acute decompensation, beta-blockers should not be initiated until hemodynamic stability is achieved. Dosage titration is required for those on beta-blocker therapy at the time of decompensation. Once treatment is initiated, cardiac oxygen consumption decreases whereas stroke volume and filling pressure remain unchanged.

Hydralazine and isosorbide dinitrate can offer relief for patients intolerant of ACE inhibitors or ARBs. Ethnopharmacologic data indicates that African American patients, may experience additional benefits when supplemented with standard treatment options. Vasodilators improve blood flow, reduce regurgitation, and increase exercise capability without compromising renal function.

Nitrates alone can relieve the symptoms related to failure and patients may be taught to initiate sublingual nitroglycerin as needed for acute dyspnea or utilize transdermal modalities for nocturnal symptoms. Nitrates are easily prescribed, cost effective and generally tolerated in individuals. Common side effects include hypotension, flushing, and headache.

Calcium channel blockers are excluded in the management of systolic dysfunction. Short-acting dihydropyridines and nondihydropyridines in fact may be lethal. Amlodipine and felodipine may be suitable alternatives in patients presenting with angina and hypertension.

Digoxin inhibits the Na-K pump, thus, lessening the positive inotropic effect reduces sympathetic activity, slows ventricular response specifically in atrial fibrillation, and limits vasoconstriction while improving renal circulation. There is no data to support effects on mortality, but when used with diuretics and an ACE inhibitor, it may produce resolution of symptoms. Providers must recognize the potential for toxicity especially in patients with renal dysfunction.

Positive inotropic drugs have been evaluated in heart failure, but except for digoxin, have a limited role because of increased mortality. Researchers are studying the effects of calcium sensitizers, cytokine blockers, endothelin blockers, matrix metalloproteinase inhibitors, and immune modulators as potential future treatment modalities in the management of heart failure.

Chest Pain

Chest tightness, pressure, discomfort, or any pain arising along the anterior aspect of the thorax may be described as chest pain. Many people with chest pain fear a heart attack. However, there are many possible causes of chest pain including cardiac diseases resulting from blockages in coronary arteries, other cardiac problems (such as pericarditis), musculoskeletal diseases of the chest wall, gastrointestinal diseases, arthritis, and neurological disease. Any organ or tissue in your chest can be the source of pain, including your heart, lungs, esophagus, muscles, ribs, tendons, or nerves. The pain may range from mildly bothersome to serious and could even be life threatening.

Angina is a type of heart-related chest pain resultant from ischemia and may present in the same manner as the pain of a heart attack. Angina is referred to as stable angina when chest pain begins at a predictable level of activity. Unstable angina is chest pain that occurs unexpectedly after light activity or occurs at rest and necessitates immediate attention. Other causes of chest pain include respiratory infection, pulmonary embolism, pneumothorax, asthma, or pleurisy. In these cases, the chest pain often worsens on deep inspiration or cough and is described as sharp and pulling or may be expressed in terms of tension between the ribs. Unstable angina results from an imbalance between oxygen supply and demand. Angina pain is a clinical manifestation of this imbalance. Because the left ventricle comprises the majority of the cardiac mass and faces the greatest pressures, it is at the highest risk for ischemia. The ischemia may be precipitated by coronary atherosclerosis, plaque rupture, coronary artery spasm, anemia, and hypoxemia, with subsequent and limited diastolic filling time secondarily produced by tachycardia and hypertension.

The term *unstable angina* denotes new pain or a departure from previous anginal pattern. Unstable angina occurs at rest or more commonly with light activity. Pain lasting for more than 15 minutes also suggests an unstable pattern after activity is discontinued. The pain of unstable angina may awaken a patient from sleep. The correlation between severe ischemia and death has heightened the need for definitive diagnostic and therapeutic intervention in individuals with chest pain. Braunwald (2000) identified 5 critical factors that lead to the diagnosis of unstable angina and increase the likelihood of survival if indeed there is an ischemic event. Careful history is essential to identify these elements. They include: (1) the nature of the symptoms, (2) a prior history of CAD, (3) age, (4) sex, and (5) the number of traditional risk factors that are present for CAD. Patients with UA should be identified quickly and access to appropriate reperfusion modalities expedited to improve outcomes.

Myocardial Infarction

The spectrum referred to as acute coronary syndrome includes ST-elevation MI (STEMI), non–ST-elevation MI (NSTEMI), and unstable angina. This categorization is valuable because patients with ischemic discomfort may or may not have ST-segment elevations on electrocardiogram. Those without ST elevations may ultimately be diagnosed with NSTEMI or with unstable angina based on the presence or absence of cardiac enzymes. In addition, therapeutic decisions, such as administering an intravenous thrombolytic or performing percutaneous coronary intervention (PCI), are often made based on these criteria.

Diagnostic testing, specifically the measurement of cardiac markers, helps to categorize myocardial infarction. Troponin is the ideal biomarker for diagnosis as it provides the greatest sensitivity and specificity. The test may be utilized in both diagnostic and prognostic aspects of care. Troponin is not found in serum except in the presence of myocardial necrosis. Troponin I is detectable in serum 3–6 hours after an AMI and its level remains elevated for 10–14 days.

CK-MB may also be utilized in diagnosing MI. Serum levels rise approximately 4 hours following injury, peak at 18–24 hours, and normalize in 3–4 days. Therefore, it is essential to note that normal findings do not exclude myocardial necrosis. Infarcts can be missed by CK-MB and should be used in addition to serial troponin levels in patients with suspected MI and negative serial CK-MBs.

Chest radiography, CT scan, or transesophageal echocardiography (TEE) may assist in the detection of MI from aortic dissection in high-risk patients. Echocardiography is helpful in evaluating wall motion abnormalities and overall ventricular function. Perfusion imaging has been used in risk stratification after MI and for measurement of infarct size to evaluate reperfusion therapies. CT scanning reveals fine details of the patient's coronary arteries. This noninvasive technology enables early diagnosis and potentially earlier treatment before coronary ischemia ensues. Improved visualization can depict the status of coronary arteries, potential plaque within the artery, or the patency of a graft.

TEE has become the single most important tool during the intraoperative course with it multifaceted indications. Commonly, it is used to determine ejection fraction, ventricular and atrial wall movement, abnormalities of flow, integrity and function of valves, determination of intravascular volume, presence of abnormal anatomy, evaluation of post valve repair/replacement, and pericardial effusion just to name a few. This tool is geared to the intraoperative arena, requiring intubation and currently only used for an examination rather than sustained monitoring. During the ICU monitoring, a TEE can be used for assessment of hemodynamic instability, assessment of unexplained respiratory failure, suspected endocarditis, suspected pulmonary embolus, diagnosis of aortic dissection, and evaluation of clot formation before cardioversion in patients with AF.

Both transthoracic echocardiography (TTE) and TEE require significant training to obtain and accurately interpret findings. The TEE determines the ventricular contraction, volume status and presence of pericardial fluid/tamponade. The echocardiogram functions by using a transducer to transmit and receive ultrasound waves into cardiac and vascular structures. Two-dimensional (2D) and M-mode imaging provide details of structure and motion based on the intensity and time delay of ultrasound waves that are reflected at the tissue interfaces. Doppler imaging provides velocity information based on the change in frequency of backscattered ultrasound waves produced by moving structures, usually blood. The classic example is that of standing still and listening to a passing train. As the train approaches and then passes, the pitch changes.

Real-time imaging or 2D imaging involves rapidly sweeping an ultrasound beam back and forth across a plane. The reflected ultrasound signals are used to generate a 2D thin slice through the structure of interest with motion displayed in real time. M-mode imaging display reflects ultrasound waves along a single scan line over time known as *motion over time*. M-mode imaging has a very high depth of resolution and therefore is ideal for measuring distances along the scan line and for observing rapidly moving structures.

There are currently 4 Doppler imaging modes in use, which include the following: (a) color flow, (b) pulsed wave (PW), (c) continuous wave (CW), and (d) tissue. The flow Doppler displays blood velocity as a color map over the 2D image. By convention, red represents flow toward the transducer whereas blue is blood flowing away. The importance is to recognize that depending on the angle of the transducer or what structure you are examining, *blue* can be arterial flow whereas *red* can be venous flow. When the velocity of the flow exceeds a certain speed, the color flows can reverse. The classic example of this, known as aliasing or exceeding the Nyquist limit, is the optical illusion of watching a wheel that goes so fast that it looks like it is going backward. The spectral Doppler, the pulse wave, continuous wave, and tissue Doppler also record velocities along a single scan line. The TTE will more reliably visualize the LV apex and the ventricular apex of a prosthetic mitral valve because of orientation. The TEE provides excellent view of the mitral and aortic views.

Interventional technologies have become essential in the reperfusion of coronary arteries. PCI are performed as a primary intervention when available or may be indicated in the individual who experiences failure of thrombolysis. PCI is more effective than thrombolysis when readily available and is indicated for confirmed STEMI in the presence of a new left bundle branch block, severe congestive heart failure. Success is correlated to early intervention specifically within hours of symptom onset.

Complications caused by hemorrhage following PCI are minimal when compared with thrombolysis. There is restoration of patency of cardiac vessels in most patients. The limiting factor is the requirement of an angioplasty suite with the required staff round the clock. On call cardiothoracic capabilities can also prohibit universal availability of PCI. Primary PCI for STEMI should be performed at hospitals with readily available cardiothoracic surgery. This is open to interpretation and may be defined as the ability to transport patients to a facility with cardiothoracic capabilities.

Patients with persistent ST elevation require evaluation for reperfusion modalities. In the presence of ST elevation, diagnosis may be driven by troponin levels. Unstable angina may be noted in the absence of cardiac marker elevation. Patients presenting with no ST-segment elevation are not candidates for emergent thrombolytics, but rather, elective angiography and PCI may be of value. For unstable angina, diagnosis may be delayed to enable diagnostic studies such as coronary angiography or imaging studies to rule out noncoronary causes of chest pain. The primary goal is identifying and intervening quickly in patients with STEMI. Treatment should be multifaceted and aimed at restoring oxygenation, minimizing ischemia, relieving pain, and preventing complications.

Patients presenting with STEMI have a different pathology and therefore a different treatment protocol. These patients generally have a thrombotic occlusion of a coronary artery. The goal is early reperfusion therapy. Studies have shown (Thrombolysis in Myocardial Infarction[TIMI]) that mortality decreases with early treatment. Initial and immediate treatment includes the aforementioned aspirin, clopidogrel, heparin, beta-blockers, nitrates, oxygen, and morphine. The next and most important step is the administration of thrombolysis therapy. Currently, alteplase, streptokinase, tenecteplase, and reteplase are available. Although potentially myocardial sparring, the reperfusion patency is only 60% of patients with the potential complication of bleeding.

Aspirin should be administered immediately to decrease mortality and reinfarction rates after MI. Aspirin inhibits cyclooxygenase-1, which prevents the formation of thromboxane A2 and thus inhibiting the ability of platelet aggregation. Clopidogrel may be an alternative in case of aspirin allergy but may also be recommended as adjunctive therapy. Clopidogrel irreversibly binds to adenosine diphosphate receptor and inhibits ADP-dependent platelet activation. Understandably, the combination of clopidogrel and aspirin increases the risks of bleeding and should be discontinued at least 5 days prior to a planned coronary artery bypass grafting (CABG). Additional treatment to inhibit platelet formation is the glycoprotein IIb/IIIa-receptor antiagonist. Currently, three agents are available, abciximab (ReoPro)<PE>, eptifibatide (Integrilin), and tirofiban (Aggrastat). Heparin, both unfractionated and low molecular weight, is also beneficial when combined with aspirin and clopidogrel for the acute treatment phase.

Traditionally, the nonischemia therapy has been nitrates with their ability to vasodilate veins, arteries, and arterioles. They augment collateral coronary blood flow, decrease preload and demand, reduce coronary artery vasospasm, and may inhibit platelet aggregation. Intravenous nitroglycerin will also cause hypotension, flushing, headaches, and has a tendency to cause tachyphylaxis after 24 hours.

Beta-blocker therapy to control rate and reduce myocardial oxygen demand are mandated unless contraindicated. Metoprolol, the most common selective beta1-adrenergic receptor blocker, decreases automaticity of contractions. Beta-blockers have been determined to reduce reinfarction rate, prevent ischemia, and ultimately reduce mortality.

Nitrates reduce preload and enhance relief of acute symptoms but do not demonstrate an impact on overall mortality in MI. These potent vasodilators are contraindicated if systolic BP <90, HR <60 or >100, and in the presence of RV infarction. Parenteral nitroglycerin may reduce ischemic discomfort, control blood pressure elevations, or assist in relieving pulmonary congestion. Men who have taken phosphodiesterase inhibitor for erectile dysfunction should be given a 24-hour time frame prior to the administration of nitrates (Kloner, 2005). Men who have been prescribed tadalafil require a 48-hour window before nitrates may be administered (Kloner, 2005).

Optimal outcomes in thrombolytic therapy are clear when administered within the initial 2 hours after MI. Thrombolysis is generally preferred when the PCI door-to-balloon time exceeds 3 hours. Administration of a platelet glycoprotein (GP) IIb/IIIa-receptor antagonist is suggested, in addition to aspirin and heparin, for patients with persistent ischemia or other high-risk features in whom PCI is anticipated is recommended. The addition of intravenous platelet GP IIb/IIIa-receptor antagonists to aspirin and heparin improves both early and late outcomes, including mortality, Q-wave MI, need for revascularization procedures, and length of hospital stay.

Consistent with AHA guidelines and clinical guidelines patients with suspected ischemia require prompt identification, intervention and possibly transfer to interventional facilities. Thrombolytics should be considered immediately upon diagnosis. Administration may serve as a bridge for those who do not have immediate access to interventional facilities. Gershlick et al., (2005) cited improved outcomes for patients undergoing rescue angioplasty to prevent death in patients who fail thrombolysis during an MI. Heparin serves as adjunctive agent in patients receiving alteplase, reteplase, or tenecteplase, but should not be used with nonselective fibrinolytic agents. Heparin is also indicated in patients undergoing primary PCI. Low–molecular-weight heparins (LMWH) may be preferred because of convenient dosing and reliable therapeutic levels. No definitive trials of LMWH in patients with STEMI are available to provide an evidence-based approach.

An ACE inhibitor is indicated in the first 24 hours of STEMI in the presence of anterior infarction, pulmonary congestion, or LV ejection fraction <40% in the absence of hypotension. An angiotensin receptor blocker (valsartan or candesartan) should be administered to patients with STEMI who are intolerant of ACE inhibitors and have either clinical or radiological signs of heart failure or LVEF <40%.

Overall community management of MI and the availability of resources for reperfusion are critical to survival after MI. Resources and protocols must proactively address a collaborative effort between emergency team, interventional providers, and cardiothoracic surgeons. The decision to administer a thrombolytic agent may be made by the emergency providers, with or without the input of a cardiologist, depending on institutional protocol. In a center with the full range of treatment options, an expeditious phone consultation with a cardiologist would be prudent to determine the most appropriate option for the patient.

Aortic Surgery

The four major diseases that present for surgical correction in the aorta are dissection, aneurysm, rupture, and coarctation. The aneurysm and dissection tend to go together as one syndrome; both of which can be progressive. There are many causes of aneurysms; however, the most common are hypertension, atherosclerosis, infections, and genetic or congenital causes, which would include Marfan syndrome. The aneurismal sac can take on several forms. Thoracoabdominal aortic aneurysms are classified based on where it is initiated and ends using the Crawford classification (see Exhibit 4.5).

Aortic aneurysms are slow to expand but have great potential to dissect or rupture. Aneurysms do not grow linearly and tend to get increase in smokers and the chronically hypertensive. Current recommendation suggests a deferral of

Exhibit

4.5   Crawford Classification

TYPE I arises distal to the left subclavian and extends to the level of the superior mesenteric artery but above the renals.

TYPE II arises distal to the left subclavian and extends to below the renal arteries.

TYPE III arises from below the level of the sixth intercostals and extends to below the renal arteries.

TYPE IV arises from the level of the twelfth intercostal space and extends to below the renal artery.

intervention until the aneurysm is over 5.5 cm in the ascending aorta and over 6 cm in the descending aorta.

Generally, aortic aneurysms are found as incidental findings from a chest x-ray or CT scan. Some aneurysms can cause vague symptoms from pressure or hoarseness with stretching of the recurrent laryngeal nerve. Accurate diagnosis is best accomplished with a CT scan with contrast and axial reconstruction.

Treatment of the aneurysm is dependent on several factors including size, location, and rapidity of growth. Conventional medical treatment is diet, blood pressure control, and smoking cessation. The advent of advanced endovascular options enables the treatment of descending aneurysms by stenting. Current options enable some ascending aneurysms to be stented, which is a remarkable shift in therapy and reduces risk of morbidity and mortality.

Aortic dissections, although still part of the continuum of disease of the aortic aneurysm, are far more abrupt, painful, and if left untreated, will result in death. The patient may describe the pain as a sharp or tearing in nature in their chest. During the dissection, the intima of the aorta is sheared off the aorta, creating a false lumen, which can spread in either direction. Most of the aortic dissections begin at the ascending aorta, 5%–10% being at the arch and 30%–35% being in the first part of the descending aorta. There are two main classifications: the DeBakey and Stanford classification. For the DeBakey type I and II (Stanford A), surgery is usually indicated to prevent aortic rupture and aortic insufficiency. DeBakey III (Stanford B) is usually managed medically (see Table 4.2).

A functional aortic regurgitation can result from the dilation of the annulus or root. A pericardial effusion may accompany the dissection. As the intima shears off and creates a false luminal passage vital organs may be compromised by ischemia. Although ECG and chest x-ray may be abnormal, they may also appear normal and may be difficult to interpret. CT scan, in contrast, has 90% sensitivity and 85% specificity. MRI provides high-quality images, but may be time prohibitive in the patient who is hemodynamically unstable. TEE offers rapid visualization of the ascending and descending aorta but requires a skilled operator and the descending aorta cannot be easily visualized. Angiography is invasive and may fail to show entry and reentry sites.

The key for the ICU practitioner is to control the blood pressure and thereby reduce shear forces against the wall

4.2 Classification of Aortic Dissections

Site of Involvement	Ascending & Descending Aorta Involved	Confined to the Ascending Aorta	Ascending Aorta not Involved
DeBakey	I	II	III
Stanford	A	A	B

and further dissection. Blood pressure targets should be adjusted based on evidence of perfusion to other vital organs (i.e., renal, cerebral). The treatment of choice is to use a combination therapy of beta-blocker and vasodilator, such as labetalol and sodium nitroprusside, respectively. The use of invasive blood pressure monitoring is essential for appropriate management.

Coronary Artery Bypass

CABG is very effective in reducing or eliminating symptoms in patients with angina pectoris and in certain subgroups, CABG improves prognosis. For stable patients with preserved LV function, the operative mortality risk is <1% and even for patients with impaired LV dysfunction, there is still a survival advantage of CABG over medical therapy in select populations. LV dysfunction increases the operative risk and the risk of difficulty of separating the patient from the bypass machine. Since PTCA has become more prevalent, the patients assigned for open CABG procedures are usually older, sicker, and have more extensive disease. Other factors that can influence the decision regarding CABG include the size of the coronary vessels and the nature of diffuse or distal coronary artery disease, which may reduce the effectiveness of grafts. Some short-term risk factors that influence mortality following a CABG include age, COPD, peripheral vascular disease, elevated creatinine, prior heart surgery, prior MI, urgency, NYHA class III or IV, and low ejection fraction. Conduits used for the bypass include the saphenous veins, the internal mammary arteries, and the radial artery from the nondominant hand. The left internal mammary artery is commonly used for a direct bypass to the left anterior descending artery. The arterial grafts, particularly the left and right internal mammary arteries have the longest patency rates.

CABG surgery is often considered for patients with unacceptable angina pectori despite medical therapy, patients with left main coronary artery disease, and triple vessel disease. CABG does not however stop coronary artery disease progression. Obstruction can occur in native vessels that were not bypassed and in the bypassed grafts themselves. Most arterial grafts have a patency of 10 years, whereas the venous grafts tend to stay patent for only 7 years, with angina reoccurring in 50% of these patients. Universal interventions in maintaining graft patency are aspirin therapy, changes in diet, smoking cessation, blood pressure control, and change in sedentary life style.

Patients with obstructive coronary artery disease are considered for percutaneous transluminal coronary angioplasty. As angioplasty and stenting with drug eluding stents becomes more advanced, the patient population that would be served well increases. Drug-eluting stents are coated with antiproliferative drugs such as sirolimus. PTCA involves threading a balloon catheter into a coronary artery, positioning the balloon across the stenotic lesion and then inflating the balloon to dilate the stenosis. The procedure disrupts the intima, splits the atherosclerotic plaque, and often results in a small local dissection. Acute coronary occlusion can complicate the PTCA and lead to acute myocardial infarction and or the need for emergency coronary bypass. The mortality rate associated with PTCA is about 1%. Restenosis rates vary dramatically and the deployment of a stent will improve the patency rate. The introduction of drug-eluting stents compared to the initial bare metal stents have shown improved long-term success rates. Patients though with a left main lesion are not typically candidates for PTCA or stenting.

Heart Transplant

United Network of Organ Sharing (UNOS) is the national U.S. organization that is responsible for control and fair distribution of donated organs. UNOS will offer organs on the basis of geography, donor–recipient compatibility, and medical urgency. UNOS is a nonprofit, scientific, and educational organization that administers the nation's only Organ Procurement and Transplantation Network (OPTN). UNOS is required to collect and manage data about every transplant event occurring in the United States. The organization facilitates the organ matching and placement process using specific data technology. Collectively, UNOS brings together medical professionals, transplant recipients, and donor families to develop organ transplantation policy.

The criteria for selection for heart recipients have evolved as the success of this procedure has improved, but the availability of donors remains limited. Candidates must have end-stage cardiac disease with limited life expectancy and have exhausted conventional therapies, including pharmacologic and bypass surgery. The primary diagnoses that are considered criteria include ischemic and nonischemic cardiomyopathy, valvular disease, congenital heart disease, and primary heart transplant failure. The exclusion criteria include older than 65 years of age, irreversible hepatic or renal failure, active infection, poor medication compliance, psychological instability, malignancy, alcohol, recreational drug abuse, obesity, cerebrovascular disease, crossmatch incompatibility, and a pulmonary vascular resistance over 5 Woods units. The placement of a healthy donor heart into a patient with pulmonary hypertension will rapidly fail, whereas the native heart with its longstanding compensation has greater ability to overcome pulmonary hypertension. The ACNP should restrict exposure to unnecessary blood transfusions that will create a higher percentage of panel reactive antibodies with the cross-matched potential donor and create a greater likelihood of a rejection. The uncomplicated heart transplant patient with short ischemic time, minimal blood loss, and good function, with or without low-dose inotropic support, should be extubated in <24 hours with a usual postoperative recovery. Chest tubes can be removed if the output is approximately <100 ml in a 24-hour period.

The new transplanted heart will have some degree of dysfunction, with the right ventricle usually being affected more than the left. This may require slightly higher filling pressures. Generally, a modest tachycardia is advisable as the ventricles tend to be stiff. This is generally achieved in several methods including dopamine and milrinone, and/or pacing. Most transplant patients need a small degree of vasopressors for a few days following surgery, secondary to the naturally occurring vasodilation. Pulmonary hypertension should be avoided and it is not uncommon to induce a moderate diuresis after the second day as these patients tend to retain fluid.

Vigilance in the use of masks, gloves, and gowns must be maintained when in contact with transplant patients as the need for scrupulous infection control measures outweighs almost any other priority. Immunosuppression protocols vary among institutions and ongoing evaluation of regimens prevails at centers of excellence.

The major cause of early mortality is primary graft failure. Ventricular failure, predominantly left sided, may be the first sign. Myocardial stunning from prolonged ischemia time and recipient pulmonary hypertension as a result of heart failure may cause the donor heart to fail. Considering temporary extracorporeal membrane oxygenation (ECMO) may supply time for the donor heart to adapt.

Despite all acceptable therapy, the possibility of rejection must always remain a consideration with any change in status. Hyperacute rejection is an uncommon cause of primary graft failure. Human leukocyte antigen (HLA) antibodies are increased with higher amounts of transfusion exposure, in particular platelets. Leukocyte depleted transfusions are recommended for the recipient if blood is needed. Furthermore, with a high percentage of panel reactive antibodies, preoperative plasmapharesis should be a consideration to prevent postoperative complications.

Other early complications for the heart transplant patient include tricuspid regurgitation (TR), respiratory failure and bleeding, renal failure with fluid overload, and gastrointestinal problems. Complications that occur after the first 5 days include acute rejection, infection, systemic embolism, and coronary artery disease, secondary to the new-onset rejection. The insidious path of acute rejections is marked by arrhythmias, hypotension, and ventricular dysfunction best seen with an echocardiogram. Planned biopsy at or near the 10th day should be a routine. Coronary artery disease may be caused by rejection and this is manifested by chronic rejection, wherein a perfectly healthy donated heart will develop rapid coronary occlusion.

Use of Devices/Ventricular Assist Device

Pharmacologic management described earlier in this chapter have improved quality of life for patients with failing hearts. However, even with the most aggressive treatments, some still require surgical intervention. Currently, there are several options, which include reduction ventriculoplasty, transmyocardial laser revascularization, and the insertion of partial or total heart assist devices.

Consideration of an assist device should not be taken lightly; one must first consider the limitations of a device and the anticipated benefit. The HeartMate left ventricular assist device (LVAD) is the only device labeled as destination therapy because it is designed to be implanted in the patient with external drive lines. What is important for the practitioner to understand is the general types of devices available, the anatomic placement, and recognition of problems in the acute care setting.

The physiology of these devices is to facilitate the patient's ability to augment or, if need be, totally rely on these devices for left, right, or biventricular output. These devices were first developed as an outcome of the initial cardiopulmonary bypass (CPB) machines when it was recognized that some patients were not able to be separated. The initial thought was that these devices would be used for short-term rest and recovery to eventually wean and separate a patient from the CPB. Initial attempts throughout the 1960s were less than successful. Eventually in 1980, the National Institute for Health (NIH) funded research that supported a long-term LV assist device.

The basic mechanisms of all the devices are similar. The devices remove blood proximal to the diseased ventricle bypass the ventricular system and return the blood distally. The two main mechanisms are pulsatile flow devices and continuous flow devices. The later includes the axial flow pumps and the centrifugal flow pumps.

Indications

The indications for the insertion of the ventricular assist device are increasing and evolving. However, the three major categories are a bridge to destination therapy, a bridge to transplant, or in rare occasion, a bridge to recovery. With experience, timing, device selection, and most importantly, appropriate patient selection, there have been improved outcomes. The indication may include cardiogenic shock or decompensated chronic heart failure as a bridge to recovery. There are also a few well-studied protocols for use of the LVAD in pulmonary transplant failure and ARDS.

The use of the LVAD as a bridge to recovery is most promising in the patient with fulminate acute myocarditis, which can cause heart failure; unfortunately, this patient population is very limited. Acute cardiogenic shock is more common and the data reflects that those requiring LVAD in cardiogenic shock as intraoperative rescue procedure, postoperative, or in the case of acute myocardial infarction have poor outcomes. The bridge to transplant population have more positive data, although the lack of available suitable donors severely restricts this indication. The insertion of a VAD in a patient already on the transplant list offers more hope. These patients represent a more robust recipient and improved outcomes. The bridge to recovery population comprises the following three subgroups: postoperative patients, individuals with shock following myocardial infarction, and those with acute myocarditis; the last group having the best prognosis.

Complications

Although positive results have been seen with the institution of the VAD, there are many complications associated with their placement. Early complications include hypoxemia, air embolism, hemorrhage, and RV heart failure. The hypoxemia occurs secondary to missed atrial defects that can cause a right to left shunt. Air embolism, like hypoxemia, can be the result of a patent foramen ovale (PFO). Hemorrhage may obviously occur with the simple placement of the device as extensive surgery may be required for proper orientation. Compounding this is the fact that most transplant surgeons are reluctant to transfuse potential recipients for fear of inducing HLA alloimmunization. Furthermore, most patients are already debilitated and recovery from such a procedure may prove an insurmountable hurdle. While most devices are placed for left heart failure, one must be cognizant that the right heart may be in failure and not sufficient to fill the left side and a subsequent biventricular device may be inserted.

Late complications include infection, thromboembolism, and primary device failure. Infection may be the primary cause. Once a device is infected, there are few options. Predisposing factors include multiple central lines, the drive lines, the surgically created pockets for devices, poor nutrition, and the need for an ICU environment despite the exposure to many pathogens. The incidence of thromboembolism may have improved with the advent of better materials, surfaces, and protocols. Lastly, there is the possibility of the devastating primary device failure.

Device Selection

Device selection tends to be based on several factors, including the need for single or biventricular assistance, size of the patient, and duration of the expected support. Generally, however, the comfort of the surgeon with a particular device seems to be the most pressing factor, particularly in the acute need as in postoperative failure.

The devices currently available can be divided by several characteristics including implantability, size, pulsatility, and need for anticoagulation. Ideally, a device should be small enough to be totally implanted, allowing mobility. The device should not need any anticoagulation, as most devices only require antiplatelet therapy, be resistant to infection, be failure free, and should have enough energy to be mobile for a prolonged period. No device meets all these criteria at this time.

The ABIOMED® AB5000 Ventricle is a short-term, external device that is used to support the heart. This device can be used as a bridge to a longer term support device, or as a cardiac assist device to allow time for the heart to rest after surgery or other reversible heart dysfunction. The ABIOMED® AB5000 Ventricle is approved by the FDA for use as a bridge to recovery for patients with potentially reversible heart failure. Patients on this device must remain in the hospital during the support phase. This device can provide right, left, or biventricular cardiac support.

The Thoratec HeartMate® XVE is an implantable LVAD that can be used as a bridge to heart transplantation or as destination therapy. The pump is implanted in the upper abdomen and is attached to the heart. This pulsatile pump assists the left ventricle. The pump is monitored and controlled by an external controller that is approximately the size of an adult's hand. The patient carries the controller in a fanny pack. Patients on this device are discharged from the hospital and can go back to work or school and resume most daily life activities. The device is powered by an AC unit or by batteries. The device is approved by the FDA as a bridge to heart transplantation.

The HeartMate® II is a new technology that utilizes rotor flow to propel blood from the left ventricle to the aorta. This device is used primarily as a LVAD and is a bridge to heart transplantation. The pump is approximately the size of a large candy bar and can be placed in smaller patients because of its smaller size. This device is an internal pump and is monitored by an external controller that is approximately the size of an adult's hand. Like the Heartmate XVE, the patient carries the controller in a fanny pack. The patient on this device is discharged from the hospital and can go back to work or school and resume most daily life activities. The device is powered by an AC unit or by batteries.

The Thoratec® IVAD can be used for left, right, or biventricular support. This device is primarily used as a bridge to heart transplantation. The pump can be used internally (IVAD) or externally (PVAD). Patients can be discharged on both devices and may resume most normal daily activities. While at home, the pumps are operated using a portable compressor system that is about the size of a piece of carry-on luggage.

The patient with a VAD should be monitored closely with regard to progress, including improved homeostasis, enhanced renal function, liver function, and, weight gain. Long-term complications may include clot formation, thrombi, infection, and to some degree, psychological disturbances.

When considering the use of a VAD in a patient, a thorough evaluation of comorbidities must be undertaken. Those with chronic irreversible end-organ disease states are poor candidates for assist devices. Other situations that would be a poor choice would include the use of a VAD for a bridge to transplant with little or no hope of succeeding on the transplant list, destination therapy with a poor prognosis, and certainly those who would be bridge to recovery, but have little hope in that regard. In addition, there are several additional relative contraindications for a VAD such as severe pulmonary dysfunction, excessive weight, and malignancy. Irreversible neurologic injury and overwhelming infection are absolute contraindications.

Outcomes of these devices have improved over the years with good results for destination therapy, bridge to recovery, and bridge to transplant. There are more devices and modifications in future development to make these options more readily available. The ultimate goal might still be considered the totally implantable, artificial heart. CardioWest does have one approved by the FDA as a bridge to transplant; therefore, it is probably only a matter of time and engineering that one is given approval as destination therapy.

Use of Devices/Intraortic Balloon Pump

Intraaortic balloon counterpulsation (IABP) is a short-term support for patients with severe myocardial ischemia or LV systolic failure. The IABP device itself is a long catheter with two lumens. One lumen is used for the flow of the helium, whereas the second lumen is used for the transducing intraaortic pressure. The catheter is connected to an external console that controls the timing of the balloon inflation and deflation, including a display for the ECG, arterial blood pressure, and balloon pressures. The balloon is fashioned as a sausage shape. The underlying purpose of the device is to inflate at the start of diastole and to deflate at the start of systole. The net effect is afterload reduction via reduction of aortic end-diastolic pressure resulting in a reduction in LV systolic wall tension. Secondarily, and perhaps most importantly, the inflation in the diastolic phase will increase coronary perfusion.

Extracorporeal Membrane Oxygenation (ECMO)

The critical element of inserting a device in the bridge to recovery population is timing and perhaps more importantly the timing of when to discontinue therapy. With all extracorporeal devices, the risk benefit needs to be addressed continually and the risk of infection, bleeding, clotting, and costs increase with each hour and day. For the patient in acute shock due to the above categories, daily evaluation of ejection function should be assessed with echocardiography. Capabilities of bridging with these devices are for a limited time frame.

Postcardiac Surgery Monitoring

The key to monitoring a postoperative cardiac patient or one with risk factors undergoing thoracic or noncardiac surgery is the measurement of cardiac performance. The cardiac output is a reflection of preload, afterload, contractility, and heart rate.

Many ICUs use the preferred method of pulmonary artery catheter (PAC) with continuous cardiac output capabilities and SVO2 measurement. There has been great discussion on the impact of survivability and possible increased risk associated with a PAC, although these catheters have not been specifically studied in postcardiac patients. New less invasive technologies are now emerging to estimate the cardiac output usually based on the Fick principle. The Fick method relates cardiac output to oxygen consumption and the arteriovenous content. The direct Fick method with the requirement of measured oxygen consumption is generally impractical. So the indirect Fick methods of using a normogram for consumption ($125ml/m^2$) is based on body surface area. When the arterial oxygen is being consumed by the body and replenished by the lungs at an equal rate, the VO^2 is the product of cardiac output and the O_2 concentration difference. The oxygen content from the systemic arterial and mixed venous (pulmonary arterial) is measured and the sample allows calculation of the flow rate (cardiac output). Under nonsteady states of oxygen consumption, these calculations could be less accurate.

Other conventional invasive methods of cardiac output measurement include the PAC with manual cold thermodilution technique (rarely used), PAC with continuous cardiac output and a warming coil, and TEE. There are several semi-invasive methods available including, transpulmonary thermodilution with arterial pulse contour analysis (PiCCO), lithium dilution curve with arterial waveform analysis (LiDCO), and the doppler method. Noninvasive techniques include pulse contour analysis (FloTrac) and bioimpedance cardiography. Dye-dilution techniques were the first methods to be used for estimation of cardiac output. The Stewart–Hamilton equation assumes that the injection of a certain quantity indicator will appear and disappear and is reflective of the cardiac output. The dye dilution technique has been supplanted by the easier thermodilution technique. The thermodilution technique was developed following the introduction of the flow directed PAC (Swan & Ganz, 1970). While initially devised to measure right-sided pressures and PAD, with the addition of thermal indicators, it became more useful for continuous and nearly continuous measurement of CO. There is great debate about the utility and safety about PAC, however in studies that sought to correlate the values from the Fick equation, there is evidence that when the cardiac output is above 5 L/min, the precision of the Swan declines.

Thermodilution technique requires a bolus of liquid into the proximal port of the catheter. The change in temperature registered at the distal thermometer is then calculates the area under the curve as the cardiac output and it is similar to dye-dilution method. Patients with shunts or TR or pulmonary regurgitation (PR) early recirculation will cause inaccurate recordings. Furthermore, rapid infusion of fluids will alter the effectiveness of this device. Continuous thermodilution cardiac output measurement is similar to the above cold bolus techniques except the catheter releases a small amount of heat to the distal thermostat then calculates the cardiac output. The correlation to the bolus method is more precise.

Lithium dilution technique has a core indictor of the dilution technique. The advantage is that it can be given through a peripheral catheter and measurement of the waves from an ion-selective electrode attached to the peripheral arterial catheter. The technique is considered safe and accurate. The only contraindication is if the patient is already taking lithium. The primary utility of this technology at this time is to calibrate the Pulse CO monitor (LiDCO) that calculates the continuous cardiac output by arterial pulse wave analysis.

Doppler-based method can be used to determine cardiac output by measuring the blood flow velocities. Placement of the probe in parallel to the flow is vital as it can lead to errors. Several technologies take advantage of this method including an endotracheal tube with an ultrasound probe mounted on the tip as this method has inherent problems, including the need for the patient to be sedated and intubated. Furthermore, there are frequent discrepancies due to positioning.

Conclusion

The entire spectrum of diagnosis and treatment of cardiovascular disease has undergone a dramatic shift and embraces an evidence-based approach. Aggressive treatment options have proven able to mitigate damage and preemptive care has decreased morbidity. The responsibility of the practitioner caring for these patients is to keep abreast of the most current therapies.

However, when we look specifically in the cardiovascular ICU and care of the cardiovascular patient, it is important to remain keenly attentive to the basics. The care of the cardiothoracic patient employs, above all, the tenets of excellent ICU care:

attention to cardiac function, EKG and rhythm identification and intervention hemodynamics, fluid and electrolyte balance, and thoughtful therapies. Vigilance, attention to detail, and judicious critical care are essential to the cardiac patient in critical care.

References

American College of Cardiology. (2008). ACC/AHA/Physician Consortium 2008 Clinical Performance Measures for Adults With Nonvalvular Atrial Fibrillation or Atrial Flutter. *Journal of the American College of Cardiology, 51,* 865–884.

ACC/AHA. (2008). ACC/AHA/Physician Consortium 2008 Clinical Performance Measures for Adults With Nonvalvular Atrial Fibrillation or Atrial Flutter. Circulation, *Circulation, 117,* 1101–1120.

Agency for Healthcare Research and Quality. (2003). *Ventricular Systolic Dysfunction: Effect in Female, Black, and Diabetic Patients, and Cost-Effectiveness* (Evidence Report/Technology Assessment No. 82). Rockville, MD: Author.

American Heart Association. (2000). AHA with the International Liaison Committee on Resuscitation. Guidelines 2000 for Cardiopulmonary Resuscitation and Emergency Cardiovascular Care. Part 7: the era of reperfusion: section 1: acute coronary syndromes (acute myocardial infarction). *Circulation, 102*(Suppl. 8), I172–203.

American Heart Association. (2007). Antiarrhythmic Drugs. Retrieved September 2, 2008 from http://www.americanheart.org/presenter .jhtml?identifier=153

Braunwald, E. (2000). Management of Patients with Unstable Angina and ST-Segment Elevation MI, A report of the ACC/AHA Task Force on Practice Guidelines.

Goldenberg, I., Moss, A. J., Maron, B. J., Dick, A. W., Zareba, W. (2005). Cost-effectiveness of implanted defibrillators in young people with inherited cardiac arrhythmias. *Annals of Noninvasive Electrocardiology, 10*(4 Suppl), 67–83.

Gregoratos, G., Abrams, J., Epstein, A. E., Freedman, R. A., Hayes, D. L., Hlatky, M. A., et al. (2002). ACC/AHA/NASPE 2002 guideline update for implantation of cardiac pacemakers and antiarrhythmia devices: Summary Article: A report of the American College of Cardiology/ American Heart Association Task Force on Practice Guidelines (ACC/AHA/NASPE Committee to Update the 1998 Pacemaker Guidelines). *Circulation, 106*(16), 2145–2161.

Klein, H. U., & Reek, S. (2000). The MUSTT Study: evaluating, testing, and treatment. *Journal of Interventional Cardiac Electrophysiology, 4*(Suppl. 1), 45–50.

Kloner, R. A. (2005). Pharmacology and drug interaction effects of the phosphodiesterase 5 inhibitors: focus on alpha-blocker interactions. *American Journal of Cardiology, 96*(12B), 42M–46M. Epub 2005 Dec 5.

Kuck, K. H., Cappato, R., Siebels, J., & Rüppel, R. (2000). Randomized comparison of antiarrhythmic drug therapy with implantable defibrillators in patients resuscitated from cardiac arrest: the Cardiac Arrest Study Hamburg (CASH). *Circulation, 102*(7), 748–754.

Moss, A. J., Zareba, W., Hall, W. J., Klein, H., Wilber, D. J., Cannom, D. S., et al., (2002). Prophylactic implantation of a defibrillator in patients with myocardial infarction and reduced ejection fraction. *The New England Journal of Medicine, 346,* 877–883.

Strickberger, S. A., Hummel, J. D., Bartlett, T. G., Frumin, H. I., Schuger, C. D., Beau, S. L., et al. (2003). Amiodarone versus implantable cardioverter-defibrillator: Randomized trial in patients with nonischemic dilated cardiomyopathy and asymptomatice nonsustained ventricular tachycardia—AMIOVERT. *Journal of the American College of Cardiology, 41*(10), 1713–1715.

Strippoli G. F., Craig, M. C., Schena, F. P., et al., (2006). Role of blood pressure targets and specific antihypertensive agents used to prevent diabetic nephropathy and delay its progression. *Journal of the American Society of Nephrology 17:*S153–5.

Swan, H. J. C., Ganz, W., Forrester, J., Marcus, H., Diamond, G., Chonette, D. (1970). Catheterization of the heart in man with use of a flow-directed balloon-tipped catheter. *New England Journal of Medicine, 243,* 443–451.

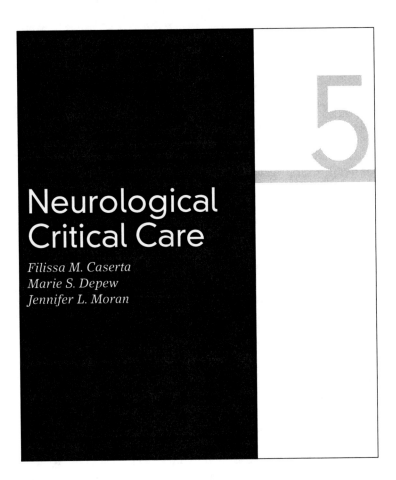

Neurological Critical Care

Filissa M. Caserta
Marie S. Depew
Jennifer L. Moran

Introduction: Initial Evaluation of the Neurologically Impaired Patient

The most critical portion of neuroscience care is the neurologic examination. When the practitioner fully understands the physiology behind the examination, a lesion can be localized by clinical findings. This chapter is designed to assist the acute care nurse practitioner to obtain a detailed, yet efficient examination. In addition, this chapter will review the main tests used to diagnose neurologic emergencies in the neurocritical care setting.

Physical Examination

Anatomy Review. When performing neurological assessment, it is important to understand basic anatomy and then use that anatomy to correlate the examination. The lobes of the brain are referred to as the cerebral cortex and include the frontal, parietal, temporal, and occipital lobes (Hickey, 2002). The key functions of the frontal lobes are the awareness portion of the level of consciousness, intelligence, judgment, attention span, memory, voluntary motor, and motor/expressive speech (Broca area). The parietal lobes are primarily responsible for sensory functions including the ability to identify objects by touch, distinguish right from left, and have awareness of one's body position in space (proprioception). Sensory/receptive speech is a function of both the parietal and temporal lobes (Wernicke area). The primary auditory receptive areas are located in the temporal lobes, as is smell interpretation and long-term memory. Occipital lobes contain the primary visual cortex and interpret visual cues. The cerebellum is responsible for coordination (Gelb, 2000). Cranial nerves III through XII have their origins in the brainstem. The III and IV cranial nerves originate in the midbrain, V through VII in the pons, and the medulla contains the origins of cranial IX through XII. Cranial nerves I and II are located in the cerebral cortex (Seidel, Ball, Dains, & Benedict, 2006). The reticular formation, which is responsible for wakefulness and arousability portion of the level of consciousness, also has its origins in the brainstem (Hickey). By performing the examination from cortex to brainstem in an orderly fashion, the examiner will obtain the main components of the neurological assessment in a concise and organized fashion. This reduces the chances of missing any key component of the examination (Gelb). Any neurological examination should include assessment of level of consciousness, memory, language, motor strength, sensory, coordination, cranial nerves, and reflexes.

Level of Consciousness/Memory/Language. When assessing the level of consciousness, the examiner gathers information regarding memory and language. Initially, level of consciousness assessment begins with three basic orientation questions of person, place, and time (Seidel, Ball, Dains, & Benedict, 2006). The examiner can then ask the patient if they know why they are in the hospital and if they know their providers name, thereby assessing short-term memory. A long-term memory question that the examiner can validate easily is asking the patient for his date of birth. While the patient is providing the answers to the examiner's questions, the examiner should be listening to the patient's speech, noting the clarity, appropriateness, and presence of any word finding difficulties. To further evaluate language, the examiner should ask the patient to repeat phrases such as "No ifs, ands, or buts" and "It's a bright and sunny day in (insert city)." It is also critical to ask the patient to identify objects and is also critical to note his or her difficulty or inability to name them. Comprehension can be assessed by asking the patient to perform a task such as "Take your left hand and touch your right ear," ensuring that no visual cues are used (Gelb, 2000).

A helpful tool that is utilized in addition to the earlier mentioned tests to assess consciousness is the Glasgow Coma Scale (GCS) (Table 5.1). This scale is divided into three parts and assesses best motor, verbal, and eye opening responses. The highest score a patient can obtain is a 15 and the lowest is a 3. It is an excellent way to trend the neurologic examination (Hickey, 2002).

Motor. The motor examination is simply performed by assessing the individual muscle groups and rating them with the motor scale as noted in Table 5.2. The strength of each muscle group should be documented with the result being expressed as a fraction, using 5 for the denominator (Seidel, Ball, Dains & Benedict, 2002). For example, a person with active movement against gravity in a particular extremity should have their strength documented as $3/5$ for that extremity.

Sensory. There are various examinations that can be performed to assess gross sensory function; however, the simplest are right and left discrimination and proprioception or position sense (Goetz, 2007). Ask patients to close their eyes and to identify where in their body they are being touched. As the examiner, first touch one arm, then the other, and then both. Repeat the same for the lower extremities. The reason for the simultaneous stimulation of upper and lower extremities is to assess for tactile extinction, which is an indication of a hemineglect. Tactile extinction is noted when the patient can feel touch in each individual extremity, but when touched on both, sides he or she

5.1 The Glasgow Coma Scale

Glasgow Coma Scale	
Eye Opening	
Spontaneous	4
To loud voice	3
To pain	2
None	1
Verbal Response	
Oriented	5
Confused, disoriented	4
Inappropriate words	3
Incomprehensible	2
Sounds	2
None	
Best Motor Response	
Obeys commands	6
Localizes	5
Withdraws (flexion)	4
Abnormal flexion	3
Abnormal extension	2
None	1

5.2 Rating of Muscle Strength

Muscle Strength	Rating
No contraction	0
Flicker or trace of contraction	1
Active movement, with gravity eliminated	2
Active movement against gravity	3
Active movement against gravity and resistance	4
Normal power	5

5.1

Dermatomes

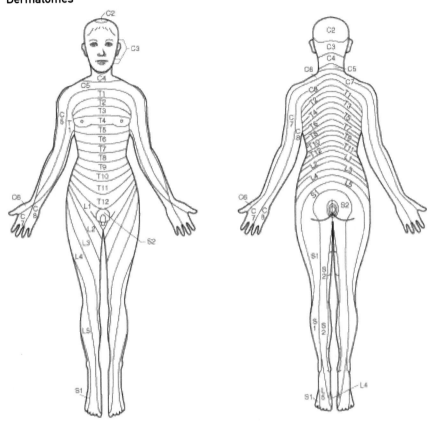

can only feel only unilateral stimulation. The presence of this finding indicates a possible lesion in the contralateral sensory cortex. A more detailed sensory examination to include superficial pain is warranted on any patient with spinal pathology. Assessing for superficial pain is done by testing the patient's ability to distinguish sharp from dull throughout the various dermatomes from C4 through S1 (Figure 5.1). In this way, a deficit can be directly correlated to an anatomical location on the spine (Devereaux, 2007). Proprioception of both the upper and lower extremities can be assessed by testing joint position sense. This is done by holding the lateral aspects of the thumb or toe in a raised or lowered position and asking the patient to state in which direction his or her toe or thumb is pointed.

Coordination. Coordination in the critical care arena is tested via assessment of rapid alternating finger-to-nose and heel-to-shin movements (Hickey, 2002). Assess rapid alternating movements by asking the patient to touch the thumb of one hand to each finger on the same hand, starting with the index finger and ending with the little finger and back. Assess this on both hands. Next, ask the patient to alternately touch his or her own nose and then touch the examiner's finger with the index finger of one hand. Have him or her repeat this with the other hand. Finally, have the patient run the heel of one foot down the shin of the other leg (Seidel, Ball, Dains, & Benedict, 2006). Again, this should be performed on both lower extremities.

Cranial Nerves. The assessment of the cranial nerves does not need to be an arduous task. In an inpatient setting, cranial nerve I (olfactory nerve) is not tested. Table 5.3 lists the basic examination for remaining cranial nerves II to XII.

Reflexes. Deep tendon reflexes (DTRs) should be a part of any initial neurological assessment and include the biceps, triceps, brachioradial, patellar, and Achilles (Seidel, Ball, Dains, & Benedict, 2006). See Table 5.4 for a rating scale of DTRs. Assess for ankle clonus by briskly dorsiflexing the patient's foot with the hand and noting any rhythmic, oscillating movements of the foot against the examiner's hand. The plantar reflex is assessed by stroking the lateral aspect of the foot from the heel to the ball then curving across the ball of the foot to the medial side (Goldberg, 2007). A normal plantar reflex is plantar flexion of all toes. An "up going" or dorsiflexion of the great toe with or without fanning of the other toes is an abnormal response, which is indicative of motor tract dysfunction.

Unconscious Patient. The assessment of a patient who is not following commands and unable to participate in a full neurological assessment is obtained by utilizing the GCS and assessing a core of cranial nerves. Assessing the pupils (CN II and CN III), corneas, (CN V and CN VII) and cough and gag

5.3 The Cranial Nerves and Their Functions

Nerve	Name	Test
II	Optic	Visual acuity—have patient read something (id badge) and ask if it is clear Visual fields—assess via confrontation of both eyes with examiner covering his eye and patient covering the opposite eye Pupils—sensory portion of pupillary response
III	Oculomotor	Pupils—motor portion of pupillary response Eyelid—assess if keeps eyelid open Extraocular movements—up, medially, and down and out
III, IV, VI	Extraocular movements (EOMs)	
III	Oculomotor	EOMs—up, medially, and down and out
IV	Trochlear	EOMs—down and in
VI	Abducens	EOMs—lateral gaze
V	Trigeminal	Facial sensation: ophthalmic, maxillary, and mandibular branches Facial motor: clenching teeth Corneal reflex on non-awake patient: sensory portion
VII	Facial	Facial motor: assess symmetry of smile Eyelid- ability to close eye tight Corneal reflex on non-awake patient: motor portion
VIII	Acoustic	Hearing
IX	Glossopharyngeal	Cough, gag, swallow and palate symmetry
X	Vagus	Cough, gag, swallow and palate symmetry
XI	Spinal Accessory	Strength of shoulder shrug and turning face against examiner's hand
XII	Hypoglossal	Tongue—ability to stick out straight

5.4	Rating of Deep Tendon Reflexes (DTRs)

Grade	DTR response
0	No response
1+	Present but sluggish or diminished
2+	Normal amplitude
3+	Increased in amplitude with spread to an adjacent site
4+	Increased in amplitude with spread to an adjacent site with intermittent clonus

(CN IX and CN X) will give the examiner a critical snapshot of brainstem function (Lower, 2002).

Imaging

The main imaging studies that are utilized in the neurocritical care population are magnetic resonance imaging (MRI) with and without gadolinium and computerized axial tomography (CT) with and without contrast. Table 5.5 lists the available modalities and the indications for each. In general, for an acute process such as trauma, stroke, severe headache, and mental status change, a noncontrast head CT is the first choice. If the findings suggest tumor or abscess, a contrast head CT should be considered. (Gunderman, 2006). Any question of acute spinal cord compression should be evaluated with an MRI of the spine. MRI of the brain is usually obtained for a process whose onset is >48 hours (Gunderman).

Other diagnostic tests that are utilized in the neurocritical care environment are the electroencephalogram (EEG) and electromyography (EMG). An EEG is used primarily to diagnose seizures and to assist with the differential diagnosis of acute encephalopathy (Praline et al., 2007). EMG is simply the electrophysiologic assessment of the neuromuscular system. It includes a needle electromyographic study and nerve conduction studies (NCS) (Warrell, Cox, Firth, & Benz, 2003). EMG and NCS both aid in the differential diagnosis of disorders of the peripheral neuromuscular system such as Guillain-Barré syndrome (GBS) and myasthenia gravis (MG).

Modality	Indications/Conditions
BRAIN	
CT: No contrast	Acute change in mental status: Hemorrhage/Edema/Mass effect/Herniation/Hydrocephalus
	Acute trauma: Skull fractures/Hemorrhage/Contusions/Mass effect/Herniation
	Acute stroke: Ischemia/Hemorrhage/Hydrocephalus
	Acute severe headache: Hemorrhage (Subarachnoid/Intracerebral/Intraventricular)
CT: Contrast	Mass: tumor/abscess
	Staging of cancers known to have brain metastasis
MRI: No Contrast	Inflammatory conditions; meningitis, encephalitis
	Posterior fossa lesions of all types
	Subacute stroke
	Subacute trauma: Diffuse axonal injury, subdural hematoma at skull base
	Anoxic brain injury
	Epilepsy
MRI: Contrast	Mass: tumor/abscess
MR angiogram (MRA)	Ischemic stroke: assess vessels
	Hemorrhagic stroke: vascular abnormalities (arteriovenous malformations, aneurysms)
CT angiogram (CTA)	Ischemic stroke: carotid arteries (neck CT) for occlusion or dissection/intracranial vascular occlusions
	Hemorrhagic stroke: vascular abnormalities (arteriovenous malformations, aneurysms)
SPINE	
Non-contrast CT	Acute Trauma: fractures/ligamentous injury (MRI superior)
	Lumbar disc disease
	Hemorrhage
	Postoperative for suspected hardware displacement
Contrast CT	Spinal abscess
CT Myelogram	When MRI contraindicated or will cause hardware artifact
	Vascular malformations of the spinal cord
MRI: No contrast	Acute trauma; first choice to assess ligamentous injury and cord compression
	Rapidly progressive paraparesis/paraplegia: cord compression; edema; tumor
	Cervical and thoracic disc disease

Adapted from Grainger, Allison & Dixon, 2008; Castillo, 2006; Gunderman, 2006.

Change in Mental Status

Introduction

Changes in mental status are daily occurrences in the acute care setting. It is important that providers are aware of the multitude of conditions that lead to altered mental status and the proper workup to rule out those conditions. Primary neurologic causes of mental status changes such as seizures, hemorrhages, ischemia, trauma, and central nervous system infections are discussed in other sections of this chapter. This segment is devoted to reviewing the non-neurologic causes of the acute confusional states of delirium and encephalopathy.

Clinical Manifestations/Symptoms

The terminology used to describe changes in mental status can be quite confusing. Table 5.6 lists the various types and definitions of altered behavior that patients in the acute care setting may exhibit. It should be noted that dementia is not an acute confusional state but rather a progressive disorder that, if present, is likely a part of the patient's medical history (Caselli, 2003).

5.6 Altered Mental Status Terminology

Term	Definition
Acute confusional state	Presents with impaired attention, logical thinking, and memory with incoherent conversation
Delirium	Type of acute confusional state characterized by agitation, autonomic disturbances (tachycardia, hypertension, diaphoresis), hallucinations, and restlessness.
Encephalopathy	Type of acute confusional state that is accompanied by a change in level of consciousness from drowsiness to stupor or coma
Dementia	An acquired and often progressive impairment of memory and at least one other cognitive function without alterations in level of consciousness or underlying psychiatric illness

Adapted from Roper & Brown, 2005.

Pathophysiology

The causes of non-neurologic changes in mental status as well as the proper diagnostic tests to rule out the individual causes are listed in Table 5.7. The etiologies are divided into toxic, metabolic, and systemic.

5.7 Common Causes of Mental Status Changes in the Acute Care Setting

Possible Cause	Findings/Diagnostic Tests
	TOXIC
Prescription Medications	Review medication list for interactions or CNS depressant side effects
Alcohol intoxication or withdrawal	Toxicology screen of blood and urine
Illicit drugs	Toxicology screen of blood and urine
Poisons	
▓ Ethylene glycol	— Fluorescent urine under UV lamp, osmolar gap >10, metabolic acidosis
▓ Methanol	— Hyperemic optic disc, osmolar gap >10, metabolic acidosis
▓ Insecticides	— Cholinergic symptoms: DUMBBELS (Diarrhea, Urination, Miosis, Bradycardia, Bronchospasm, Emesis, Lacrimation, Salivation)
▓ Carbon monoxide	— Carboxyhemoglobin levels (Stone, 2008)
Systemic infections/Sepsis	— Complete blood count with differential
	— Culture and sensitivity blood, urine and sputum
	— Urinalysis
	— Chest x-ray
	METABOLIC
Electrolytes: high or low	Electrolyte studies
▓ Sodium	
▓ Calcium	
▓ Magnesium	
▓ Phosphate	
Hypercapnia	Arterial blood gas
Hypoxemia	Arterial blood gas

(continued)

| 5.7 | Common Causes of Mental Status Changes in the Acute Care Setting *(continued)* |

Possible Cause	Findings/Diagnostic Tests
Hyperglycemia or Hypoglycemia	Blood glucose
Hyperthyroid or Hypothyroid	Thyroid function tests
Hyperadrenalism	— Dexamethasone suppression test, 24-hour urine "free" cortisol level
Hypoadrenalism Nutritional	— ACTH stimulation test
▨ Wernicke's encephalopathy (thiamine deficiency)	— Classic triad of clinical findings: opthalmoplegia (usually horizontal gaze paralysis), ataxia and confusion, thiamine (B_1) level, macrocytic anemia on peripheral blood smear
▨ Vitamin B12 deficiency	— B_{12} level
▨ Folate deficiency	— Folate level (Aminoff, 2005)
	SYSTEMIC
Hypertensive encephalopathy	Vital signs
Cardiac failure	— Cardiac enzymes
	— Pro-Brain Naturetic Peptide
	— Transthoracic echocardiogram
Liver failure	— Liver function tests
	— Serum ammonia levels
Renal Failure	— Serum Creatinine
	— Creatinine clearance
	— Fractional excretion of sodium (FENa)

Adapted from Stone & Humphries, 2008; Roper & Brown, 2005; Tintanelli et al., 2004.

Diagnostic Criteria

When a patient presents with a change in mental status, it is key to remember the ABCs. If there is any question of oxygenation or ventilation status, an arterial blood gas should be performed (Stone & Humphries, 2008). If a noninfectious neurologic cause has been ruled out via a noncontrast head CT and EEG, the following tests should be performed: lumbar puncture, chemistry panel to include liver function studies, complete blood count with differential, and ammonia (Aminoff, Greenburg, & Simon, 2005). If the results of those preliminary tests are inconclusive, then further studies as listed in Table 5.7 should be obtained.

Treatment

Treatment depends on the underlying cause of the mental status alteration. Because many of the causes of the change in mental status are life-threatening, prompt recognition and appropriate diagnostic workup are critical in order for the proper treatment to be initiated.

Prognosis and Outcomes

Patients with delirium have a 1-month mortality rate of 14% and a 6-month mortality rate of 22% (McAvay et al., 2006). This is partially related to patients having concomitant dementia as well as significant comorbid diseases. The prognosis and outcome for patients with encephalopathy are highly dependent on the underlying cause, the expeditious nature of identifying, and treating the cause as well as comorbidities.

Cerebral Edema and Intracranial Hypertension

Definition and Types of Cerebral Edema

Cerebral edema, simply defined, is an increase in the normal brain water content of approximately 80%. It is usually a response to a primary brain insult, which includes traumatic brain injury (TBI), subarachnoid hemorrhage (SAH), central nervous system (CNS) infection, and ischemic and hemorrhagic strokes (Raslan & Bhardwaj, 2007). Cerebral edema has traditionally been classified into two major subtypes: cytotoxic and vasogenic. Cytotoxic brain edema is characterized by sustained intracellular water accumulation involving both astrocytes and neurons, which occurs independently from the blood–brain barrier (BBB) integrity (Unterberg, Stover, Kress, & Kiening, 2004). The most common cytotoxic edema occurs as the result of cerebral ischemia/infarction.

This edema type is conventionally thought to be resistant to any known medical treatment. Vasogenic edema is defined as fluid originating from blood vessels that accumulates around cells (Marmarou, 2007). Vasogenic edema that results from the breakdown of the BBB because of increased vascular permeability, as commonly encountered in TBI, neoplasms, and inflammatory conditions, predominately affects the white matter. This edema subtype is responsive to steroid administration (in the setting of neoplasm) and osmotherapy (Raslan & Bhardwaj). Most brain insults involve a combination of these fundamental subtypes of edema, although one can predominate depending on the type and duration of injury. Cytotoxic and vasogenic edema are greatest between 24 and 72 hours after the initial insult. (Marmarou, 2007). Most cases of brain injury that results in elevated intracranial pressure begin as focal cerebral edema (Raslan & Bhardwaj).

Cerebral Dynamics

The Monro-Kellie doctrine provides the framework for reviewing physiology and treatments for elevation in intracranial pressure (ICP). It states that the intracranial compartment is a rigid container and consists of three components: brain tissue (80%), blood (10%), and cerebrospinal fluid (CSF) (10%). Under normal physiologic conditions, these components are balanced in a state of dynamic equilibrium. When an increase occurs in the relative volume of one component, such as brain tissue, the volume of one or more of the other components decreases to maintain a normal ICP (Arbour, 2004). Once the compensatory mechanisms are exhausted, even a subtle increase in one component may result in large increases in ICP. This phenomenon is referred to as a loss of intracranial compliance.

In adults, normal ICP range is 5–15 mmHg. Intracranial hypertension (HTN) is defined as ICP >20 mmHg (Rangel-Castillo & Robertson, 2007). Sustained increases in ICP are of great importance to the practitioner because intracranial hypertension decreases cerebral perfusion, which leads to ischemia, infarction, and ultimately, death. The brain requires 50–55 ml of blood per 100 g of brain tissue to maintain a normal metabolic state. Cerebral perfusion pressure (CPP) is an approximation of global cerebral blood flow (Arbour, 2004). CPP is equal to the mean arterial pressure (MAP) minus the ICP. As a result, CPP (and thus cerebral perfusion) can be reduced from an increase in ICP, a decrease in blood pressure or a combination of both factors. Through a regulatory process called cerebral autoregulation, the brain is able to maintain a normal cerebral blood flow (CBF) with CPP ranging from 50–150 mmHg. If CPP falls below 50 mmHg, the brain may not be able to compensate adequately and CBF will passively follow changes in CPP. In addition, after a brain insult, cerebral autoregulation may be absent or impaired. As a result, even with a normal CPP, CBF will passively follow changes in CPP (Figure 5.2) (Rangel-Castillo & Robertson).

$$CPP = MAP - ICP$$

5.2

Cerebral Autoregulation

The solid line represents normal cerebral autoregulation between a CPP of 50 and 150 mmHg. The dotted line represents how in an injured brain, how CPP can be passively pressure dependent.

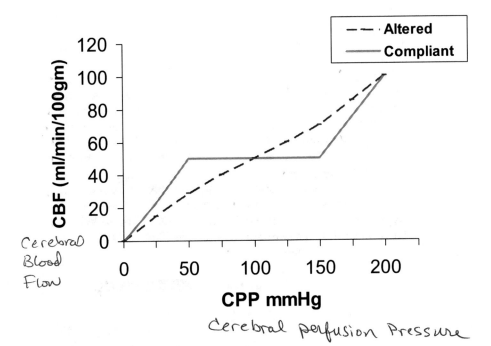

Cerebral Blood Flow

Cerebral perfusion Pressure

Increased ICP

Elevation in ICP beyond 20 mmHg for an extended period of time can rapidly lead to brain damage or death through the following two principal mechanisms: (a) global hypoxic-ischemic injury caused by a reduction in CPP and (b) mechanical compression, distortion, and herniation of brain tissue (Mayer, Coplin, & Raps, 1999). Each of these mechanisms represents a means of secondary brain injury. The primary injury represents the initial damage to the brain such as brain tumor, intracranial hemorrhage (ICH), ischemic stroke, and TBI. The detrimental sequelae that follows, anywhere from hours to days post injury, is known as secondary brain injury. There are intracranial as well as extracranial processes, which lead to secondary brain injury. Intracranial processes include cerebral edema, hydrocephalus, increased ICP, and cerebral herniation. Extracranial processes that promote secondary brain injury include airway obstruction, hypoxia, hypercapnia, hypertension or hypotension, hyperpyrexia, and seizures.

Secondary Brain injury

Neurologic Examination. An accurate assessment of a patient with a neurologic injury is challenging from the onset and with the additional complications of cerebral edema and subsequent intracranial HTN, it becomes a challenging endeavor. In terms of physical examination, the neurologic indicators for intracranial HTN are varied, not necessarily found in all patients, and defined as early and late signs. *Early signs* of increased ICP include decreased level of consciousness (LOC), confusion, lethargy, agitation, changes in mental status, headache, seizures, unequal or sluggish pupillary responses, hippus, and cranial nerve defects—CN III paresis (difficulty with upward gaze) and CN VI paresis (difficulty with looking outward, seizures, and sensory changes). *Late signs* of increased ICP include continued decrease in LOC, flexor/extensor posturing, headache, vital sign variation (Cushing triad—widening pulse pressure, bradycardia, respiratory variation), dilated fixed pupil(s), vomiting (without nausea), coma, and loss of protective reflexes—cough, gag, and corneal reflexes. Because of the inconsistency at which these signs present themselves, the only real way to accurately assess ICP is to insert an ICP monitor.

Herniation Syndromes. When elevations of ICP are severe and sustained, there is risk for herniation, which is defined as abnormal protrusion of an organ or other body structure through a defect or natural opening in a covering membrane, muscle, or bone (Hickey, 2002). In general, cerebral herniation syndromes are classified into two major types: supratentorial and infratentorial. Supratentorial herniations occur above the meningeal layer of the tentorium cerebelli and include central, uncal, and subfalcine herniation. Infratentorial herniation occurs below the tentorium and includes tonsillar herniation (Hickey). See Table 5.8 and Figure 5.3 on page 157 for a review of the herniation syndromes.

ICP Monitoring Techniques. ICP cannot be reliably estimated from any specific clinical feature or CT finding; it must be directly measured. The decision as to when to utilize an ICP monitor has only been specifically outlined in the TBI literature; however, it is used for various brain injuries. In general, a patient is suspected to be at risk for increased ICP if a CT shows cerebral edema or intracranial mass effect (midline shift or effacement of basal cisterns) as well as having rating of <8 on the Glasgow Coma scale (Arbour, 2004). Several methods, which include intraventricular catheter (external ventricular drain [EVD] and ventriculostomy), subarachnoid bolt, subdural/epidural catheter, and intraparenchymal insertion of a fiber-optic transducer-tipped catheter, are used to monitor ICP (Figure 5.4).

The intraventricular catheter is currently the standard for ICP measurement (Arbour, 2004). It is usually inserted into the nondominant ventricle and is attached to an external fluid-filled drainage system where pressure is transduced using the foramen of Munroe (external auditory meatus) as the reference point. This system allows accurate, continuous ICP monitoring as well as the ability to drain and sample CSF and to evaluate cerebral compliance. The main disadvantage to the intraventricular catheter is infection, but it may also become obstructed by a clot or brain matter and needs to be recalibrated often. The subarachnoid bolt (SAB) is another fluid-filled system. It is inserted through a burr hole, which perforates the dura and comes in contact with the subarachnoid space. The bolt, which is primed with preservative free saline, transduces pressure through the external system. The main advantage of the SAB is that it is easily placed and has

Intraventricular catheter
risk- Infection, needs recalibration.

5.8 Herniation Syndromes

	Anatomical Changes	Signs of Herniation
Supratentorial		
Cingulate/ Subfalcine	—Cingulate gyrus is forced under the falx cerebri, displacing it toward the opposite side	Contralateral lower extremity weakness
Central	—Downward displacement of one or both cerebral hemispheres	—Stupor to coma —Gradual loss of vertical gaze —Contralateral hemiplegia —Bilateral small reactive pupils progressing to dilated & fixed —Rigidity developing into flexor/extensor posturing —Elevated ICP —Cushing's triad
Uncal	—Herniation of mesial temporal lobe, uncus and hippocampal gyrus through the tentorial incisura —Compression of oculomotor nerve, midbrain, and posterior cerebral artery	—Decreased LOC —Ipsilateral papillary dilation —Contralateral hemiparesis —Decerebrate posturing —Central neurogenic hyperventilation —Elevated ICP
Infratentorial		
Tonsillar	—Herniation of cerebellar tonsils through the foramen magnum, medullary compression	—Precipitous changes in blood pressure & HR —Small pupils —Ataxic breathing —Disturbance of conjugate gaze —Quadraparesis

Adapted from Hickey (2002), Raslan & Bhardwaj (2007).

5.3

Types of Herniation

This diagram shows four types of herniation. 1) The brain squeezes under the falx cerebri in cingulate herniation 2) The brainstem herniates caudally 3) The uncus and the hyppocampal gyrus herniate into the tentorial notch 4) The cerebellar tonsils herniate through the foramen magnum in tonsillar herniation

Reprinted with permission from Wikipedia.

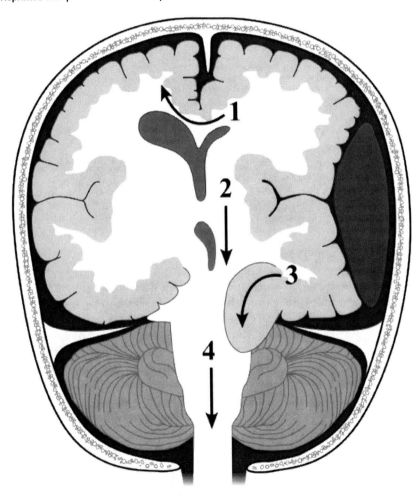

5.4

ICP Monitoring Devices

This figure depicts the anatomical placement of each of the ICP monitoring device (Arbour. 2004).

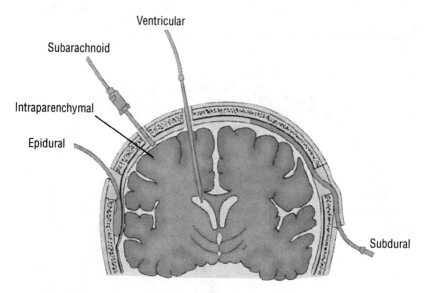

a low risk of infection. The main disadvantages of the SAB are that CSF cannot be drained, it tends to be less accurate at higher ICPs, frequent recalibration is required and it has the potential for dampened waveform because of debris (Arbour). The placement of subdural or epidural catheters is accomplished via a small-twist drill hole through the skull. Advantages to these monitors are that they have a low infection rate, that they are easily placed, and that they are less invasive. However, they are prone to malfunction, displacement, and drift as well as inaccuracy caused by a wedge effect from the catheter and the adjacent dura (Arbour). Lastly, the intraparenchymal fiber-optic transducer-tipped catheter is placed through a bolt into the brain tissue. The benefits of the fiber-optic catheters are ease of insertion, maintenance of quality waveforms, single calibration upon insertion, minimal drift, and no required transducer adjustment when there is a change in patient position. The disadvantages are that it provides no access for CSF drainage and that it is easily damaged (Arbour).

Treatment

General Measures to Reduce ICP. The overall treatment goals for management of cerebral edema and intracranial HTN are to optimize CBF and prevent further ischemic injury. These are achieved by reducing and controlling increases in ICP (<20 mmHg), maintaining an adequate CPP (>60 mmHg), and promoting oxygenation and venous drainage as well as minimizing cerebral metabolic demands (Raslan & Bhardwaj, 2007). The following general care measures help achieve these goals.

To optimize venous outflow and promote displacement of CSF from the intracranial compartment, finding the optimal neutral head position is essential for avoiding jugular compression. The head of bed should be maintained at 30 degrees and the neck should remain in neutral position (Hickey, 2002). It is also important to avoid devices that impede venous outflow, so circumferential devices to secure endotracheal tubes should be avoided.

Hypoxia and hypercapnia are potent cerebral vasodilators and should be avoided in patients with cerebral edema. It is recommended that any patients with GCS scores less than or equal to 8 or those with poor upper airway reflexes be intubated preemptively for airway protection (Raslan & Bhardwaj, 2007). Levels of $PaCO_2$ should be maintained in the low normal range (35–40 mmHg) in the absence of active increases in ICP. Prophylactic hyperventilation should be avoided unless one is actively treating increases in ICP, seeing that this may actually worsen ischemia, especially in the first 48 hours. Avoidance of hypoxemia and maintenance of PaO_2 at about 100 mmHg is also recommended (Raslan & Bhardwaj). Positive pressure ventilation can also have deleterious effects and delivery of positive end expiratory pressure (PEEP) at levels >10 cm H_2O should be monitored closely as it can also increase ICP.

Systemic dehydration and the use of hypotonic solutions (such as dextrose-containing solutions or half-normal saline) should be avoided at all costs unless treating a symptomatic hypertonic state (Mayer et al., 1999). To maintain adequate CPP of >60 mmHg, euvolemia or mild hypervolemia with the use of isotonic fluids (0.9% saline) should be maintained. Avoidance of hypotension should also be paramount and means should be taken to keep MAP elevated enough to maintain adequate CPP (>60 mmHg). In the absence of an available ICP monitor and known ICP value, a systolic blood pressure (SBP) <100 mmHg or MAP <60 mmHg should be actively treated with fluid and vasoactive agents if necessary.

In terms of controlling cerebral metabolic demands, it is important to avoid hyperthermia, treat seizure activity, and control agitation. Fever increases metabolic rate by 10% to 13% per degree Celsius and is a potent vasodilator. Fever should be controlled with antipyretic and cooling blankets (Rangel-Castillo & Robertson, 2007). Seizures increase cerebral metabolic demand and also counterproductively cause profound elevation of CBF, blood volume, and ICP even in patients who are sedated and paralyzed (Mayer et al., 1999). Routine seizure prophylaxis is controversial and is not recommended for all patients but is recommended for TBI patients for the 1st week. It is important to consider seizures (nonconvulsive status epilepticus) in comatose patients and to treat seizures promptly. Lastly, agitation and pain may significantly increase blood pressure and ICP. The goal in treatment of agitation is to keep the patient quiet and nearly motionless but with ability to be aroused (if possible) for neurologic examination. The choice of agent is important with an optimal agent causing minimal hemodynamic changes. If the need be vasoactive agents may need to be added to maintain CPP. Some common agents used in the intensive care unit (ICU) for sedation include fentanyl, remifentanil, propofol, midazolam, and lorazepam.

Specific Treatment to Reduce Refractory ICP

Controlled Hyperventilation. For patients with sustained elevations in ICP of >20–25 mmHg, additional measures are needed to control ICP. Based on the principles of cerebral pathophysiology associated with brain injury, controlled hyperventilation remains the most efficacious therapeutic intervention for cerebral edema (Raslan & Bhardwaj, 2007). A decrease in $PaCO_2$ by 10 mmHg produces a proportional decrease in CBF (and decreases cerebral blood volume (CBV) in the cranial vault) resulting in rapid and prompt ICP reduction. A common clinical practice is to lower and

$\downarrow PaCO_2 \rightarrow \downarrow CBF \rightarrow \downarrow ICP$

maintain $PaCO_2$ by 10 mmHg to a target level of approximately 30–35 mmHg. The vasoconstrictive effects of hyperventilation has been shown to last for 10–20 hours. It should be noted that controlled hyperventilation is to be used as a rescue or resuscitative measure for a short duration until more definitive therapies are instituted. Prolonged hyperventilation has been shown to worsen outcomes in TBI and overaggressive hyperventilation may actually result in cerebral ischemia (Raslan & Bhardwaj, 2007).

Steroids. Steroids are commonly used for primary and metastatic brain tumors to decrease vasogenic cerebral edema. Dexamethasone (Decadron) at a dose of 4 mg intravenously (IV) every 6 hours is a common regimen with higher doses required in the setting of increased ICP (Gomes, Stevens, Lewin, Mirski, & Bhardwaj, 2005). However, this is the only setting in which steroids are indicated for increased ICP. The corticosteroid randomization after significant head injury (CRASH) trial in patients with TBI showed no benefit with a significant increase in death (Rangel-Castillo & Robertson, 2007). Therefore, steroids are *not* indicated in TBI. They have also shown to be ineffective in treating cytotoxic edema and therefore have no role in the treatment of SAH or stroke.

Osmotherapy. The fundamental goal of osmotherapy is to create an osmotic gradient to egress water from the brain extracellular (and possibly intracellular) compartment into the vasculature, thereby decreasing intracranial volume and improving compliance (Raslan & Bardwaj, 2007). An ideal osmotic agent is one that produces a favorable osmotic gradient, is inert and nontoxic, is excluded from an intact BBB, and has minimal systemic side effects (Raslan & Bhardwaj). The two main agents used in osmotherapy are mannitol and hypertonic saline. Mannitol is the most commonly used hyperosmolar agent for intracranial hypertension. IV bolus administration of mannitol lowers the ICP in 1–5 minutes with a peak effect at 20–60 minutes. The effect of mannitol on ICP lasts 1.5–6 hours depending on the clinical condition. Mannitol is usually given as a bolus of 0.25–1 g/kg, with a dose of 1g/kg given in cases when urgent reduction of ICP is needed (Rangel-Castillo & Robertson, 2007). Hypertonic saline (HS) is available in various formulations (2%, 3%, 7.5%, 10%, and 23.4%). It produces increasing osmotic gradients with higher

[handwritten margin note: • mannitol • hypertonic saline]

concentrations although there is little clinical evidence for choosing one concentration over another in terms of attenuating brain water content (Quereshi & Suarez, 2000). It is postulated that HS produces this diuretic effect from stimulation of atrial natriuretic peptide (ANP) release rather than direct osmotic diuresis, which accounts for its ability to augment intravascular volume and cardiac performance, avoiding hypotension and hypovolemia (Ziai, Toung, & Bhardwaj, 2007). HS in the form of 2% or 3% is administered as a continuous drip and can also be given in boluses of 250–500 cc in a controlled setting. A desired sodium goal of 145–155 mEq/L (or higher) is set and the drip is titrated over 24–48 hours to meet the desired goal. Larger concentrations of HS (e.g., 23.4%) are often given as a bolus doses in the emergent setting of cerebral herniation to quickly control ICP (this must be given via central line over several minutes to avoid further hemodynamic compromise). Overall HS has shown to be as efficacious as mannitol in reducing ICP. Although a large scale trial that is randomized and controlled, which directly compares equiosmolar doses of mannitol and HS has yet to be undertaken, several clinical studies suggest that HS solutions may be more effective in lowering elevated ICP than mannitol (Ziai et al., 2007).

Pharmacological Coma. Induced pharmacologic coma is used in the setting of retractable ICP where other methods of ICP reduction have failed. Traditionally, high-dose barbiturates (pentobarbital) have been used to induce coma and decrease cerebral metabolic activity, resulting in reduction in CBF, CBV, and ultimately, ICP. The recommended regimen entails a loading IV bolus of pentobarbital (3–10 mg/kg) followed by continuous infusion of (0.5–3 mg·kg^{-1}·hr^{-1}). The infusion is titrated to a reduction of ICP or burst suppression on EEG as well as targeted levels of 30–50 mcg/ml (Raslan & Bhardwaj, 2007). The barbiturate coma is maintained for 48–72 hours during which time, daily pentobarbital levels are obtained. After 48–72 hours, the drip is slowly withdrawn and the ICP is monitored closely to assess for persistent intracranial HTN. Barbiturate therapy is not without controversy. Barbiturates carry with them a list of unwanted side effects including hypotension (lowering CPP), cardiac depression, immunosuppression, and risk of ileus (Raslan & Bhardwaj).

As a result, propofol has emerged as an appealing alternative especially because of its extremely short half-life (Bratton et al., 2007). Propofol is loaded at 3–5 mg/kg with continuous infusion starting at about 30 mcg·kg^{-1}·min^{-1} and titrated to either ICP control or burst suppression. Hypotension is the major side effect of propofol, and vasoactive agents are often needed to maintain CPP during the coma period. Propofol infusion syndrome is also of concern in patient is characterized by severe metabolic acidosis, rhabdomyolysis, and cardiovascular collapse frequently leading to death. Some data suggests that this disorder is caused by interference with mitochondrial respiration (Marik & Varon, 2004). It is currently recommended that the dosage not exceed 100 mcg·kg^{-1}·min^{-1} and measurements of daily creatinine kinase (CPK) a marker of rhabdomyolysis and triglycerides to identify failure of free fatty acid metabolism in the form of hyperlipidemia be done to monitor for the syndrome.

Hypothermia. Although it is very clear that hyperthermia has deleterious effects on the brain, the role of hypothermia is controversial in terms of translation to neurological outcomes. The setting of out-of-hospital cardiac arrest and the induction of hypothermia to 32°C within 8 hours and maintained for 12–24 hours has improved mortality and functional outcomes (Raslan & Bhardwaj, 2007). A hypothermia trial in patients with TBI did not improve long-term outcomes. However, in the setting of intractable ICP, a trial of adjunctive, controlled hypothermia may be considered. The mainstay of treatment, as discussed previously, is a focus on normothermia via the use of antipyretics and cooling devices.

Surgical Decompression. The surgical decompression of part of the calvaria to create a window in the cranial vault is the most radical intervention for intracranial hypertension. Decompressive craniotomy has been used to treat uncontrolled intracranial hypertension of various origins, including cerebral infarction, trauma, SAH, and spontaneous hemorrhage. Patient selection, timing of operation, type of surgery, and severity of clinical and radiologic brain injury all are factors that determine the outcome of the procedure (Rangel-Castillo & Robertson, 2007). The size of the craniotomy is of critical importance. In small craniotomies there is risk of brain herniation with venous infarction and increased edema at the bone margins. It is also recognized now that the dura must be opened to achieve decompression (Hutchinson, Timofeev, & Kirkpatrick, 2007). The role of decompressive craniotomy is accepted in the TBI population, but data still remains controversial in the setting of stroke, mainly in terms of improvement in functional outcomes. As a result, many institutions have established strict criteria on which patients receive this life-saving procedure.

Prognosis

Overall prognosis in the setting of cerebral edema and increased ICP is dependent on the underlying primary injury (stroke, tumor, TBI, infection) and the degree of secondary injury endured.

Traumatic Brain Injury

Definition and Epidemiology

Traumatic brain injury (TBI) is a nondegenerative, noncongenital insult to the brain from an external mechanical force, possibly leading to permanent or temporary impairments of cognitive, physical, and psychosocial functions with an associated diminished or altered state of consciousness (Segun, 2007). TBI is commonly categorized by means of the GCS, as severe (GCS ≤8), moderate (GCS 9–13) and minor (GCS 14–15). TBI is usually the consequence of impact to the head, which undergoes sudden acceleration, deceleration, or rotation. Injuries are divided into two subcategories: (a) primary injury that occurs at the moment of trauma and (b) secondary injury that evolves hours or days after injury as a consequence of systemic or intracranial complications (Toyama et al., 2005).

An estimated 1.1 million patients are evaluated each year in emergency departments for acute TBI. It occurs most often in young people, with peak incidence at 15–24 years of age (Heegaard & Biros, 2007). High-risk populations include low income individuals, unmarried individuals, members of ethnic minority groups, residents of inner cities, men, and individuals with history of substance abuse (Segun, 2007). Although the most common mechanism for TBI has changed from assaults to motor-vehicle–associated injuries, TBI remains the single largest cause of trauma morbidity and accounts for nearly one third of all trauma deaths (Heegaard & Biros).

Pathophysiology and Types of Primary Brain Injury

As previously mentioned, primary brain injury occurs at the moment of trauma and is irreversible. The physical mechanisms of brain injury are classified using the following categories: acceleration/deceleration injury and rotational injury. Acceleration–deceleration trauma is the most common result of a closed head injury. This occurs when the head is accelerated and then stopped suddenly, as in a motor vehicle collision, and this causes discrete, focal lesions to two areas of the brain. The brain will suffer contusions at the point of direct impact (coup) and at the site directly opposite the point of impact because of the oscillation of the brain within the skull (contra coup). Rotational trauma occurs when impact causes the brain to move within the cranium at a different velocity than the skull. This results in a shearing of axons by the bones of the skull. Because this type of injury damages neural connections rather than gray matter, it can affect a wide array of cerebral functions and should therefore be considered a type of diffuse injury (Hickey, 2002).

Common types of primary TBI include skull fractures, concussion, diffuse axonal injury, epidural hematoma, subdural hematoma, traumatic subarachnoid hemorrhage, cerebral contusion, and penetrating head injury.

Skull Fractures. A skull fracture is a break in one or more of the bones in the skull caused by a head injury. Isolated skull fractures are not very serious injuries, but the presence of a skull fracture may indicate that significant enough impact occurred to cause brain trauma (Graham & Gennareli, 2000). Linear skull fractures are the most common type of skull fracture and occur in 69% of patients with severe head injury. They occur when the impact causes the area of the skull that was struck to bend inward, making the area around it buckle outward (Graham & Gennareli). Linear fractures are highly associated with extradural hematomas. Temporal linear skull fractures with laceration of the middle meningeal artery are commonly seen (Davis & Briones, 1998).

Comminuted skull fractures, those in which a bone is shattered into many pieces, can result in bits of bone being driven into the brain causing lacerations to the parenchyma (Graham & Gennareli, 2000). They can be depressed or non-depressed as well as open or closed. The depressed skull fracture has a characteristic "step off" where the skull fragment is resting on the brain structures below. In a closed-type fracture, the dura remains intact, allowing no communication between the brain and the environment whereas open fractures permit communication with the outside environment (Davis & Briones, 1998).

Basilar skull fractures are those that involve the anterior, middle, and/or posterior fossas of the skull. Anterior fossa skull fractures are easily recognizable by the classic "raccoon's eyes" caused by bleeding into the periorbital space. Middle fossa skull fractures typically display "Battle sign," which is ecchymosis of the mastoid process and may also have associated conductive hearing loss and Bell's palsy. Dural tears often accompany these types of fractures and leaking of cerebral spinal fluid either from the nose (rhinorrhea) or ear (otorrhea) is common (Hickey, 2002). Posterior fossa skull fractures, in the form of an occipital condyle fracture, are rare and are usually accompanied by cervical spine injury, lower cranial nerve injury, and limb paresis/plegia (Graham & Gennareli, 2000).

Concussion. A concussion is a transient brief interruption of neurologic function after minor head trauma, with or without a loss of consciousness, usually a result of acceleration-deceleration forces to the head (Heegaard & Biros, 2007). Although anyone can sustain a concussion, it is most often a consequence of a sports-related minor head injury. The most common complaints after concussion are headache, confusion, and amnesia; the neurologic examination is nonfocal. Various theories have been proposed to explain the physical and functional signs and symptoms following a concussion. These include shearing or stretching of white matter fibers, temporary neuronal dysfunction, transient alterations in levels of neurotransmitters, or temporary changes in cerebral blood flow and oxygen use (Heegaard & Biros). Vague symptoms, such as headaches, sensory sensitivity, memory or concentration difficulties, irritability, sleep disturbances, or depression may persist for prolonged periods after a concussion. These constitute the postconcussive syndrome (PCS). For years, it was believed that PCS was psychosomatic, but functional imaging and sophisticated neuropsychometrics have documented structural abnormalities, which offer an explanation for the symptoms associated with the syndrome (Heegaard & Biros).

Diffuse Axonal Injury. Diffuse axonal injury (DAI) is now widely accepted as one of the most common types of primary brain lesions in patients with severe head trauma. Patients with DAI usually present with severe impairment of consciousness from the moment of impact, presenting with a GCS ≤ 8. The mechanism is one of widespread tearing of axons caused by shearing forces during acceleration, deceleration, and rotation of the brain (Toyama et al., 2005). A component of DAI is believed to be present in all motor vehicle collisions where the patient has lost consciousness (Meythaler, Peduzzi, Eleftheriou, & Novack, 2001). The predominant anatomic sites of injury seen with DAI are the parasagittal white matter of the cerebral cortex, basal ganglia, corpus callosum, and the pontine–mesencephalic junction adjacent to the superior cerebellar peduncles. Injury to the tracts leading in and out of the hypothalamus and/or direct injury to the pituitary stalk and gland, results in many of the common medical complications noted after TBI including dysautonomia, hormonal changes, disorders of salt and water metabolism, and altered temperature regulation (Meythaler et al., 2001).

CT and MRI scans taken initially after injury are often normal. Only 10% of DAI patients demonstrate the classic CT findings associated with DAI characterized by hemorrhagic punctate lesions of the corpus callosum, the gray-white matter junction of the cerebrum, and the pontine–mesencephalic junction adjacent to the cerebellar peduncles (Meythaler et al., 2001). The Adams classification is used to categorize the degree of DAI as mild, moderate, or severe. Mild (Grade 1) DAI is characterized by microscopic changes in the white matter of the cerebral cortex, corpus callosum, brainstem, and occasionally, the cerebellum. Moderate DAI (Grade 2) is defined by grossly evident focal lesions isolated to the corpus callosum. In severe DAI (Grade 3), there are additional focal lesions to the dorsolateral quadrants of the rostral brainstem (Meythaler et al.). Overall, DAI is the most common cause of vegetative state and severe disability after injury (Toyama et al., 2005).

Epidural Hematoma. Epidural hematoma (EDH) is the accumulation of blood between the dura and the inner table of the skull. Normally because the periosteal surface of the dura is densely adherent to the inner table of the skull, no epidural space exists. Blunt trauma to the head, with or without skull fracture, may cause the dura to separate from the inner table. The separation may occur on the side of the trauma (coup) or the contralateral side (contra-coup). EDH into the traumatically created epidural space may result from laceration of the middle or posterior meningeal artery, meningeal emissary veins, or venous sinus (Harris, 2000). The most common locations are the temporal, frontal, and occipital regions. On CT, the hematoma has a biconvex or lenticular shape with sharp margination as a result of the fact that the dura remains adherent at both edges. EDH tends not to cross cranial sutures where the dura is tightly adherent. Because they lie outside the dura, EDH may cross the falx or displace the dural venous sinuses (Toyama et al., 2005).

Classically, there is an initial period of unconsciousness followed by a lucid interval after which rapid neurological deterioration develops (Toyama et al., 2005). The lucid interval is a delay between the trauma and the moment the EDH enlarges and becomes symptomatic. However, this classic lucid interval is seen in only 40% of patients with acute EDH. The mass compresses the brain and may cause compression or obliteration of the ipsilateral lateral ventricle and uncal herniation with midline shift. Surgery to evacuate the clot and ligate the ruptured vessel is the mainstay of treatment for EDH (Toyama et al., 2005).

Subdural Hematoma. Subdural hematoma (SDH) represents a collection of blood located between the dura and arachnoid membrane. The blood comes principally from torn superficial cortical veins separating the arachnoid from the dura but may also arise from the venous sinus or by bleeding cerebral contusions. SDH is classified into three categories based on the clinical timeline and radiographic findings—acute: immediate to 72 hours, subacute: 72 hours–2 weeks, chronic: >2 weeks (Toyama et al., 2005).

Underlying cerebral injuries are more frequent with acute SDH than acute EDH. Associated contusions are present in 50% of patients with SDH. Swelling of the underlying hemispheres is common, so that mass effect is greater than expected based on the size of the clot alone. The classic CT appearance of an acute SDH is a crescent-shaped, extra-axial collection that is homogeneously and hyperdense and that spreads diffusely over the affected hemisphere. The usual management of acute SDH is surgical (Toyama et al., 2005). However, the use of early surgery has not always improved outcomes. Other factors including age, GCS on presentation, amount of blood, and absence/presence of midline shift often weigh in on whether surgery is pursued or the patient is to be watched clinically.

Traumatic Subarachnoid Hemorrhage. Traumatic subarachnoid hemorrhage usually arises from hemorrhagic contusion with bleeding into the subarachnoid space and is a frequent occurrence in severe head injury. The most frequent location is over the convexity, followed by the fissures and basal cisterns (Toyama et al., 2005). Despite the severity of injury noted to the brain, mortality doubles in the presence of traumatic SAH. If there is blood in the basal cisterns, there is a 70% positive predictive value of a poor outcome. The volume and extent of traumatic SAH is related to outcome, independent of the other injuries noted in TBI patients (Chestnut et al., 2007).

Cerebral Contusion. Contusions are focal injury of the brain surface caused by direct impact with the calvarium. Contusions are most common at sites of bony protuberances of the skull base and therefore, are seen in the frontal poles, orbital surface of the frontal lobes, temporal poles, and inferior surface of the temporal lobes and adjoining the anterior sylvian fissure near the lesser sphenoid wing (Toyama et al., 2005). On a noncontrast CT, hemorrhagic contusions appear as heterogeneous, hyperdense lesions (hemorrhage) surrounded by an irregularly margined hypodense component (edema and necrosis). Lesions that are small on initial head CT have the potential to "blossom" within 24–48 hours into larger, more extensive hemorrhages with increased surrounding edema. Given this fact, patients with a TBI associated with a loss of consciousness and any evidence of contusion should be monitored in the hospital and undergo repeat imaging in 24–48 hours (Toyama et al., 2007).

Penetrating Head Injury. The definition of a penetrating head trauma is a wound in which a projectile breaches the cranium but does not exit it (Vinas & Pilitsis, 2006). Despite the prevalence of these injuries, the morbidity and mortality of penetrating head injury remains high. Penetrating head injuries can be the result of numerous intentional or unintentional events, including missile wounds, stab wounds, and motor vehicle or occupational accidents (nails, screwdrivers). The pathological consequences of penetrating head wounds depend on the circumstances of the injury, including the properties of the weapon or missile, the energy of the impact, and the location and characteristics of the intracranial trajectory. In missile wounds, the amount of damage to the brain depends on numerous factors including (a) the kinetic energy imparted, (b) the trajectory of the missile and bone fragments through the brain, (c) ICP changes at the moment of impact, and (d) secondary mechanisms of injury (Vinas & Pilitsis).

Stab wounds represent a smaller fraction of penetrating head injuries. The causes may be from knives, nails, spikes, forks, scissors, and other assorted objects. Penetrations most commonly occur in the thin bones of the skull, especially in the orbital surfaces and the squamous portion of the temporal bone. The mechanisms of neuronal and vascular injury caused by cranial stab wounds may differ from those caused by other types of head trauma. Unlike missile injuries, no concentric zone of coagulative necrosis caused by dissipated energy is present. Unlike motor vehicle accidents, no diffuse shearing injury to the brain occurs. Unless an associated hematoma or infarct is present, cerebral damage caused by stabbing is largely restricted to the wound tract (Vinas & Pilitsis, 2006).

Pathophysiology and Types of Secondary Injury

Secondary brain injury may occur in minutes, hours, to days after injury as a consequence of systemic or intracranial complications. Examples of systemic secondary brain insults include hypotension, hypoxia, anemia, hypercapnia, and hypocapnia. Intracranial secondary brain insults include intracranial hypertension (increased ICP), seizures, cerebral edema, hydrocephalous, and herniation (Hickey, 2002).

The degree and type of secondary brain insults are major determinants in the final neurologic outcome. For a review of cerebral physiology and the impact of cerebral edema and intracranial HTN on secondary brain injury, please see the increased ICP section of this chapter.

Diagnosis

The diagnosis and categorization of TBI (mild, moderate, severe) is made on the basis of the clinical examination, which includes a comprehensive neurologic examination with GCS scoring and radiographic findings on CT. It is also imperative as the practitioner to get an accurate account of the events (mechanism of injury, loss of consciousness, any vomiting, seizures, presence of severe headache, or any amnesia since the injury) from the patient or a reliable bystander (New Zealand Guideline Group [NZGG], 2006). Often the patient is unable to give specific details as to the manner at which the injury occurred due to a loss of consciousness. The physical examination is also vital and must include neurologic examination (including GCS), inspection for signs of skull fracture (otorrhea/rhinorrhea) or other overt injuries. Noncontrast CT is the gold standard for diagnosing TBI. CT scans should be immediately requested for adults who have sustained a head injury if they have any one of the following risk factors: (a) any deterioration in condition, (b) a GCS of <13 when assessed (irrespective of the time elapsed since the injury), (c) a GCS of 13 or 14 two hours after the injury, (d) a suspected open or depressed skull fracture, (e) any sign of basal skull fracture (raccoon eyes, cerebrospinal fluid otorrhoea/rhinorrhea, Battle sign), (f) posttraumatic seizure, (g) focal neurological deficit, (h) more than one episode of vomiting, or (i) amnesia for more than 30 minutes for events before the injury (NZGG, 2006). In addition, CT scanning should be immediately obtained for adults with any of the following risk factors who have experienced an injury to the head with some loss of consciousness or amnesia since the injury: (a) age 65 years or older, (b) coagulopathy (history of bleeding, clotting disorder, current treatment with warfarin), (c) high-risk mechanism of injury (a pedestrian struck by a motor vehicle, (d) an occupant ejected from a motor vehicle, (e) or a fall from a height of >1 m or five stairs (NZGG, 2006).

[handwritten margin note: TBI DX – Non-Contrast CT – gold Standard]

Treatment of TBI

The treatment of TBI depends on the type of primary injury as well as the presence and extent of any secondary injury. For the purposes of this review, we will focus on the treatment of moderate and severe TBI. The Brain Trauma Foundation has released its newest set of guidelines regarding the Surgical Management of Traumatic Brain Injury as well as Guidelines for the Management of Severe, Traumatic Brain Injury, 3rd edition. The recommendations from those guidelines are summarized in Tables 5.9 and 5.10.

Prognosis

Approximately 52,000 U.S. deaths per year has resulted from TBI. Local factors in the United States may influence this mortality rate; it is lowest in the Midwest and Northeast and is highest in the South. The initial GCS score, and therefore, the severity of the TBI help to predict likelihood of death from the injury. The mortality rate is high in severe TBI and low for moderate TBI (Segun, 2007). Overall, the type of primary injury incurred (concussion, contusion, hemorrhage, DAI) and the development and severity of secondary brain injury are the factors in morbidity and mortality.

Spinal Cord Injury

Introduction

Acute spinal cord injury (ASCI) is a devastating diagnosis that is encountered in the acute neurosciences arena. There are approximately 11,000 new cases of ASCI per year and it is estimated that there are about 250,000 people in the United States living with spinal cord injury. The average age of injured individuals is 38 and men are more likely to sustain an ASCI than woman. The number one cause of traumatic ASCI is motor vehicle accidents, number two is falls followed by violent acts (gunshot wounds), and third is sports injuries (National Spinal Cord Injury Statistical Center, 2006)

5.9 Surgical Management of TBI

Type of Injury	Is Surgery Indicated?/Criteria	Timing & Methods
Depressed Skull fracture	Patients with open (compound) cranial fractures depressed greater than the thickness of the cranium should undergo operative intervention to prevent infection	Elevation and débridement is recommended as the surgical method of choice. Replacement of bone is a surgical option in the absence of wound infection at the time of surgery. All management strategies for open (compound) depressed fractures should include antibiotics
Basilar skull fracture	No	Manage ICP and CSF leak
Concussion	No	Observation
Contusion	Patients with contusions AND ▨ Signs of progressive neurological deterioration referable to the lesion ▨ Medically refractory increased ICP ▨ Signs of mass effect on computed tomography (CT) ▨ GCS 6–8 with frontal or temporal contusions >20 cm^3 in volume with midline shift of at least 5 mm and/or cisternal compression on CT scan, ▨ Any lesion >50 cm^3	Craniotomy with evacuation of mass lesion ▨ Is recommended for those patients with focal lesions and the surgical indications listed Bifrontal decompressive craniectomy ▨ Within 48 hours ▨ Treatment option for patients with diffuse, medically refractory posttraumatic cerebral edema and resultant increased ICP. Decompressive procedures (subtemporal decompression/temporal lobectomy/hemispheric decompressive craniectomy) ▨ Refractory increased ICP and diffuse parenchymal injury ▨ Clinical and radiographic evidence for impending transtentorial herniation

(continued)

5.9 Surgical Management of TBI *(continued)*

Type of Injury	Is Surgery Indicated?/Criteria	Timing & Methods
Diffuse Axonal Injury	No	Supportive Care
Subdural Hematoma	▨ Thickness >10 mm OR ▨ Midline shift >5 mm on CT scan ****Regardless of GCS**** IF GCS ↓ between time of injury and hospital admission by 2 or more AND/OR ▨ The patient presents with asymmetric or fixed and dilated pupils ▨ ICP >20 mmHg	Timing: ▨ If meet criteria as defined ▨ ASAP Methods: ▨ Craniotomy with/without bone flap removal AND ▨ Duraplasty
Epidural Hematoma	INDICATIONS ▨ >30 cm^3 should be evacuated regardless of GCS	TIMING ▨ If acute EDH in coma (GCS score <9) WITH ▨ Anisocoria (unequal pupils) ▨ ASAP METHODS ▨ Craniotomy ▨ There are insufficient data to support one surgical treatment method, however provides a more complete evacuation of the hematoma
Traumatic SAH	No	Medical management If hydro- EVD
Penetrating	Varies	Removal of object I&D

Adapted from from Bullock et al. (2006).

5.10 Management for Severe TB

Intervention	Level of Evidence*	Recommendation
Blood Pressure & Oxygenation	Level II Level III	▓ Goal SBP >90 ▓ Goal Sats >90% ▓ PaO$_2$ >60 mmHg
Hyperosmolar Therapy ▓ *Mannitol* ▓ *Hypertonic saline*	Level II Level III Insufficient evidence	▓ 0.25–1 g/kg ▓ Avoid hypotension (SBP <90) ▓ No evidence to suggest that a bolus is better than continuous ▓ Only use BEFORE placing ICP monitor if patients is actively herniating or has progressive neurological deterioration ▓ Need randomized controlled trial to determine benefits of mannitol versus hypertonic saline
Prophylactic Hypothermia	Level III	▓ Suggest a decrease in mortality risk when hypothermia is maintained for >48 hours (32–35° C)
Infection Prophylaxis *General Care*	Level II	▓ Periprocedural antibiotics for intubation should be used to decrease the incidence of pneumonia ▓ Early tracheostomy will decrease number of ventilator days (but not mortality or pneumonia).
External Ventricular Device (EVD)	Level III	NOT Recommended ▓ To do routine EVD exchange ▓ To give prophylactic antibiotics for EVD placement

(continued)

5.10 Management for Severe TB *(continued)*

Intervention	Level of Evidence*	Recommendation
Deep Vein Thrombosis (DVT) Prophylaxis	Level III	▨ SCDs are recommended until patient is ambulatory ▨ Low molecular weight heparins or low dose unfractionated heparin should be used in combo with SCDS. However, there is an increase risk of ICH expansion ▨ No data for preferred agent or timing

ICP Monitor	Level II
	
	Level III
		▨ Severe TBI (GCS 3–8)
		▨ Abnormal Head CT
		▨ Severe TBI (GCS 3–8) with normal CT and 2 or more of
		   - >40 years old
		   - Posturing
		   - SBP <90

ICP Monitoring Technology	No Level listed	▨ EVD is most accurate, lowest cost device ▨ Fiber-optic/microstrain gauge placed in EVD provides greater benefit but costs more. ▨ Subarachnoid, subdural, and epidural are not as accurate
ICP Threshold	Level II Level III	▨ Initiate treatment for ICP >20 mmHg ▨ Combo of ICP, clinical picture, and head CT findings should be used to determine need for treatment
CPP Threshold	Level II Level III	▨ AVOID aggressive attempts to get CPP >70 with fluid and pressors caused by ↑ risk ARDS ▨ AVOID CPP <50 mmHg ▨ CPP target 50–70 mmHg

		▓ Using monitors for cerebral blood flow, oxygenation, or metabolism facilitate CPP management
Brain Oxygen Monitoring and Thresholds	Level III	Treatment thresholds ▓ Jugular venous saturation <50% OR ▓ Brain tissue oxygen tension <15 mmHg

* Level I: Good quality randomized controlled trial (RCT), Level II: Moderate quality RCT, Good quality cohort, Good quality case control, Level III: Poor quality RCT, moderate or poor quality cohort, moderate or poor quality case control, case series, databases or registries. Adapted from Bratton et al. (2007).

Pathophysiology   Acute Spinal Cord Injury

An ASCI is caused when there is direct physical force that damages either the ligaments, vertebrae, or disks of the spinal column causing bruising, crushing, or tearing of the spinal cord (Beers, Porter, Jones, Kaplan, & Berkwits, 2006). Just as with traumatic brain injury, there is primary injury, which occurs at the moment of trauma and then secondary injury, which occurs hours to days after the initial insult. Secondary injury of the spinal cord is the result of many pathologic processes including ischemia, hemorrhage, and inflammation. The ultimate expression of secondary injury is spinal cord edema. Cord edema peaks at 3–5 days postinjury and lasts for weeks after the trauma (Stevens, Bhardwaj, Kirsh, & Mirski, 2003). The types of ASCI are complete or incomplete. A complete spinal cord injury is defined as total loss of motor and sensory below the level of the injury caused by a complete transection of the cord. Most complete injuries are the result of penetrating injuries such as a gunshot or knife wound. The damage to the cord with both complete and incomplete injuries is the result of either flexion, extension rotation, and/or compression of the spine (Sekhon & Fehlings, 2001). The types of incomplete spinal cord injuries are Brown–Séquard, anterior cord, and central cord syndrome.

Clinical Manifestations/Symptoms

A complete ACSI causes immediate, complete, flaccid paralysis with loss of all sensory function and reflexes and causes autonomic dysfunction below the level of the injury (Beers et al., 2006). Within hours to days, the flaccid paralysis becomes spastic paralysis and if the injury has spared the lumbosacral region, DTRs will return and will be hyperreflexic. With incomplete ASCI, there are various degrees of motor and sensory dysfunction. Brown–Séquard syndrome is hemisection of the cord usually caused by a penetrating injury, which results in results in loss of motor (spastic paralysis), vibration, and proprioception below the level and on the same side as the injury and contralateral loss of pain and temperature. On the same side of the lesion, the pain and temperature are spared and contralateral to the lesion, motor, vibration, and proprioception are spared (Tintanelli, Kelen, Stapczynski, Ma, & Cline, 2004) Anterior cord syndrome occurs as the result of injury to the anterior spinal artery causing ischemia to the anterior two thirds of the spinal cord. As a result, only vibration, light touch, and proprioception remain intact and motor and sensory below the level of the injury are lost. Central cord syndrome is a type of incomplete ASCI that is seen with cervical trauma usually in patients with preexisting cervical spondylosis who sustain a hyperextension injury. The classic presentation of central cord syndrome is motor weakness more severe in the arm than the legs and varying sensory dysfunction depending on which sensory tracts are injured (Tintanelli et al.). Spinal shock, the loss of all spinal cord function, including reflexes, occurs immediately after the ASCI and can last hours to days (Ditunno, Little, Tressler, & Burns, 2004). Most often spinal shock is seen with injuries occurring at T6 and above. Bradycardia and hypotension are seen during this stage because of the loss of sympathetic outflow, vasodilatation, and vagal stimulation to the heart (Hall, Schmidt, & Wood, 2005). Autonomic dysreflexia, a syndrome characterized by paroxysmal hypertension, headache, and bradycardia, is rarely seen in the acute care setting. It is usually seen in patients with injury above T6 and occurs weeks to months after the initial injury (Branco, Cardenas, & Svircev, 2007).

Diagnostic Criteria

The imaging guidelines for the cervical spine (c-spine) are outlined in Table 5.11. "Clearing" the cervical spine is the priority in ASCI to avoid a potentially devastating injury if the c-spine is unstable and not properly immobilized. The initial imaging for suspected thoracic and lumbar ACSI is a noncontrast CT to assess bony involvement. MRI is superior in assessing the spinal cord itself (Castillo, 2006).

Treatment

In May 2000, the Section on Disorders of the Spine and Peripheral Nerves of the American Association of Neurological Surgeons and the Congress of Neurological Surgeons began the painstaking process of developing guidelines for the management of acute spinal cord injuries. After an exhaustive review of the published scientific evidence, this group published the Guidelines for the Management of Acute Cervical Spine and Spinal Cord Injuries in 2002 (Hadley, et al.). The recommendations are identified as a *Practice Standard, Practice Guideline,* or a *Practice Option.* Practice Standards have the highest degree of clinical certainty as they are backed by the strongest scientific evidence. Practice Guidelines have a moderate degree of clinical certainty because the data to support them were extracted from less stringent clinical studies. Finally, Practice Option reflects unclear clinical certainty as these recommendations were taken either from case series, case reports, flawed randomized controlled trials, or expert opinion (Hadley et al.). Table 5.12 summarizes the guidelines as they relate to the management of the cervical spine immobilization, radiographic assessment and surgical intervention, the need for intensive respiratory and cardiovascular monitoring, blood pressure management, pharmacologic interventions, DVT prophylaxis, and nutritional support.

An area that may be underrecognized in this population is pain. Patients with ASCI may experience pain, due to postsurgical manipulation, as well as muscle spasm and neuropathic pain. Nonsteroidal anti-inflammatory drugs (NSAID), opiates, antispasmodic medications, antidepressants, and anticonvulsant are all possible options for pain control depending on the type of pain the patient is experiencing (Ullrich, 2007).

5.11 Imaging Guidelines for the Management of Acute Cervical Spine and Spinal Cord Injuries Summary

Intervention	Recommendation Level	Details Recommended	Not Recommended
C-spine* immobilization before admission to hospital on all trauma patients with an actual or suspected c-spine injury	Option	▨ Immobilize at the scene and during transport ▨ Use a combination of a rigid cervical collar with supportive blocks on a rigid backboard with straps	▨ Use of sand bags and tape alone
Radiographic assessment of c-spine in asymptomatic, awake, alert and not intoxicated trauma patients with no other significant injury** to distract from the physical examination	Standard	▨ Clinical examination to include assessment of neck pain or mid line tenderness on palpation	▨ Radiographic assessment
Radiographic assessment of c-spine in symptomatic ***, trauma patients	Standard	▨ Anteroposterior, lateral and odontoid "3-view" c-spine films ▨ C-spine CT to further define suspicious or poorly visualized areas	
Discontinuing C-spine immobilization: Awake, symptomatic patient	Option	▨ Normal "3-view" c-spine series ▨ Normal c-spine CT if needed AND	

		ONE of the following ■ Normal adequate dynamic flexion/extension radiographs OR ■ Normal MRI within 48 hours of injury
Discontinuing C-spine immobilization: Unconscious or uncooperative	Option	■ Normal "3-view" c-spine series ■ Normal c-spine CT if needed AND ONE of the following ■ Normal adequate dynamic flexion/extension radiographs OR ■ Normal MRI within 48 hours of injury OR ■ At the discretion of the treating physician
Closed-reduction of c-spine fracture-dislocation injuries	Option	■ Early closed-reduction with craniocervical traction in AWAKE patients (to continually assess neurologic function) ■ Obtain a c-spine MRI prereduction on non-awake patients to assess for disc herniation ■ Obtain a c-spine MRI for patients who fail closed reduction ■ For patients with additional rostral injury

5.12 Guidelines for the Management of Acute Cervical Spine and Spinal Cord Injuries Summary

Intervention	Recommendation Level	Details	
		Recommended	Not Recommended
Management in an intensive care unit or other monitored setting	Option	Patients with ASCI are best managed in the ICU setting for 7–14 days post injury due to increased susceptibility to cardiac and respiratory instability	
Blood Pressure	Option	Avoid and correct systolic blood pressure <90 mmHg Maintain mean arterial blood pressure >85–90 mmHg for 7 days postinjury	
Pharmacological Therapy: Corticosteroids	Option: only undertaken with the knowledge that evidence suggests more harmful side effects than benefit	Methylprednisolone (30 mg/kg IV for 1 hour and then 5.4 mg/kg × 23 hours) given within 8 hours of injury for either 24 or 48 hours	
Pharmacological Therapy: GM-1 ganglioside	Option without clinical benefit	GM-1 ganglioside (300 mg loading dose and then 100 mg/day for 56 days) after administration of methylprednisolone	

VTE**** Prophylaxis	Standard	Prophylactic treatment VTE with either:
		- LMWH*****
		- Rotating beds
		- Adjusted dose heparin to maintain APTTr 1.5 × control
		- Combination of modalities
		- Low dose heparin (5000 units sq BID or TID) in combination with PCS***** or electrical stimulation)
	Guidelines	Low-dose heparin alone
	Options	Diagnostic tests with lower extremity Doppler ultrasound, impedence plethysmography and venography

(continued)

5.12 The Guidelines for the Management of Acute Cervical Spine and Spinal Cord Injuries Summary (continued)

Intervention	Recommendation Level	Details	
		Recommended	Not Recommended

		▨ 3 month duration of prohylaixs
		▨ Vena cava filters if
		  — patient does not respond to anticoagulation
		     OR
		  — patient is not a candidate for anticoagulation and/or other mechanical devices including	

Nutritional Support	Option	▨ Nutritional support to meet caloric and nitrogen needs via enteral route if functional gut and parenteral route for nonfunctional gut ▨ Energy expenditure assessment via indirect calorimetry rather than the less accurate equation estimates	

*C-spine: cervical spine
**Significant injury is defined as long bone fractures, visceral injuries requiring surgical evaluation, large lacerations, deglovings, crush injuries, large burns
***Symptomatic patient is defined as either an awake patient complaining of neck pain and/or c-spine tenderness, a patient with a neurologic deficit associated with the c-spine, an unconscious, uncooperative, intoxicated patient, or a patient with other significant injuries
****VTE: venous thromboembolism
*****LMWH: low molecular weight heparins
******PCS: pneumatic compression stockings

Treatment of spinal shock is primarily aimed at managing the dysautonomia. Treatment of hypotension should start with ensuring adequate volume status with IV crystalloids. If IV fluids alone does not assist with meeting the blood pressure goals, vasoactive drugs should be used. The choice of vasoactive drip depends on the patient's heart rate and cardiac function. (Stevens et al., 2003) Bradycardia should be treated per advanced cardiac life support guidelines (American Heart Association, 2005).

Prognosis and Outcomes

The predictor of survival of ACSI is age, level of injury, and neurologic grade per rating scales like American Spinal Injury Association Scale (American Spinal Injury Association, 2002). Early death rates vary between 4% and 20% (Sekhon & Fehlings, 2001). Within the cervical cord injury population, there is anywhere from a 1.5- to 6.6-fold increased risk of death depending on level of injury.

Postoperative Elective Neurosurgical Patients

Introduction

Elective neurosurgical surgery comprises approximately 60% of the patients admitted to the neurocritical care setting. Although these cases are not emergent, they require an ICU stay given the high risk of neurologic devastation if a postoperative complication occurs and is not identified quickly. Most patients require less than a 24-hour ICU stay for close monitoring and can transfer to a nonmonitored setting on postoperative day 1 (Nitahara, Valencia, & Bronstein, 1998). The predominant elective surgical procedures admitted in this setting are craniotomy and major spinal surgery (Bhardwaj, Mirski, & Ulatowski, 2004). Craniotomy is most often done for tumor resection, unruptured intracranial aneurysm clipping, arteriovenous malformation resection, seizure focus resection, and repair of an Arnold–Chiari malformation. Major spinal surgeries include multilevel, complicated spinal fusions, and tumor resection (Bhardwaj et al.). In many hospital settings, these patients are admitted directly to the neurosciences ICU with no recovery room stay (Nitahara, et al.).

Pathophysiology

The major neurologic complications postcraniotomy, regardless of the anatomical location of the surgery, are intracranial hemorrhage, edema, and infection (Brell, Ibanez, Caral, & Ferrer, 2000). Other possible postcraniotomy complications vary, depending on the anatomical location of the surgery as well as the type of surgical procedure. Patients undergoing resection of a pituitary adenoma via a craniotomy or transphenoidal approach carry the risk of diabetes insipidus as well as visual field deficits (Loh & Verbalis, 2008). After the resection of a vestibular schwannoma, there is the risk of facial nerve damage as well as hearing loss (Bennett, & Haynes, 2007). The risks of postspinal surgery are bleeding, infection (Boakye et al., 2007; Zak, 2003), and hardware failure (Brantigan, Steffee, Lewis, Quinn, & Persenaire, 2000; Brkaric et al., 2007). A summary of the neurologic complications that the clinician must anticipate when caring for the neurological patient postoperatively are listed in Table 5.13.

Diagnostic Criteria

The best diagnostic tool the clinician has in the neuroscience population is the neurologic examination (Lower, 2002). Therefore, it is key for the clinician to know the preprocedure baseline examination to be able to identify subtle changes in the postoperative course. Communication with the neurosurgical team during the immediate postoperative period regarding any anticipated neurologic deficits based on the surgical procedure is crucial. To ensure the best chance of identifying a significant neurologic change, the initial postprocedure examination should be done with all providers and nurses of the neurocritical care team present (Bhardwaj et al., 2004). Thereafter, the nursing staff should perform the neurologic assessment every 1–2 hours. If there is a change in the examination, an emergent noncontrast head CT is warranted for the craniotomy patients (Castillo, 2006). If the head CT findings do not explain the neurologic deterioration, an EEG should be considered to rule out subclinical seizures (Praline et al., 2007). Unanticipated motor or sensory changes

5.13 Potential Neurologic Complications after Elective Neurosurgery

Procedure	Potential Complications
Supratentorial Craniotomy (cerebral cortex)	Cerebral edema Ischemic stroke Intracranial hemorrhage Meningitis Seizures
Infratentorial Craniotomy (cerebellum and brainstem)	Cerebral edema Ischemic stroke Intracranial hemorrhage Meningitis Brainstem injury Cranial nerve injury Hydrocephalus
Pituitary Adenoma Resection	Cerebral edema Ischemic stroke Intracranial hemorrhage Meningitis Cerebrospinal fluid (CSF) leak Visual field deficit Diabetes Insipidus (DI)
Vestibular Schwannoma Resection	Cerebral edema Ischemic stroke Intracranial hemorrhage Meningitis Cerebrospinal fluid (CSF) leak Brainstem injury Cranial nerve injury (especially VII, VIII)
Spine Surgery	Epidural hematoma/Epidural abscess Meningitis Myelopathy Cranial nerve deficits (high cervical)

in the postoperative spine patient warrants emergent imaging, such as an MRI, CT, or CT myelogram, depending on the procedure (Gunderman, 2006).

Clinical Manifestations/Symptoms

As previously mentioned, it is key to have strong neurological assessment skills to be able to detect subtle changes in the neurological examination. Often, the earliest indication that a patient may be experiencing a complication after craniotomy is a change in level of consciousness (Hickey, 2002). Other signs include a subtle motor weakness such as a pronator drift, new speech difficulties, or a cranial nerve deficit (Lower, 2002). Transient increases in blood pressure with concomitant bradycardia (Cushing reflex) are a later finding indicative of increased intracranial pressure and impending herniation (Morgan, Mikhail, & Murray 2006).

Treatment

The interventions in this patient population are aimed at preventing postoperative complications. Common medications patients given in the postoperative period are summarized in Table 5.14.

All patients with brain tumors are prescribed corticosteroids during the preoperative and postoperative period. The exact mechanism by which steroids work is not clearly understood; however, there are multiple studies describing their benefit for the reduction of peritumoral edema (Gomes et al., 2005). Dexamethasone is the steroid of choice because of its nominal mineralocorticoid activity and long half-life (Drappatz, Schiff, Kesari, Norden, & Wen, 2007). Low doses of 4–8 mg daily are effective at decreasing edema and mass effect, although higher doses (80–100 mg daily) are utilized (Gomes et al.). Patients with tumors of the spinal cord may also benefit from the use of dexamethasone to decrease swelling (Koehler, 1995). A patient with a brain tumor who has experienced a seizure will be placed on an antiepileptic drug (AED). Although there is no data to support the efficacy of seizure prophylaxis in individuals with brain tumor, most providers prescribe AEDs for patients who have never had a seizure after resection of a cortically based brain lesion (Glantz et al., 2000). A loading dose of the AED is often administered intraoperatively.

5.14 Suggested Medications to Prescribe Postoperatively by Procedure

Procedure	Recommended Post-op Meds

Supratentorial craniotomy for tumor	Dexamethasone
	AED
	Proton pump inhibitor or H2 blocker
	Sliding scale regular Insulin
	Antiemetic: nondrowsy
	    Metoclopromide
	    Ondansetron
	    Dolasetron
	Narcotics
	    Fentanyl IV while NPO
	    Oxycodone once taking po
	Antibiotic $\times$ 24 hours

Infratentorial Craniotomy	Dexamethasone
	Proton pump inhibitor or H2 blocker
	Sliding scale regular Insulin
	Anti-emetic: nondrowsy
	    Metoclopromide
	    Ondansetron
	    Dolasetron
	Narcotics
	    Fentanyl IV while NPO
	    Oxycodone once taking po
	Antibiotic $\times$ 24 hours

Transphenoidal hypophysectomy	Proton pump inhibitor or H2 blocker
	Sliding scale regular Insulin
	Anti-emetic: nondrowsy
	    Metoclopromide
	    Ondansetron
	    Dolasetron
	Narcotics
	    Fentanyl IV while NPO
	    Oxycodone once taking po
	Antibiotic $\times$ 24 hours

Spine Surgery	Dexamethasone for tumor only Proton pump inhibitor or H2 blocker Sliding scale regular Insulin

(continued)

5.14 Suggested Medications to Prescribe Postoperatively by Procedure *(continued)*

Procedure	Recommended Post-op Meds
	Anti-emetic: nondrowsy
	Metoclopromide
	Ondansetron
	Dolasetron
	Narcotics
	Fentanyl IV while NPO
	Oxycodone once taking po
	Antibiotic $\times$ 24 hours

Blood Pressure Control. Acute postoperative hypertension (APH) is common in the neurosurgical patient and is often caused by pain, anxiety, or a prior history of hypertension. The sequela of APH can lead to bleeding at the surgical site and cardiovascular stress There is no consensus concerning the treatment threshold for the management of non-cardiac surgery patients with APH. Treatment is frequently a bedside decision by the anesthesiologist or surgeon that takes into consideration the baseline BP, concomitant disease, and the perceived risk of complications (Marik & Varon, 2007). Medications used to manage postoperative hypertension that can be safely given as an intravenous bolus, include hydralazine and labetalol (Aggarwal & Khan, 2006). Restarting preadmission blood pressure medications is prudent once the patient is able to take medications by mouth.

Pain Control. Practitioners must be mindful of the narrow index between effective analgesia and the consequences of oversedation. Masking neurological deficits due to excessive medication prevents timely intervention and can result in death or disability. Both the spinal surgery and craniotomy patient populations have significant pain postoperatively and it is key to initiate pain management as soon as reasonable. This is usually after the initial neurological assessment has been performed by the team. For the patients undergoing a craniotomy, small (25–50 mcg) intermittent (every 25 minutes) IV boluses of the short-acting opioid fentanyl provides excellent pain control without oversedation (Frakes, Lord, Kociszewski, & Wedel, 2006). Once the gastrointestinal tract is functioning and bowel sounds have returned, transitioning to an enteral opioid such as oxycodone 5–10 mg by mouth should be initiated in preparation for transfer to a nonmonitored setting. There is limited data available assessing the safety of intravenous patient-controlled analgesia (IV PCA) for postoperative craniotomy pain. This is an area that warrants further investigation because the steady narcotic dose provided with IV PCA provides optimal pain control (Ortiz-Cardona & Bendo, 2007). However, the risk of oversedation masking a neurologic complication is a major concern.

Pain from spinal procedures in the neurointensive care arena is best managed with IV PCA. Using longer-acting opioids such as morphine or hydromorphone tend to offer better pain control than fentanyl, due to fentanyl's short duration of action (Ornstein & Berko, 2006). Because many patients who undergo spine surgery have chronic pain, the provider should be familiar with the patient's prior narcotic use because this is key to ensuring adequate opiate dosing postoperatively (Ortiz-Cardona & Bendo, 2007). There have been studies demonstrating the benefit of ketorolac in pain control after spinal surgery, however, NSAID have been associated with a decrease in spinal fusion rates (Ornstein & Berko, 2006).

Nausea/Vomiting. Postoperative nausea and vomiting (PONV) is common after both craniotomy and spine surgery. Choosing an antiemetic with minimal central nervous system depression is optimal for patients postcraniotomy. Ondansetron 4 mg IV intraoperative has been proven to decrease PONV in patients undergoing craniotomy for supratentorial tumors (Wig, Chandrashekharappa, Yaddanapudi, Nakra, & Mukherjee, 2007). Metoproclamide 10 mg IV q 6 is also effective in relieving PONV without causing sedation.

Antibiotic Prophylaxis. The consensus of the National Surgical Infection Prevention Project on antibiotic prophylaxis is that antibiotics should be given within 60 minutes before surgical incision and that prophylactic antimicrobial agents should be discontinued within 24 hours of the end of surgery

(Bratzler & Houck, 2005). A meta-analysis of the data on the use of prophylactic antibiotics prior to craniotomy by Barker (2007) revealed that this practice reduces the rate of postoperative meningitis by approximately 50%.

Venous thromboembolism (VTE) Prophylaxis. The recommendations for VTE prophylaxis postcraniotomy are intermittent pneumatic compression (IPC) initiated intraoperatively with or without graduated compression stockings (Geertz et al., 2004). Use of either low-dose unfractionated heparin (LDUH) or low molecular weight heparin (LMWH) in addition to IPC and/or graduated compression stockings is indicated in those patients that are high risk for VTE formation (prior VTE, >40 years old, malignancy) (Geertz et al.). Most providers prefer to deter pharmacologic prophylaxis until 24 hours postoperatively to decrease the risk of bleeding into the operative bed. The recommendation for patients undergoing major spine surgery as those seen in the neurocritical care arena is to institute either postoperative LMWH alone or LDUH alone or perioperative IPC alone. Patients with multiple risk factors should receive a combination of LDUH or LMWH with graduated compression stockings and/or IPC (Geertz et al.).

Stress Ulcer Prophylaxis. Stress ulcer prophylaxis with H2 receptor agonists or a proton pump inhibitor is appropriate in the postoperative patient in the neurocritical care arena, especially because those patients with tumors will be on high-dose steroids (Allen, Kopp, & Ersted, 2004).

Glycemic Control. Studies have demonstrated that tight glucose control can reduce morbidity and mortality in patients with critical illness (Van den Berghe et al., 2001). Utilizing rapid-acting or short-acting insulin during the postoperative period while patient is NPO is ideal for maintaining normoglycemia. Once the patient is eating, prescribing a basal dose with an intermediate-acting insulin as well as with correctional and prandial insulin is recommended (Hassan, 2007).

Prognosis and Outcomes

The rate of postoperative complication for craniotomy and major spine procedures varies depending on the reason for the surgery, location of the lesion, patient's age, and comorbidities (Boakye et al., 2008; Brell et al., 2000; Petrozza, 2002; Zak, 2003).

Stroke

Stroke is the leading cause of disability and loss of productive years in the United States and is the third leading cause of death (Adams, del Zoppo, & von Kummer, 2006). There are two main categories of stroke: hemorrhagic and ischemic. Distinguishing between the two is important because it influences the care given. Intracerebral hemorrhage comprises 9% of all strokes and the majority of hemorrhagic strokes. Subarachnoid hemorrhage is less common and comprises 3% of all strokes. Ischemic strokes account for the remaining 88% of strokes (American Heart Association Statistics Committee and Stroke Statistics Subcommittee, 2006).

Hemorrhagic Stroke

Pathophysiology. Intracerebral hemorrhage is the type of hemorrhagic stroke that is typically seen in patients older than 55 years of age and has a higher incidence of morbidity and mortality than ischemic stroke. The patient with an intracerebral hemorrhage is more unstable, has a greater need for neurocritical care and possible neurosurgery than the patient with an ischemic stroke (Bhardwaj et al., 2004). Risk factors for intracerebral hemorrhage include hypertension, anticoagulation, underlying vascular abnormalities, alcohol use, liver dysfunction, use of aspirin, use of cocaine or amphetamines, smoking, diabetes, prior ischemic stroke, and hematologic disorders (Adams et al., 2006). SAH accounts for a small portion of all total strokes, but it is a devastating event that affects a relatively young population (Feigin et al., 2005). SAH is discussed fully later in this text and is excluded from the discussion that follows.

Presenting Symptoms/Diagnosis. Obtaining an accurate history is key in determining if a stroke is hemorrhagic or ischemic. The patient with an ICH is more likely to have a headache that begins while they are active, focal neurological deficits that progressively worsen over minutes to hours and an associated change in level of consciousness. Increased blood pressure and vomiting are common (Broderick et al., 2007).

Treatment. Early recognition of ICH and rapid treatment are keys to reducing morbidity and mortality associated with this disease. Determining the underlying etiology of the hemorrhage and preventing further bleeding are essential; radiographic imaging helps to guide further treatment (Broderick et al., 2007). If a cerebellar hemorrhage is found on head CT, then transferring the patient to a tertiary care center that has the ability to provide neurosurgical intervention is reasonable (Jensen & St. Louis, 2005). Other treatment for ICH includes reversing any coagulopathy, controlling hypertension, and providing supportive care (Adams et al., 2006). Table 5.15 summarizes the guidelines for management of spontaneous ICH in adults.

Ischemic Stroke

Pathophysiology. Ischemic stroke, a clinical syndrome of rapid onset of focal cerebral deficit, comprises the majority of all strokes and can occur for various reasons (Bandera et al., 2006). There are three main causes: thrombotic, embolic, and hypoperfusion strokes. Risk factors associated with all ischemic stroke subtypes include current smoking, hypertension, diabetes, lower high-density lipoprotein cholesterol, and lower education level (Ohira et al., 2006). Thrombotic strokes are usually caused by an obstruction of the artery caused by artherosclerosis, whereas embolic strokes are more likely to occur from a cardiac source and are common in patients with atrial fibrillation and valvular heart disease. Patients that present with strokes related to hypoperfusion have relative systemic hypoperfusion and may have intracranial or extracranial stenosis (Bhardwaj et al., 2004).

Presenting Symptoms/Diagnosis. The patient with an acute stroke usually presents with a change in neurological status. The timing and progression of the symptoms are important in helping to differentiate between the types of stroke and other diseases. It is important to rule out other disease states that mimic ischemic stroke including masses, encephalitis, seizures or postictal state, metabolic derangement (hypoglycemia or hyperglycemia), and migraines (Bhardwaj et al., 2004). An ischemic stroke can at times be precipitated by a transient ischemic attack (TIA). Most TIAs last <30 minutes but the definition of TIA is transient loss of neurological function that lasts <24 hours (Lerner, 1995).

5.15 Guidelines for the Management of Spontaneous Intracerebral Hemorrhage in Adults

	Intervention	Recommendation Level*
Recommendations for Emergency Diagnosis and Assessment of ICH	ICH should be promptly recognized and diagnosed with either a head CT or MRI	Class I
Recommendations for Initial Medical Therapy	Monitoring and management of patients should take place in an ICU	Class I
	Appropriate antiepileptic therapy should always be used for treatment of clinical seizures	Class I
	Sources of fever should be treated and antipyretic medications administered to lower temperatures in febrile patients	Class I
	Early mobilization and rehabilitation are recommended in patients with ICH who are clinically stable	Class I
	Treatment of elevated ICP ▓ elevate head of bed ▓ provide analgesia and sedation The following generally require monitoring of ICP and BP; CPP >70 mmHg must be maintained. ▓ osmotic diuretics (Mannitol and hypertonic saline) ▓ CSF drainage via EVD ▓ Neuromuscular blockade ▓ Hyperventilation	Class IIa
	Tight glycemic control, treat glucose >185 mg/dL	Class IIa

(continued)

5.15 Guidelines for the Management of Spontaneous Intracerebral Hemorrhage in Adults (continued)

	Intervention	Recommendation Level*
	Blood pressure control with bolus doses or continuous infusions of Labetalol, Nicardipine, Esmolol, Enalapril, Hydralazine, Nipride, or Nitroglycerin	Class IIb
	▪ If SBP >200 mmHg or MAP >150 mmHg → aggressive reduction of BP	
	▪ If SBP >180 mmHg or MAP >130 mmHg and evidence of elevated ICP → monitor ICP and reduce BP to keep CPP >60 mmHg to 80 mmHg	
	▪ If SBP >180 mmHg or MAP >130 mmHg and no elevated ICP → modest reduction of BP, goal MAP 110 mmHg or target BP 160/90 mmHg	
	Treatment with recombinant activated factor VII within first 3–4 hours after onset of bleed	Class IIb
	Use of prophylactic antiepileptic therapy may reduce risk of early seizures in patients with lobar hemorrhage	Class IIb
Recommendations for Prevention of Deep Vein Thrombosis and Pulmonary Embolism	Use of intermittent pneumatic compression devices on patients with hemiparesis/ hemiplegia	Class I
	Long-term treatment of hypertension	Class I
	After cessation of bleeding, low-dose subcutaneous low-molecular-weight heparin or unfractionated heparin in patients with hemiplegia after 3–4 days from onset	Class IIb

	Patients who develop acute proximal venous thrombosis should be considered for placement of vena cava filter	Class IIb
	Adding long-term antithrombotic therapy several weeks after placement of vena cava filter → cause of hemorrhage must be taken into consideration and associated conditions with increased arterial throm-botic risk (atrial fibrillation and overall health and mobility of patient)	Class IIb
Recommendations for the Man-agement of ICH Related to Coagulation and Fibrinolysis	Protamine sulfate should be used to reverse heparin-associated ICH, dose dependent on time from ces-sation of heparin	Class I
	Treatment with IV vitamin K to reverse warfarin-associated ICH and treatment to replace clotting factors	Class I
	Prothrombin complex concentrate, factor IX complex concentrate and rFVIIa normalize elevated INR levels rapidly but have greater risk of thromboembolism. FFP can be used but is associated with greater volumes and longer infu-sion times	Class IIb
	Decision to restart antithrombic therapy after ICH ▪ Antiplatelet therapy may be a better choice for patients with a lower risk of cerebral infarction and a higher risk of amyloid angiopathy or with very poor overall neurological function	Class IIb

(continued)

5.15 Guidelines for the Management of Spontaneous Intracerebral Hemorrhage in Adults *(continued)*

	Intervention	Recommendation Level*
Recommendations for Surgical Approaches	▪ Restart warfarin therapy 7–10 days after onset of original ICH in patients with very high risk of thromboembolism	
	Treatment of patients with ICH related to thrombolytic therapy includes urgent empirical therapies to replace clotting factors and platelets	Class IIb
	In patients with cerebellar ICH >3 cm who are deteriorating neurologically or who have brainstem compression and/or hydrocephalus from ventricular obstruction should have surgical removal of hemorrhage	Class I
	Stereotactic infusion of urokinase into clot cavity within 72 hours of ictus reduces clot burden and risk of death, but rebleeding is more common and functional outcome is not improved → usefulness unknown	Class IIb
	Minimally invasive clot evacuation using mechanical devices or endoscopy→ usefulness unknown	Class IIb
	Evacuation of supratentorial ICH by standard craniotomy might be considered for patients presenting with lobar clots within 1 cm of surface	Class IIb
	Routine evacuation of supratentorial ICH by standard craniotomy within 96 hours of ictus is NOT RECOMMENDED	Class III

Recommendations for Timing of Surgery	No clear evidence shows that ultra-early craniotomy improves functional outcome or mortality rate; very early craniotomy may be associated with increased risk of recurrent bleeding. Operative removal within 12 hours, when performed by less-invasive methods has the most supportive evidence	Class IIb
	Delayed evacuation by craniotomy appears to offer little if any benefit; in patients presenting in coma with deep hemorrhages, removal of ICH by craniotomy may actually worsen outcome and is NOT RECOMMENDED	Class III
Recommendations for Decompressive Craniectomy	Too few data exist to comment on the potential of decompressive craniectomy to improve outcome in ICH	Class IIb
Recommendation for Withdrawal of Technological Support	Careful consideration of aggressive full care during the 24 hours after ICH onset and postponement of new DNR orders during that time	Class IIb
Recommendations for Prevention of Recurrent ICH	Treating hypertension in the non-acute setting	Class I
	Discontinuation of smoking, heavy alcohol use, and cocaine use	Class I

*Class I Recommendation, Benefit >>>Risk
Class IIa Recommendation, Benefit >>Risk
Class IIb Recommendation, Benefit > or equal to Risk
Class III Recommendation, Risk > or equal to Benefit
Adapted from Broderick et al., 2007.

Treatment. There are many different modalities that are available for stroke treatment. Intravenous tissue plasminogen activator (tPA), intra-arterial thrombolysis, and clot extraction by mechanical methods are some of the more advanced treatments that are available at tertiary care centers that are designated as stroke centers. Rapid brain imaging, including noncontrast head CT and MRIs, are tools that aid the clinician in rapid assessment and management options for stroke patients (Hill, Demchuk, Tomsick, Palesch, & Broderick, 2006). Treatment options are time sensitive and only a small portion of patients who suffer from ischemic stroke actually receive thrombolysis or clot extraction (Weintraub, 2006). If any of the aforementioned modalities are used to treat an ischemic stroke, the patient will need to be admitted to the intensive care unit for supportive care. After the acute phase of the ischemic stroke has passed, it is essential to focus on the rehabilitation and modification of risk factors for the stroke patient (Bhardwaj et al., 2004). Guidelines for the early management of the adult with acute ischemic stroke are summarized in Table 5.16. Class III recommendations guide the provider regarding activities that may place the patient with an acute ischemic event at greater risk based on existing data. The Class III recommendations for ischemic stroke are summarized in Table 5.17.

Prognosis and Outcomes. Stroke is the leading cause of disability and the third leading cause of death in the United States (Adams et al., 2006). The majority of functional recovery after stroke occurs in the first 3 months and prognosis after stroke is dependent on the type of stroke suffered and on the anatomical location of the lesion. (Aronen, Laakso, Moser, & Perkio, 2007).

Subarachnoid Hemorrhage

Definition and Etiology

Subarachnoid hemorrhage, defined as bleeding between the arachnoid and pia mater layers of the meninges (McQuillan, Von Reuden, Hartsock, Flynn, & Whalen, 2002), is a subtype of stroke that accounts for 10% of all strokes. The main cause of SAH is trauma; nontraumatic SAH is usually caused by

5.16 Guidelines for the Early Management of Adults with Ischemic Stroke

	Intervention	Recommendation Level*
Designation of Stroke Centers	Creation of primary stroke centers (PSC)	Class I
	Development of a comprehensive stroke center (CSC)	Class I
	For patients with suspected stroke, EMS should bypass hospitals that do not have resources available to treat acute stroke and go to closest facility capable of treating acute stroke	Class I
Emergency Evaluation and Diagnosis of Acute Ischemic Stroke	Have an organized protocol for the emergency evaluation of patients with suspected stroke ▓ Goal = complete evaluation in 60 minutes ▓ Careful clinical assessment, including neurological examination	Class I
	Use of stroke rating scale, preferably NIHSS	Class I
	A limited number of hematologic, coagulation, and biochemistry tests are recommended during initial emergency evaluation	Class I
	Patients with clinical evidence of acute cardiac or pulmonary disease may warrant a chest x-ray	Class I
	Obtain an ECG because of high incidence of heart disease in patients with stroke	Class I
Early Diagnosis: Brain and Vascular Imaging	Imaging of brain is recommended before initiating any therapy to treat ischemic stroke ▓ Head CT is usually sufficient ▓ Imaging should be interpreted by physician with expertise in reading CTs or MRIs	Class I

(continued)

5.16

Guidelines for the Early Management of Adults with Ischemic Stroke *(continued)*

	Intervention	Recommendation Level*
General Supportive Care and Treatment of Acute Complications	Vascular imaging is needed as a preliminary step for intra-arterial administration of phar-macological agents, surgical procedures, or endovascular interventions	Class IIa
	Airway support and ventilatory as-sistance if patient has decreased level of consciousness or bulbar dysfunction	Class I
	Hypoxic patients should receive supplemental oxygen	Class I
	Treat sources of fever and adminis-ter antipyretic medications	Class I
	Use of cardiac monitors to screen for atrial fibrillation and other serious arrhythmias for first 24 hours	Class I
	Cautious management of arterial hypertension	Class I

	Treat BP in patients that are otherwise eligible for rtPA
	   ■ SBP <185 mmHg
	   ■ DBP <110 mmHg before lytic therapy is started.
	Maintain BP below 180/105 mmHg for the first 24 hours after rtPA is given.
		Class I

	In patients undergoing acute interventions to reopen occluded vessels, the rtPA BP guide-lines should be followed	Class I

	Treat underlying cause of arterial hypotension	Class I
	▪ Treat hypovolemia with normal saline	
	▪ Correct cardiac arrhythmias that may reduce cardiac output	
	Treat hypoglycemia, goal = normogylcemia	Class I
Intravenous Thrombolysis	Intravenous rtPA (0.9 mg/kg, maximum dose 90 mg) recommended for select patients who are treated within 3 hours of onset of ischemic stroke	Class I
	Physicians should be aware of potential complications with rtPA	Class I
	▪ Bleeding	
	▪ Angioedema, causing airway obstruction	
Intra-Arterial Thrombolysis	Intra-arterial thrombolysis is a treatment option for selected patients who have major stroke symptoms <6 hours duration due to occlusions of the MCA; these patients are not candidates for intravenous rtPA	Class I
	Treatment must take place at an experienced stroke center that has immediate access to cerebral angiography and qualified interventionalists	Class I
	Intra-arterial thrombolysis is reasonable in patients who have contraindications to intravenous thrombolysis such as recent surgery	Class IIa
Antiplatelet Agents	Administration of aspirin 325 mg within 24–48 hours after stroke onset	Class I

(continued)

5.16 Guidelines for the Early Management of Adults with Ischemic Stroke (continued)

	Intervention	Recommendation Level*
Volume Expansion, Vasodilators, and Induced Hypertension	In exceptional cases vasopressors may be used to augment cerebral blood flow	Class I
Endovascular Interventions	Use of MERCI device is a reasonable intervention for extraction of intra-arterial thrombi	Class IIb
Admission to the Hospital and General Acute Treatment	Use of stroke units incorporating rehabilitation	Class I
	Use of standardized stroke care order sets	Class I
	Early mobilization and measures to prevent subacute complications of stroke	Class I
	Swallow assessment before eating or drinking	Class I
	Treat patients with suspected urinary tract infections or pneumonia with antibiotics	Class I
	Prevent deep vein thrombosis in immobilized patients with subcutaneous injections of anticoagulants	Class I
	Treat concomitant medical diseases	Class I
	Prevent recurrent stroke by promoting early interventions	Class I
Treatment of Acute Neurological Complications	Patients with large areas of infarction are at high risk for brain edema and increased ICP.	Class I
	▆ Close neurological monitoring during first few days	

▦ Take measures to lessen cerebral edema	
▦ Consider transfer to institution with neurosurgical expertise	
Treat patients with acute hydrocephalus with placement of ventricular drain	Class I
Decompressive surgical evacuation of space-occupying cerebellar infarct	Class I
Treat recurrent seizures after stroke	Class I
Decompressive surgery for malignant edema may be life-saving, but impact of morbidity is unknown. Family should be informed about potential outcomes including severe disability	Class IIa

*Class I Recommendation, Benefit >>>Risk
Class IIa Recommendation, Benefit >>Risk
Class IIb Recommendation, Benefit > or equal to Risk
Class III Recommendation, Risk > or equal to Benefit
Adapted from Adams et al., 2007.

the rupture of a saccular aneurysm. There are several risk factors that contribute to the incidence of aneurysmal subarachnoid hemorrhage, including cigarette smoking, heavy alcohol consumption, hypertension, oral contraceptive use, cocaine/amphetamine use, and familial history (Feigin et al., 2005). This section focuses on the diagnosis and management of aneurysmal SAH.

Diagnosis

One of the keys to accurately diagnosing SAH is a comprehensive clinical history. The patient with aneurysmal SAH will typically complain of "the worst headache of life" or describe a headache with a sudden, "thunderclap" onset. Noncontrast head CT is essential to the diagnosis of SAH (Liebenberg, Worth, Firth, Olney, & Norris, 2005). On a noncontrast head CT, blood is seen in the subarachnoid space

5.17 Ischemic Stroke CLASS III Recommendations

	Intervention	Recommendation Level
Early Diagnosis: Brain and Vascular Imaging	Emergency treatment of stroke should NOT be delayed to obtain multimodal imaging studies	Class III
	Vascular imaging should NOT delay treatment of patients whose symptoms started <3 hours ago and who have acute ischemic stroke	Class III
Intra-arterial Thrombolysis	The availability of intra-arterial thrombolysis should NOT preclude the intravenous administration of rtPA if the patient is eligible for rtPA	Class III
Anticoagulants	Urgent anticoagulation with the goal of preventing early recurrent stroke, halting neurological worsening, or improving outcomes is NOT recommended in patients with acute ischemic stroke	Class III
Antiplatelet Agents	Aspirin should NOT be considered a substitute for other acute interventions for treatment of stroke	Class III
	Do NOT administer aspirin as an adjunctive therapy within 24 hours of thrombolytic therapy	Class III
	Do NOT administer clopidogrel alone or in combination with aspirin for treatment of stroke	Class III
	Do NOT administer antiplatelet agnets that inhibit the glycoprotein IIb/IIIa receptor	Class III
Volume Expansion, Vasodilators, and Induced Hypertension	Hemodilution and volume expansion is NOT recommended	Class III
	Do NOT administer medications such as pentoxifyline	Class III

Admission to the Hospital and General Acute Treatment	Nutritional supplements are NOT needed	Class III
	AVOID placement of indwelling bladder catheters	Class III
Treatment of Acute Neurological Complications	Corticosteroids are NOT recommended	Class III
	Prophylactic administration of anticonvulsants to patients who have NOT had seizures is NOT recommended	Class III

*Class I Recommendation, Benefit >>>Risk
Class IIa Recommendation, Benefit >>Risk
Class IIb Recommendation, Benefit > or equal to Risk
Class III Recommendation, Risk > or equal to Benefit
Adapted from Adams et al., 2007.

in 92% of cases if the head CT is performed within the first 24 hours of presentation. After 24 hours, the sensitivity of CT to detect the SAH decreases. Once subarachnoid blood is seen on a head CT, then no further workup is needed to diagnose the SAH. However, if the clinical history is suspicious for SAH and head CT is negative for blood, then a lumbar puncture (LP) must be obtained (Al-Shahi, White, Davenport, & Lindsay, 2006). In the setting of SAH, the opening pressure on LP will be elevated and there would be red blood cells (RBCs) present in all tubes. The LP can only be considered a traumatic tap if the last collection tube has no RBCs. If both head CT and LP are performed within a few days after initial headache and are negative, then the diagnosis of SAH can be eliminated. However, if the clinical history is still highly suspicious for aneurysmal SAH, then a cerebral angiogram should be performed (Liebenberg et al.).

Once the diagnosis of SAH has been established, it is necessary to determine the etiology of the SAH. Saccular aneurysm rupture is the most common cause of nontraumatic SAH. The golden standard for diagnosing and determining the etiology of SAH is the four-vessel cerebral angiogram. In about 20% of cases, the initial angiogram may be negative because of vasospasm, poor technique, compression of the vessel caused by extravascular clot, or thrombus in the aneurysmal pouch. If the initial angiogram is negative, it should be repeated in 2 weeks. The aneurysm location, size, and presence of neck are factors that can be seen on angiogram which help determine the best course of treatment (Bhardwaj et al., 2004).

Grading Scales. There are different grading systems for classifying SAH that aid clinicians in guiding management decisions and providing prognostic data for patients and family members, although there is no one accepted standard. The most commonly used scale is the Hunt and Hess Scale (see Table 5.18) but it has many inherent faults; it is subjective and it is difficult to assign patients to a grade when they have an atypical presentation. The other commonly used scale is the Fisher scale (see Table 5.19), which grades the severity of SAH on radiographic appearance. The Fisher scale provides an excellent prediction of risk of vasospasm (Rosen & MacDonald, 2005).

Treatment

Aneurysms can be either clipped surgically or coiled with endovascular intervention. Smaller aneurysms (<4 mm) that have a narrow neck are favorable for endovascular coiling. There is some controversy regarding the timing of the treatment of aneurysms after SAH. Early aneurysm treatment after hemorrhage may be more challenging because of edema and vasospasm; whereas the risk of later aneurysm repair is

5.18 Hunt and Hess Scale

Grade	Neurological Status
1	Asymptomatic or mild headache and slight nuchal rigidity
2	Severe headache, stiff neck, no neurologic deficit except cranial nerve palsy
3	Drowsy or confused, mild focal neurologic deficit
4	Stuporous, moderate, or severe hemiparesis
5	Coma, decerebrate posturing

Based on initial neurologic examination; adapted from Hunt, W, Hess, R. (1968). *J Neurosurgery* 28: 14.

5.19 Grading Scale Based on Radiographic Information*

Group	Appearance of Blood on Head CT Scan
1	No blood detected
2	Diffuse deposition or thin layer with all vertical layers <1 mm thick
3	Localized clot and/or vertical layers 1 mm or more in thickness
4	Intracerebral or intraventricular clot with diffuse or no subarachnoid blood

*Used to Determine Vasospasm Risk, not Clinical Outcome
Adapted from Fisher, C. M., Kistler, J. P., Davis, J. M. Relation of cerebral vasospasm to subarachnoid hemorrhage visualized by CT scanning. *Neurosurgery* 1980, 6:1.

greater if hypervolemic and hypertensive therapies are initiated in the setting of vasospasm (Bhardwaj et al., 2004).

Patients with aneurysmal SAH patients should be admitted to an intensive care unit for continuous cardiac monitoring and frequent neurological assessments. Prior to securing the aneurysm; blood pressure should be controlled, lights should remain low, and loud noises avoided to reduce the risk of further rupture of the aneurysm. A systolic blood pressure of <140 mmHg is suggested prior to securing the aneurysm and can be achieved with intravenous medications such as labetalol, hydralazine, or a nicardipine gtt. Agents that have vasodilatory effects (nitroprusside and nitroglycerin) increase intracranial pressure by increasing cerebral blood volume and should be avoided (Bhardwaj et al., 2004).

Complications and Management

After aneurysm repair, SAH patients continue to be managed in the ICU because of the high rate of complications including seizures, cerebral edema, hydrocephalus, vasospasm, and hyponatremia.

Seizures. Seizures are more common in SAH patients that have aneurysms clipped versus those repaired with endovascular coiling. During the first 7 days after SAH, if seizures are not present, then likelihood of developing seizures is low and antiepileptic therapy is discontinued. For SAH patients that do have a seizure, antiepileptic therapy is continued for at least 6 months after SAH. Prophylactic antiepileptic therapy has not been studied and remains controversial (Naval, Stevens, Mirski, & Bharwaj, 2006).

Cerebral edema. SAH patients are at risk for cerebral edema therefore it is important to keep them well-hydrated with isotonic or hypertonic fluids. Hypotonic fluids will lead to increased cerebral edema (Bhardwaj et al., 2004).

Hydrocephalus. Hydrocephalus associated with SAH can be acute, occurring within the first 24 hours after aneurysmal bleed. This obstructive hydrocephalus occurs due to impedance of cerebrospinal fluid (CSF) by blood clots in the ventricular system. Hydrocephalus seen later in SAH is usually communicating. Communicating hydrocephalus, also known as non-obstructive hydrocephalus, is caused by impaired cerebrospinal fluid resorption in the absence of any CSF-flow obstruction. Management of acute hydrocephalus may require the placement of an external ventricular drainage (EVD) catheter. Care must be used when placing an EVD in the patient with acute hydrocephalus as a large change in the transmural pressure may cause rerupture of an unsecured aneurysm (Springborg, Frederikson, Eskesen, & Olsen, 2004). Patients that develop hydrocephalus later in their disease course may need EVDs or serial LPs to relieve increased ICP until the ventricular system is able to reabsorb CSF normally. Among patients with SAH, 20% need long-term diversion of CSF with placement of shunts (Dehdashti, Rillet, Rufenacht, & de Tribolet, 2004).

Vasospasm. Vasospasm, the constriction of cerebral blood vessels caused by the presence of blood in the subarachnoid space occurs in 60% to 75% of patients with SAH. The actual incidence of clinical vasospasm (patients with change in mental status or a focal neurological deficit) is somewhat lower. Vasospasm can occur up to 21 days after the initial bleed but the peak incidence is days 7 through 11 (Kassab et al., 2007). Nimodipine has been shown to improve outcomes in SAH, although the exact mechanism of action is not fully understood (Brown & Carley, 2004). Medical management of vasospasm includes nimodipine 60 mg every 4 hours for 21 days after SAH. When signs of clinical or symptomatic vasospasm are noted, then hypervolemic, hypertensive, hemodilutional therapy (triple-H therapy) is initiated. Triple-H therapy consists of aggressive fluid repletion with the goal of euvolemia to positive fluid balance. Isotonic to hypertonic IV solutions are ordered to avoid hyponatremia, which can result in cerebral edema (Naval et al., 2006). The target hematocrit for the SAH patient is 30 and aggressive fluid repletion with hypervolemic therapy helps to achieve this goal. Blood pressure is augmented with vasopressors to increase cerebral perfusion pressure. Because not all SAH patients have an EVD with the ability to monitor CPP, a mean arterial pressure goal is set based on correlation with patient's clinical examination (Bhardwaj et al., 2004). Severe vasospasm may be refractory to all medical management and require further interventions. Transcranial Doppler (TCD) studies are obtained daily as one method of monitoring for vasospasm (Kassab et al., 2007). When blood flow velocities are visualized as increased via TCDs and the patient has an associated change in neurological examination, an angiogram may be warranted to further assess for vasospasm. With severe vasospasm, the patient has a high risk of ischemic stroke due to constriction of cerebral blood vessels. Large vasospastic vessels may be opened with balloon angioplasty. When vasospasm is seen in smaller, distal vessels then intra-arterial injections of vasodilators such as papaverine, verapamil, nicardipine, or nimodipine may be used (Feigin & Findlay, 2006).

Hyponatremia. Many SAH patients develop hyponatremia during the course of their illness. There are two main reasons for SAH patients to become hyponatremic—syndrome of inappropriate secretion of antidiuretic hormone (SIADH) and cerebral salt wasting (CSW). Diagnosing SAH accurately is imperative as the treatments for SIADH and CSW are very different (see Table 5.20) (Naval et al., 2006).

5.20 Hyponatremia Treatment

Disorder	Serum Na Level	Fluid Balance	Urine Output	Treatment
SIADH	Low	Hypervolemic or euvolemic	Low	Fluid restriction (contraindicated in SAH)
CSW	Low	hypovolemic	High	Aggressive fluid resuscitation with hypertonic saline

Prognosis and Outcomes

SAH outcomes have not improved significantly over the last few years; death or dependence is usually associated with complications surrounding SAH and have rates as high as 70% (Feigin & Findlay, 2006). This disease process has a relatively young age of onset and can dramatically affect quality of life.

Seizures

Definition

A seizure is an event of altered brain function as a result of abnormal hypersynchronous paroxysmal cortical neuronal discharge with either motor (convulsion), sensory, or cognitive dysfunction (Varelas & Mirski, 2001). Clinical manifestations of seizures occur when enough neurons are excited. The resultant seizure activity reflects the area of the brain involved. Epilepsy is defined as a condition of recurrent (two or more) unprovoked seizures (Krumholz et al., 2007).

Pathophysiology

Abnormal neuronal excitability is thought to occur as a result of disruption of the depolarization & repolarization mechanisms of the cell (termed "excitability"). Aberrant neural networks that develop abnormal synchronization can result in the development and propagation of an epileptic seizure (termed "synchronization"). Epileptic seizures originate in a setting of both altered excitability and synchronization of neurons. The excitability of individual neurons is affected by cell membrane properties, intracellular processes, structural features of neuronal elements, and interneuronal connection (Nair, 2003).

Classification of Seizures

The International League Against Epilepsy (ILAE) has developed a generally accepted classification system for seizures (Commission on Classification and Terminology of the International League Against Epilepsy, 1982). This classification of seizures is divided into two specific categories—partial and generalized. A *partial* seizure involves only a portion of the brain at onset, whereas a *generalized* seizure involves the entire brain at onset (Holmes, 1997).

Partial seizures can be divided into simple partial and complex partial subtypes. During simple partial seizures, consciousness remains intact. The signs or symptoms of simple partial seizures depend on the location of the seizure focus. Examples include focal motor (rhythmic activity of arm, leg, or face), somatosensory (visual, auditory, olfactory signs), autonomic (sweating, pallor, flushing), or psychic symptoms (hallucinations, illusions) (Holmes, 1997).

The complex partial seizure is progression to another area of the brain. A person's level of awareness or consciousness is impaired, although they do not lose consciousness. The patient either does not respond to commands or responds in an abnormally slow manner. An example of a complex partial seizure is an automatism (involuntary motor activity) characterized as facial grimacing, chewing, lip smacking, or repeating phrases. The patient does not recall this activity after the seizure. Complex partial seizures usually last from 30 seconds to several minutes and may be preceded by a simple partial seizure (aura), which serves as a warning that more seizures are to come as well as aids the practitioner to the seizure's initial focus. Both types of partial seizures can spread to the entire brain; this is referred to as secondary generalized seizures (Holmes, 1997).

Primary generalized seizures arise simultaneously in both cerebral hemispheres. They generally involve impairment of consciousness and may range from barely noticeable to tonic–clonic convulsion. Types of generalized seizures include absence, myoclonic, tonic, clonic, tonic–clonic, and atonic (Holmes, 2007).

Absence seizures are generalized seizures, which usually start abruptly without an aura, last from a few seconds to a half a minute, end abruptly, and may be associated with motor, autonomic, and behavioral phenomena such as automatisms. They are often difficult to distinguish from complex partial seizures. *Myoclonic* seizures are characterized by sudden, brief (<350 milliseconds), shock-like contractions. These may be generalized, confined to face/trunk/limb or to an individual muscle group. Because of the brevity of seizures, it is not possible to determine if consciousness is impaired. *Tonic* seizures are brief seizures (usually <60s) consisting of the sudden onset of increased tone in the extensor muscles. *Clonic* seizures consist only of rhythmic or semirhythmic contraction of muscle groups (without increase in tone/stiffening). *Generalized tonic–clonic* (formerly called grand mal) seizures occur with the onset of generalized stiffening (tonic phase) followed by generalized jerking of the muscles (clonic activity). A loss of consciousness usually occurs simultaneously with the onset of the tonic phase and is followed by a deep postictal phase. *Atonic* seizures, or drop attacks, are characterized by a sudden loss of muscle tone, they begin suddenly and without warning. Atonic seizures are rare and are usually confined to childhood (Holmes, 1997).

Diagnostic Criteria

Seizures are often a symptom of an underlying disorder, which may be genetic, traumatic, metabolic, infectious, malignant, or pharmacologic. Table 5.21 summarizes common etiologies of seizures. The underlying disorder must be identified and treated to control the seizure in most cases (Browne & Holmes, 2001). Evaluation of seizures begins with a history and physical exam with focus on the comprehensive neurologic examination. Metabolic abnormalities may be responsible for up to 30% to 35% of seizures in patients with critical illness (Varelas & Mirski, 2001). Therefore, it is imperative to send laboratory work to include complete blood count (CBC), electrolytes, liver function tests, glucose, and toxicology. The patient with a known seizure disorder, should have serum antiepileptic drug levels obtained to determine compliance. Noncontrast CT or MRI should be performed immediately in the setting of new focal neurologic deficit, trauma, fever, persistent headache, history of cancer, or anticoagulant therapy (Browne & Holmes, 2001). LP should also be considered in the setting of fever, nuchal rigidity, and altered mental status to rule out meningitis or encephalitis. The LP should be done after imaging has been completed to avoid precipitation of cerebral herniation in the setting of increased ICP. EEG can be helpful and should be considered especially in those patients who are comatose because nonconvulsive status epilepticus is often undiagnosed in the ICU (Praline et al., 2007).

Treatment

Most commonly, seizures manifest as single episodes that serve to alert the practitioner that a metabolic or structural abnormality exists (Varelas & Mirski, 2001). Often, a patient

5.21 Common Etiologies of Seizures

Metabolic Causes
- Hypoglycemia, hyponatremia, hypocalcemia, hypophosphatemia
- Fluid balance: dehydration/water intoxication
- Hypoxia, ischemia (postcardiac arrest)

Toxins (poisons)
- Carbon monoxide
- Lead

Alcohol / Drug Withdrawal
- Barbiturates, Opioids, Benzodiazepines

Drug Overdose
- Isoniazid

Medications (Lower Seizure Threshold)
- Bronchodilators (*Theophylline*)
- Antibiotics (*Beta Lactams, Flagyl*)
- Antidepressants (*Wellbutrin, Tricyclics*)
- Local anesthetics (*Lidocaine*)
- Psychostimulants (*Cocaine*)

Abrupt Withdrawal of CNS Depressants

Sepsis, Infection, Fever

Renal/ Hepatic Dysfunction

Idiopathic

Neurovascular
- Ischemic stroke
- Intracerebral hemorrhage
- Subarachnoid hemorrhage
- Vascular malformations

Tumors/Lesions

CNS Infection
- Meningitis, Encephalitis

Inflammatory Disease
- Vasculitis

Head Trauma
- Contusion
- Subdural Hematoma
- Epidural Hematoma

Birth Trauma

Neurofibromatosis

Primary Epilepsy

Low-Antiepileptic Levels (noncompliance)

who has had a single seizure with no evidence of structural lesion or electroencephalographic abnormalities may be monitored but not given medication (Browne & Holmes, 2001). However, if an underlying etiology, such as mass lesion or diagnosis of epilepsy is made, medication is initiated depending on the type of seizure. Table 5.22 summarizes the usual dosages for common antiepileptic drugs used in patients 16 years of age and older. There are instances in which medical therapy via antiepileptic drugs fails and a person's seizures become intractable. For intractable seizures, there are surgical options to remove a portion of the patient's brain

5.22 Antiepileptic Drugs in Patients 16 Years and Older*

Drug	Starting Dose (mg/day)	Dose Frequency	Dose Increase	Maintenance Dose (mg/day)	Therapeutic Range of Plasma Concentrations (μg/ml)
Carbamazepine (Carbatrol, Tegretol, Tegretol-XR)	400	Carbatrol or Tegretol-XR. twice a day; Tegretol or generic, three times a day	200 mg/day at 1-wk intervals	600–1200	4–12
Divalproex sodium (Depakote)	500–1000	Twice a day	250 mg/day at 1-wk intervals	1000–3000	50–150
Ethosuximide (Zarontin)	500	Twice a day	250 mg/day at 1-wk intervals	1000–2000	40–120
Gabapentin (Neurontin)	900	Three times a day	300 mg/day at 24-hr intervals	900–3600	Not established
Lamotrigine† (Lamictal)	50	Twice a day	50 mg/day at 2-wk intervals‡	300–500	Not established
Levetiracetam (Keppra)	1000	Twice a day	1000 mg/day at 2-wk intervals	1000–3000	Not established
Oxcarbazepine (Trileptal)	600	Twice a day	600 mg/day at 1-wk intervals	600–2400	Not established

Phenobarbital	90	Daily	30 mg/day at 4-wk intervals	90–120	10–40
Phenytoin (Dilantin)	300	Daily	100 mg/day at 4-wk intervals§	300–500	10–20
Primidone (Mysoline. Neurosyn)	100–125	Three times a day	Days 1–3, 100–150 mg daily at bedtime: days 4–6, 100–125 mg twice a day: days 7–9, 100–125 mg three times a day: day 10, 250 mg three times a day	750–1000	5–12
Tiagabine (Gabitril)	4	Twice a day to four times a day	4–8 mg/day at 1-wk intervals	32–56	Not established
Topiramate (To-pamax)	25–50	Twice a day	25–50 mg/day at 1-wk intervals	200–400	Not established
Zonisamide (Zone-gran)	100	Twice a day	100 mg/day at 2-wk intervals	400–600	Not established

*Data are from Browne and Holmes.[5] Information on dosages for younger patients is also available from this source.
†The information shown is for persons who are taking lamotrigine in combination with an enzyme-inducing antiepileptic drug (carbamazepine. phenobarbital. phenytoin, or primidone) and who are not taking valproic acid. For persons who are not taking an enzyme-inducing antiepileptic drug or who are taking valproic acid. the dose schedule is different. Consult the package insert.
‡After four weeks, the daily dose can be increased by 100 mg every two weeks.
§The dose should be increase at a rate of 30 to 50 mg per day at four-week intervals when the phenytoin plasma concentration is higher than 10 μg per milliliter.

Reprinted with permissions from Browne & Holmes, 2001.

(usually a portion of the temporal lobe) where the seizure focus originates. This is done after cortical mapping of the brain to localize the dominant language centers. Discontinuation of therapy may be considered for epilepsy syndromes if the patient is seizure free after 2 years of therapy (Browne & Holmes, 2001).

Prognosis

Overall prognosis for patients with seizure disorders is linked to the underlying etiology of the seizure. Many times those with primary epilepsy grow out of their seizures or may be well controlled by medications. However, a subgroup develops intractable epilepsy for which their quality of life is severely affected. Others present with seizures as a clinical manifestation of severe underlying pathology and prognosis is often poor or uncertain (Browne & Holmes, 2007).

Status Epilepticus

Definition

Status epilepticus (SE) is usually defined as continuous seizure activity lasting 30 minutes or as two or more discrete seizures between which consciousness is not fully regained (Dodson, DeLorenzo, & Pedley et al., 1993). In 1999, modifications to this definition were proposed by Lowenstein, Bleck, and Macdonald to consider SE as a continuous, generalized, convulsive seizure lasting >5 minutes, or two or more seizures during which the patient does not return to baseline consciousness. The rationale behind this revision is that a generalized tonic–clonic (GTC) seizure rarely lasts >5 minutes, and clinical experience suggests that the likelihood of spontaneous termination decreases after this time period.

Pathophysiology

The emergence of SE requires a pool of neurons capable of initiating and sustaining abnormal firing (Noe & Manno, 2005). This abnormal discharge is facilitated by the loss of inhibitory synaptic transmission mediated by -aminobutyric acid (GABA) and sustained excitatory transmission mediated by glutamate (Nandhagopal, 2006).

Classification of SE

In general SE can be classified broadly into generalized convulsive status epilepticus (GCSE) and nonconvulsive status epilepticus (NCSE). In GCSE, generalized convulsive activity presents as prolonged tonic or clonic activity of the extremities, and is associated with complete loss of consciousness. With prolonged seizure activity, clinical manifestations may become less apparent and prolonged seizures may evolve into subtle findings such as ocular deviation, fine nystagmus, or subtle jaw, lip, finger, or eyelid twitching before progressing to only electrical activity without physical correlation (Manno, 2003). NCSE refers to continuous or near continuous generalized electrical seizure activity for at least 30 minutes without physical convulsion (Towne et al., 2000). It constitutes approximately 20% to 25% of SE cases and some suggest that it is a more benign condition (Marik & Varon, 2004). However, patients may progress to NCSE after initially presenting in GCSE or may actually present in a coma because of the absence of outward signs of NCSE. Both have a significant mortality rate and therefore, both types of SE should be aggressively treated.

Diagnosis

Status epilepticus, in particular GCSE, should be considered a medical emergency. Treatment is focused on early termination of seizures; however the *most important* initial assessments and interventions should be centered on ensuring an adequate airway and vascular access. Once this is accomplished, a full diagnostic evaluation should be initiated including pertinent history, physical findings, recent changes in medications, alcohol or drug use, trauma, history of previous epilepsy, or neurologic insult. A full neurologic examination should be performed with the goal of identifying any focal neurologic deficits which could reveal underlying pathology. Laboratory studies should be sent to include a complete blood count, arterial blood gas, serum electrolytes, liver/kidney function, toxicology, and serum antiepileptic drug levels if applicable. In the absence of a known seizure disorder, a noncontrast head CT should be performed once the patient is stabilized and seizures are controlled. Lumbar puncture may yield important diagnostic information especially in the setting of fever and nuchal rigidity (Manno, 2003). The role of EEG is most helpful when a patient presents in a comatose state or does not regain consciousness after treatment. EEG can help determine whether the patient is in nonconvulsive status verses a prolonged postictal state (Praline et al., 2007).

The primary causes of SE include stroke, CNS tumor, epilepsy, toxic–metabolic encephalopathy (i.e., renal failure, alcohol withdrawal, sepsis), CNS infection, hypoxic–ischemic injuries, and trauma (Lowenstein, 2006). The identification and treatment of the underlying cause for SE is paramount and should be promptly pursued and reversed. When the practitioner suspects chronic alcoholism or if hypoglycemia exists, then the use of 100 mg of thiamine followed by 50 gm of 50% dextrose should be administered. The thiamine is required as correcting the hypoglycemia in the presence of a thiamine deficiency may cause Wernicke encephalopathy (Manno, 2003).

Initial Management of Status Epilepticus

First-Line Treatment. The goals for treatment of SE include rapid termination of seizures and preservation of neurologic function with minimal systemic complications. Once an adequate airway is secured (endotracheal intubation if necessary), respiratory support provided, and vascular access are obtained then medications can be initiated. First line pharmacologic treatment for SE includes administration of fast acting benzodiazepines such as lorazepam, diazepam, or midazolam. Benzodiazepines are a class of drugs that act at the $GABA_A$ receptor. Stimulation of this subunit leads to inhibition of neural transmission through hyperpolarization of the resting cell membrane (Manno, 2003). Lorazepam, dosed at 0.1 mg/kg, given at a rate of 2 mg/min, has been the preferred initial agent by many due to longer duration of action and pharmacokinetic profile. Many times initial benzodiazepine administration is enough to break the seizures, however when resistant to first-line treatment, a reevaluation of airway protection must be completed (because of sedating effects of the benzodiazepines) and second-line treatment initiated (see Figure 5.5).

5.5

Algorithm for Status Epilepticus

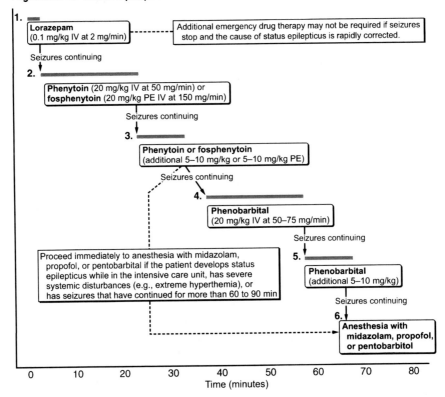

1. Lorazepam (0.1 mg/kg IV at 2 mg/min) ---- Additional emergency drug therapy may not be required if seizures stop and the cause of status epilepticus is rapidly corrected.

Seizures continuing

2. Phenytoin (20 mg/kg IV at 50 mg/min) or fosphenytoin (20 mg/kg PE IV at 150 mg/min)

Seizures continuing

3. Phenytoin or fosphenytoin (additional 5–10 mg/kg or 5–10 mg/kg PE)

Seizures continuing

4. Phenobarbital (20 mg/kg IV at 50–75 mg/min)

Seizures continuing

Proceed immediately to anesthesia with midazolam, propofol, or pentobarbital if the patient develops status epilepticus while in the intensive care unit, has severe systemic disturbances (e.g., extreme hyperthemia), or has seizures that have continued for more than 60 to 90 min.

5. Phenobarbital (additional 5–10 mg/kg)

Seizures continuing

6. Anesthesia with midazolam, propofol, or pentobarbitol

0 10 20 30 40 50 60 70 80
Time (minutes)

Second-Line Treatment. Second-line treatment should be initiated if treatment of SE fails. Following failure of benzodiazepines then loading the patient with phenytoin (Dilantin) dosed at 20 mg/kg and infused at a maximum rate of 50 mg/min is indicated. Phenytoin is a barbiturate-like drug that is effective in controlling seizure activity by limiting the repetitive firing of action potentials and slowing of the rate of recovery of voltage-activated sodium channels (McNamara, 2001). Phenytoin is highly protein bound, making only the free portion metabolically active. Phenytoin has a pH of 12, making it very caustic to peripheral veins and must be given no faster than 50 mg/min. Phenytoin should be used judiciously as it may cause hypotension, QT prolongation, and other cardiac dysrhythmias, which can be alleviated by reducing the infusion rate (McNamara). Given the limitations of phenytoin, fosphenytoin, which is water soluble, is an alternative in the setting of SE where rapid administration is desired. Fosphenytoin is measured in phenytoin equivalents (PE) and similarly loaded at 20 PE/mg at a maximum rate of 150 mg/min. The cardiovascular side effects are less with fosphenytoin and it can be infused at a much higher rate. When seizures do not respond to an initial bolus of either phenytoin or fosphenytoin, and additional 5–10mg/kg or 5–10 PE/kg may be given (Manno, 2003).

Another antiepileptic drug used as a second line agent is valproic acid (VPA), with a mechanism that is similar to phenytoin. VPA is loaded at a dose of 20 mg/kg in SE at a rate of administration of 3–6 mg·kg·min without adverse affects. The role of VPA in SE is not clearly defined; however, this has been advocated by some as an initial second line therapy after benzodiazepines because of its ease of administration and safety profile (Manno, 2003).

Phenobarbital has also been used for treatment of SE. This barbiturate prevents seizure activity by increasing $GABA_A$ mediated cellular inhibition. The use as of this medication as a second line therapy has decreased because of serious adverse effects including respiratory depression, decreased level of consciousness, hypotension, and decreased cardiac contractility. Phenobarbital has a half-life of as long as 96 hours and is now considered third line treatment for SE or deferred in favor of continuous IV administration midazolam, propofol, or pentobarbital (see Figure 5.5).

Refractory Status Epilepticus

There is no universally accepted definition of refractory status epilepticus (RSE). However, in general it is defined as SE that fails to respond to first- and second-line therapy. RSE occurs in 9% to 31% of patients with SE and is associated with a high morbidity and mortality (Claassen, Hirsch, Emerson, & Mayer, 2002). Continuous intravenous infusions with anesthetic doses of midazolam, propofol, or high-dose barbiturates for 24–48 hours are common therapies for RSE. These patients require ICU monitoring, an advanced airway, and continuous EEG monitoring. The goal of titration of these agents is either seizure suppression or burst suppression on EEG, which remains a matter of debate. There is no prospective collected data that shows one more efficacious than the other. Many believe that titration to seizure suppression is adequate to break RSE because higher doses of drug are needed to achieve electrographic burst suppression that may lead to deleterious systemic effects for the patient. These agents are administered initially for 24 hours at which time their dose is reduced and the patient is closely monitored for clinical or EEG signs of continued SE (Claassen et al., 2002).

Midazolam, a short-acting benzodiazepine, is given at a loading dose of 0.2 mg/kg and maintained at a continuous infusion of 0.1 to 2 mg·kg·hr titrated to either burst suppression or seizure suppression. Induction is rapid, effective, and well tolerated being a favorable intervention in the setting of alcohol withdrawal seizure for example, when one agent can serve two functions. The main limitation to midazolam is the fairly rapid development of tachyphylaxis that often requires persistent escalation of the dose (Manno, 2003).

Propofol, a short-acting nonbarbituate hypnotic, has been used extensively for the induction and maintenance of anesthesia and for sedation in the ICU. This global CNS depressant directly activates the GABA receptor. Propofol has the advantage of rapid induction and elimination, making it easy and practical in the treatment of RSE. A loading dose of 3–5 mg/kg is recommended, followed by an infusion of 30–100 mcg/kg/min titrated to EEG seizure suppression (Marik & Varon, 2004). Propofol does cause hypotension, which may need to be supported with vasoactive medications during the infusion. However, the most severe complication associated with propofol is the "propofol infusion syndrome," a very rare complication reported primarily in pediatric patients associated with *high-dose* propofol infusion. This syndrome is characterized by severe metabolic acidosis, rhabdomyolysis, and cardiovascular collapse frequently leading to death. Some data suggests that this disorder is caused by interference with mitochondrial respiration (Marik & Varon). The current recommended dosage should not exceed 100 mcg/kg/min and measurements of daily creatinine kinase (a marker of rhabdomyolysis) and triglycerides (a marker of failure of free fatty acid metabolism in the form of hyperlipidemia) need to be done to monitor for the syndrome.

High-dose barbiturate therapy using pentobarbital is also used for the treatment of RSE. Pentobarbital has a loading dose of 5–15 mg/kg over 1 hour and is maintained at an infusion dosage of 0.5–10 mg·kg·hour. This therapy is usually used after midazolam or propofol therapies have failed because of the profound hemodynamic and immunosuppressive effects of pentobarbital (Manno, 2003).

Prognosis

The overall mortality of SE is about 20% but varies widely on the basis of age, etiology, and duration of SE. Mortality is higher in elderly patients with some data suggesting mortality as high 76% for this population (Logroscino, Hesdorffer, & Cascino, 2002). Mortality is also higher when SE is secondary to an acute insult (i.e., acute stroke, anoxia, trauma, infections, metabolic disturbances). Most notably, the presence of myoclonic SE after acute anoxic brain injury carries a poor prognosis. SE secondary to previous strokes, alcohol or anticonvulsant withdrawal, tumors, or epilepsy has a more benign prognosis (Manno, 2003).

Myasthenia Gravis

Definition

Myasthenia gravis (MG) is the most common autoimmune disorder of the neuromuscular junction. MG is characterized by the production of antiacetylcholine receptor antibiotics, which impairs neuromuscular transmission. Treatment for MG has improved dramatically resulting in a relatively low mortality rate (Thanvi & Lo, 2004).

Diagnosis

Clinical Features. The patient with MG commonly presents with visual symptoms, including ptosis and diplopia. Patients may also present with dysphagia, difficulty chewing or speaking, and may complain of muscle fatigue and weakness (Kothari, 2004). Approximately 20% of patients who have MG will present with myasthenic crisis at some point during their disease course. Many times there is no precipitating factor for the crisis but more frequently, infection and medication changes will precipitate a crisis. Patients in myasthenic crisis may present with ptosis, muscular weakness (especially upper extremities), and respiratory distress. The patient in myasthenic crisis may require intubation and supportive care until the myasthenic crisis is resolved. The primary factor is to differentiate myasthenic crisis from cholinergic crisis, in which the patient may present with increased salivation, bradycardia, abdominal cramps, and miosis. Cholinergic crisis usually occurs after a dosage adjustment of medication (Bhardwaj et al., 2004).

Tensilon Test. One way of diagnosing MG is with the Tensilon test and can be easily performed at the bedside. The patient's blood pressure and heart rate must be closely monitored and the test should not be performed on patients in respiratory distress. A dose of 10 mg of edrophonium (Tensilon) is administered slowly through an intravenous line; atropine should be at the bedside during the test. An improvement in ptosis or muscular strength should be seen for the test to be considered positive; a patient's subjective report that strength or fatigue improves should not be considered a positive result (Kothari, 2004).

Laboratory Studies. The presence of acetylcholine receptor antibodies (AChR-Ab) aid in confirming the diagnosis of MG, but the absence of AChR-Ab does not exclude the diagnosis. The presence of antimuscle-specific kinase (MuSK) antibodies should be tested if AChR-Ab are not detectable then the diagnosis of MG is suspected (Conti-Fine, Milani, & Kaminski, 2006)

Electrophysiologic Testing. The two main electrophysiologic tests that are used in diagnosing MG are repetitive nerve stimulation and single-fiber EMG. Single-fiber EMG is the most sensitive test, although it is not specific for MG and is not widely available (Meriggioli & Sanders, 2004).

Treatment

Thymectomy. When patients are initially diagnosed with MG, they should be screened for a thymoma and if found, a thymectomy is indicated. Symptomatic improvement in MG usually occurs 6 months to 1 year after the thymectomy. When a thymectomy is performed on medically stable patients younger than 60 years old and no thymoma is found, approximately 80% of these patients experience improvement in their MG symptoms after surgery (Thanvi & Lo, 2004).

Anticholinesterase Agents, Corticosteroids, Immunosuppressants. Anticholinesterase agents provide symptomatic relief for MG, but symptoms rarely resolve completely with these agents. Corticosteroids are frequently used and are effective at reducing the levels of anti-AChR-Ab levels during the first few months. Patients are maintained on low-dose steroids for years, but they frequently encounter steroid-related complications. Other agents that are effective in treating MG include azathioprine, cyclophosphamide, cyclosporine, tacrolimus, and mycophenolate (Kothari, 2004). Many of these agents have undesirable side effects or have a delayed clinical response. In patients that do not respond to these treatments, plasma exchange or intravenous immunoglobin (IVIG) are additional options (Lehmann, Hartung, Hetzel, Stuve, & Kiesier, 2006, Part II).

Plasma Exchange and Intravenous Immunoglobulin. Plasma exchange, an extracorpeal blood purification technique that removes autoantibodies, is a therapy that is used for patients in myasthenic crisis with acute severe muscular weakness. This procedure is also used prethymectomy and postthymectomy in patients with severe MG. Plasma exchange is performed 3–5 times and 1–1.5 plasma volumes are exchanged per procedure per day (Lehmann, Hartung, Hetzel, Stuve, & Kiesier, 2006, Part I). IVIG involves administering 0.4 g/kg immunoglobulin per day from pooled human plasma for 3–5 doses. IVIG can be given in lieu of plasma exchange for MG patients in myasthenic crisis (Dalakas, 2004).

Relevant Monitoring

The most significant risk for a patient in myasthenic crisis is respiratory failure. Indicators of impeding respiratory failure include worsening negative inspiratory force and forced vital capacity. Knowing the patient's baseline values are helpful (Mehta, 2006). Ptosis time can be monitored to aid in determining if the patient's condition is improving or deteriorating. Ptosis is elicited by asking the patient to sustain an upgaze for >1 minute. Proximal muscles will weaken more quickly than distal muscles; a change in muscular strength can be determined by testing arm abduction (Roper & Brown, 2005).

Guillain-Barré Syndrome

Definition

Guillain-Barré syndrome is an eponym for a heterogeneous group of immune-mediated peripheral neuropathies. A feature common in all GBS variants is a rapidly evolving polyradiculopathy preceded by a triggering event, most often an infection. GBS generally manifests as a symmetric motor paralysis with or without sensory and autonomic disturbances (Newswanger & Warren, 2004).

Subtypes and Pathophysiology

The 4 most commons subtypes of GBS include: 1) Acute inflammatory demyelinating polyradiculopathy (AIDP), Acute motor axonal neuropathy (AMAN), Acute motor and sensory neuropathy (AMSAN) & Miller Fisher Syndrome (MFS). They differ in their pathophysiology and immunological profiles. AIDP is the most common type of GBS where the macrophages invade the myelin sheath and denude the axons mediated by both humoral and cellular immunity. Axons can be involved as a "bystander" when the inflammation is severe. Characteristic electrophysiological features reflect segmental demyelination (Seneviratne, 2000). In AMAN and AMSAN the pathological process is different: antibodies directed against ganglioside antigen may damage the axons at the node of Ranvier or at the nerve terminals, thus leaving the myelin sheath intact. Nerve conduction is impaired due to the damage induced by either a conduction block or an axonal severage and degeneration. When the ventral root is damaged a motor dysfunction in the form of AMAN is the result. AMAN is characterized by rapidly progressive weakness, often with respiratory failure but usually good recovery. When the dorsal, as well as the ventral roots are affected AMSAM results (Hughes & Cornblath, 2005). The motor and sensory dysfunction in AMSAN is characterized by marked muscle wasting and poor recovery, the disease course is typically fulminant, generally with slow and incomplete recovery. The pathology of Fisher's syndrome is not as clear. This syndrome consists of a triad of symptoms ataxia, areflexia and opthalmoplegia. Mild limb weakness, ptosis, facial palsy, and bulbar palsy may also occur. This form accounts for only about 5% of patients with GBS (Seneviratne). The primary electrophysiological finding in Fisher's syndrome is an abnormality of sensory conduction.

Diagnosis

Most patients with GBS will have an acute neuropathy reaching a peak in under 4 weeks, symmetric weakness (usually ascending), hyporeflexia or areflexia, and raised protein concentrations in CSF (Hughes & Cornblath, 2005). Other common associated symptoms include pain, dysautonomia, and cranial nerve involvement.

The acute care nurse practitioner should prioritize a thorough history and physical to accurately diagnose GBS. About two thirds of GBS patients have an infection within a 6-week period prior to the diagnosis, generally either a flu-like episode or gastroenteritis. The organisms that are most likely to be involved in the infections are Campylobacter jejuni, cytomegalovirus (CMV), Epstein–Barr virus (EBV) and Mycoplasma pneumonia (Cosi & Versino, 2006). Therefore, it is imperative to ask about any recent illnesses, how the symptoms presented and progressed. The differential diagnosis for GBS includes brainstem disorders, spinal cord, and conus lesions as well as basilar artery thrombosis, myasthenia gravis, metabolic myopathies, and transverse myelitis.

The actual diagnosis of GBS is based on clinical features (progressive motor weakness and areflexia), electrodiagnostic examination (Electromyography [EMG]) and examination of the cerebrospinal fluid (CSF). EMG findings suggestive of GBS include an absent H reflex, low amplitude or absent sensory nerve potentials, an abnormal F wave and other less frequent abnormalities (Newswanger & Warren, 2004). Characteristic CSF findings consist of elevated protein without pleocytosis (abnormal number of cells in the CSF). CSF is often normal for <48 hours following initial symptoms, but by the end of 1 week CSF protein levels are elevated. The evaluating of CSF prior to treatment with IVIG is imperative as IVIG may cause aseptic meningitis and skew the results. Other laboratory tests that can corroborate the diagnosis and may be helpful include stool culture for C. jejuni, antibodies to C. jejuni, CMV, EBV, M. pneumoniae, CBC, electrolytes and liver enzymes to rule out other causes.

Treatment

Treatment for GBS is multidisciplinary with a focus on both supportive and disease specific therapy. Supportive therapy has been the cornerstone of treatment for GBS for many years. Respiratory failure occurs in about 25% and is common in rapidly progressive GBS with upper limb involvement and/or bulbar palsy (Cosi & Versino, 2006). Intubation should be considered when the FVC falls below 15–20ml/kg. Close monitoring for dysautonomia is also essential. Dysautonomic symptoms are quite common and potentially harmful; they include cardiac arrhythmias, hyper or hypotension, ileus and urinary retention. The dysautonomia is largely responsible for the mortality associated with GBS. The goal is to provide hemodynamic support and prevent sudden cardiac death from fatal arrhythmias or wide swings in blood pressure or heart rate (Cosi & Versino, 2006). Pain is a frequent symptom associated with GBS which may be under diagnosed as patients are not often able to make their needs known. The team needs to be aware of this fact and use various communication tools and behavioral pain scoring systems to assess the patients pain level. Narcotics should be used with caution due to their risk of ileus. Medications such as gabapentin (neurontin) and carbamazepine (tegretol) have been used in conjunction with narcotics for treatment of neuropathic pain associated with GBS. These medications are targeted to treat neuropathic pain and help reduce the amount of narcotic needed for adequate control (Cosi & Versino, 2006). Prophylaxis for venous thromboembolism (VTE) should also be initiated according to the guidelines for VTE prophylxis in the critically ill patient (Geertz et al., 2004). These guidelines recommend low dose unfractionated heparin (5000 units BID) or low molecular weight heparin (<3,400 units/day) as well as graduated compression stockings and intermittent pneumatic compression devices.

Disease specific therapy in the form of plasma exchange or intravenous immunoglobulin (IVIG) is used to halt progression and promote recovery. Plasma exchange became accepted as the gold standard treatment for GBS almost 20 years ago as this process removes or dilutes the circulating immune factors implicated in the pathogenesis of GBS. The usual regimen is a total exchange of about five plasma volumes during 1–2 weeks. Complications include septicemia, hypotension, hypocalcemia and abnormal clotting (Seneviratne, 2000).

IVIG produces a modulation of the immune system through multiple mechanisms including anti-idiotypic suppression of autoantibodies. In recent years, a randomized control trial showed treatment with high dose IVIG was equally as efficacious as plasma exchange for the treatment of GBS. Another multicenter trial also showed that there was no benefit to combined treatment. As a result IVIG has become utilized in more hospitals due to its easier administration, increased comfort for the patient and less complications. American Academy of Neurology practice parameters recommend either plasma exchange or IVIG for the treatment of GBS, but questions about best regimen still remain (Hughes & Cornblath, 2005).

Prognosis

Approximately 85% of patients with GBS achieve a full and functional recovery within 6–12 months. However some patients have persistent minor weakness, areflexia and paresthesia. Approximately 7% to 15% of patients have permanent neurologic sequelae including bilateral footdrop, intrinsic hand muscle wasting, sensory ataxia, and dyesthesia. In tertiary care centers with specialists familiar with GBS the mortality rate is <5%; however, this can be as high as 20% in a community hospital setting. Several factors during the acute phase of the illness predict poor recovery. These factors include age greater than 60, severe rapidly progressive disease and low nerve conduction amplitudes which suggest axonal loss. In general, a poor long-term prognosis is directly related to the severity of the acute episode and delay in onset of specific treatment (Newswanger & Warren, 2004).

Neuro-Infections: Meningitis, Encephalitis

Differential diagnoses due to alteration in mental status must include an infectious process of the brain. The most common infections seen in the neurocritical care environment are meningitis and encephalitis.

Meningitis

Pathophysiology. Meningitis is an infectious process of the meninges of the brain, specifically the arachnoid mater, and the cerebrospinal fluid in the ventricles and subarachnoid space. Meningitis is categorized as bacterial or aseptic. The most common bacterial pathogens are *Streptococcus pneumoniae* and *Neisseria meningitidis*. Because of the introduction of childhood vaccinations, infections secondary to *Haemophilus influenzae* have markedly decreased (Goetz, 2003). Aseptic meningitis refers to any meningitis that is associated with clinical and laboratory evidence of meningeal inflammation with negative routine bacterial cultures (Roper & Brown, 2005). Infections such as mycobacterium tuberculosis, mycoplasma, and spirochetes fall into this category. Viral causes of meningitis are most commonly the enteroviruses coxsackie, echovirus, and herpes simplex virus (HSV). The immunocompromised patient, has a risk of fungal invasion with *Cryptococcus neoformans, Coccidioide immitis,* and *Histoplasma capsulatum* (Fitch, Lord, Kociszewski, & Wedel, 2008). Meningitis can develop through either colonization of the nasopharynx leading to a bloodstream infection and subsequent CNS invasion or a localized infection (urinary tract infection, endocarditis, tooth abscess) causing bacteremia that leads to invasion of the CNS. Infections of the mastoid or sinuses can cause direct entry into the CNS as can infections from neurosurgical procedures, cerebrospinal fluid (CSF) leak, and hardware (shunt, extraventricular drain) placement (van de Beek et al., 2004).

Diagnostic Criteria. Diagnosis of meningitis is made via analysis of the CSF. There is data that shows that obtaining a noncontrast head CT prior to performing the LP is only required in the following circumstances: new onset seizures, change in mental status, papilledema, or a focal neurological deficit (cranial nerve deficit, motor/sensory deficit) (Tunkel et al., 2004). However, given the minimally invasive nature and the immediacy of findings in noncontrast head CT, the risk of missing a critical pathological finding which may result in cerebral herniation outweighs the benefit of delaying CT prior to the LP. The noncontrast CT will not show any abnormal findings in a patient with meningitis. A noncontrast MRI is nondiagnostic as well. On a contrast MRI, there may be enhancement of the meninges and ventricular lining, however, as it is does not yield significant data this test is not routinely obtained (Gunderman, 2006).

At a minimum, CSF should be sent for Gram stain, bacterial, acid-fast bacilli, fungal cultures, glucose, protein, cell count, and differential (Tunkel et al., 2004). Viral testing, including HSV, although depending on the history, the CSF may also be sent for West Nile virus (WNV), varicella–zoster virus (VZV) or Cytomegalovirus (CMV) (Roper & Brown, 2005). The presence of white blood cells, high protein, and low glucose in the CSF are hallmarks of bacterial meningitis (Goetz, 2007). Table 5.23 provides the normal CSF profile as well as the findings with bacterial and viral meningitis. Additional laboratory tests should include blood cultures and a CBC with differential.

Clinical Manifestations/Symptoms. The classic triad of meningitis symptoms is altered mental status, fever, and neck stiffness. Absence of these symptoms does not preclude the diagnosis, although one of the three symptoms is usually present (Bloch, 2006; van de Beek, et al., 2004). Incidentally, the sensitivity of the Brudzinski sign (passive flexion of patient's neck causes hip flexion) and the Kernig sign (passive hip flexion followed by knee extension causes pain in back and leg) is quite low (Fitch et al., 2008) in diagnosing meningitis. Patients with *N. meningitidis* (meningococcal) meningitis may have skin manifestations of petechiae and palpable purpura as part of their presentation. Seizures occur in 30% of patients with bacterial meningitis (Bloch, 2006)

5.23 CFS Profile in Bacterial and Viral Meningitis

Parameter	Normal	Viral	Bacterial
Glucose	CSF: Serum ratio >50%	Normal	<45 mg/dL CSF: Serum ratio <40%
Protein	23–38mg/dL	50–250 mg/dL	>250 mg/dL
White Blood Cells*	0–5 cells/mm3	100–500 cells/mm^3 Lymphocytes Predominate	>1000 mg/dL PMNs** Predominate
Opening Pressure	<20 cm H$_2$O	<20 cm H$_2$O	20–50 cm H$_2$O

*For a traumatic tap, subtract 1 white blood cell for every 700 red blood cells (Goetz, 2003)
** PMNs: polymorphonuclear leukocytes

Treatment. Rapid recognition of meningitis is key to survival in meningitis. Rapid intervention minimizes the disease progression and increases, the chance of a full recovery (van de Beek et al., 2004). Common practice is to empirically initiate broad spectrum antimicrobials after the LP and then narrow coverage once culture and sensitivities are available. For adults younger than 50 years old, the recommendation is vancomycin plus a third-generation cephalosporin and for patients older than 50 years of age, ampicillin is added to the regimen of vancomycin and cephalosporin (Tunkel et al., 2004). The addition of dexamethasone (0.15 mg/kg q 6 hrs for 2–4 days) prior to or during the first antibiotic dose has been shown to decrease morbidity and mortality in patients with pneumococcal meningitis. Therefore, dexamethasone is recommended as an adjunctive treatment for suspected or proven meningitis (de Gans & van de Beek). Once the Gram stain and culture results are back, the dexamethasone should be continued only in patients with Gram-positive diplococci or *S. pneumoniae* in CSF or blood. The patient who has already received the first dose of antibiotic should not have the dexamethasone initiated (de Gans & van de Beek, 2002). Once the CSF cultures are negative generally after 24–48 hours, and the patient's clinical condition is improving, the most likely cause considered is viral and antibiotics should be discontinued without the need to repeat the LP (Ziai & Lewin, 2006). The patient whose symptoms are worsening and the diagnosis is unclear warrants a repeat LP.

Prognosis and Outcomes. The mortality rate with bacterial meningitis ranges from 13% to 27% depending on the pathogen (van de Beek et al., 2004). Viral meningitis is a self-limiting course that usually resolves within 2 weeks and is associated with low morbidity and mortality (Aminoff, Greenberg, & Simon, 2005).

Encephalitis

Pathophysiology. Encephalitis is primarily caused by a viral infection, with HSV-1 being the most common pathogen. There are many more possible viral pathogens and obtaining a detailed history will offer clues to other viral etiologies (Goetz, 2007). Because there are more viruses than there are diagnostic tests viruses, often the specific pathogen is never identified (Kupila, Vuorien,Vainionpaa, Hukkanen, Marttila, & Kotilainen, 2006). The routes of transmission are virus specific. Herpes simplex encephalitis (HSE) is thought to be caused by the reactivation of the HSV lying dormant in the trigeminal ganglia. Mosquitoes or ticks are responsible for the transmission of the arbovirus and the rabies virus is transferred via animal bite. The immunocompromised patient is at risk for VZV and CMV encephalitis (Roper & Brown, 2005). The virus replicates outside the CNS and then gains entry into the CNS either via the olfactory nerve pathways or neural pathways.

Diagnostic Criteria. Encephalitis is diagnosed via examination of the CSF as well as imaging. CSF characteristics are the same as viral meningitis (Table 5.23). As noted before, often a virus is not isolated given the many viruses that have no diagnostic test. HSV, the most common form of encephalitis, has very distinguishing characteristics on CT and MRI. CT will be normal until 3–5 days after onset and in 50% of cases, hypodensity of involved cortex will develop. MRI is the imaging of choice with any form of encephalitis and with HSV there will be signal changes with surrounding edema and possible scattered hemorrhage in inferior parts of the frontal and temporal lobes (Roper & Brown, 2005). EEG is indicated to rule out seizures.

Clinical Manifestations/Symptoms. The main difference in clinical presentation between meningitis and encephalitis is related to consciousness. Patients with encephalitis will present with a change in level of consciousness ranging from sleepiness to unresponsiveness as well as a focal neurologic deficit such as sensory, motor, or speech dysfunction (Peters, 2008). Seizures are common with both encephalitis and meningitis.

Treatment. Although there are many viruses that can cause encephalitis, the only current available antiviral treatment is for HSV-1 encephalitis. Therefore, if viral etiology is suspected, empiric treatment for HSV-1 infection with acyclovir (10 mg/kg IV Q8h) should be initiated as soon as possible because early therapy is associated with a significant decrease in mortality and morbidity. Acyclovir is also an option if VZV encephalitis is likely (Whitley, 1990). However, if the HSV or VZV results are negative, the acyclovir should be discontinued. As previously described, seizures are possible with encephalitis and control of seizures is necessary with anticonvulsant therapy. The anticonvulsants should be continued for at least a year and then discontinued as long as there is no clinical or EEG evidence of continued seizures (Roper & Brown, 2005). When a large volume of brain tissue is affected by the encephalitis, there may be cerebral edema and increased ICP. Treatment should include the measures describe in the ICP management section of this chapter. Cardiovascular support may be required due to the presence of dysautonomia (Kleiter, Steinbrecher, Bogdahn, & Schulte-Mattler, 2006). Depending on the degree of decreased level of consciousness, airway protection initially with endotracheal intubation and eventually a tracheostomy may be necessary as well as ventilatory support (Aminoff et al., 2005). Pulmonary toileting that includes suctioning and chest physiotherapy may be required for patients with increased secretions and or atelectasis. Venous thromboembolism (VTE) is a significant concern for this population since most patients will initially be immobile and the guidelines for VTE prophylaxis in the patient with critical illness (Geertz et al., 2004)

Prognosis and Outcomes. Death occurs in 5% to 20% of these patients and residual signs such as mental deterioration, amnesic defects, personality change, recurrent seizures, and hemiparesis are seen in about another 20% (Roper & Brown, 2005).

Brain Death

Definition

Brain death is the irreversible cessation of all functions of the entire brain including the brainstem. There are strict, well-defined criteria that must be present for the diagnosis of brain death to be made. These include irreversible coma, absence of cortical activity, absence of motor response to pain, loss of brainstem reflexes, and apnea (Hickey, 2002). In 1968, an ad hoc committee at Harvard Medical School developed the criteria that are currently used to determine brain death. In 1980, the Uniform Determination of Death Act (UDDA) was passed and adapted into legislation in each state. Specific policies on brain death testing may differ from institution to institution. However, the UDDA defines that "for legal and medical purposes, an individual who has sustained irreversible cessation of all functioning of the brain, including the brain stem, is dead." (http://www.nccusl.org/nccusl/uniformact_factsheets/ uniformacts-fs-udda.asp, assessed April 12, 2008)

Brain Death Criteria

The diagnosis of brain death is a clinical diagnosis that consists of three cardinal findings: coma, absence of brainstem reflexes, and apnea. Two clinical evaluations are performed 6 hours apart. Patients who meet brain death criteria should have no motor response to painful stimuli. The patient may have reflexic responses, such as triple-flexion, and spontaneous movement of the limbs should not be misinterpreted for motor responses (Young, Shemie, Doig & Teitelbaum, 2006). Central pain should be given by performing a trapezius squeeze or sternal rub, or by applying supraorbital pressure; if no motor response is elicited, then cranial nerve function should be assessed. Pupillary response is examined by darkening the room and checking for pupillary reaction with a bright light. The oculocephalic reflex, more commonly known as doll's eyes, assesses cranial nerves III and VI. The patient's eyes are held open and the head is turned side to side while a change in position of eyes is noted, if there is no change in position, then the reflex is absent. This test should not be performed when a cervical spine injury is suspected. The vestibuloocular reflex, known as cold calorics, assesses cranial nerves III, VI, and VIII. This test is completed by instilling 50 ml of cold water in each ear while the eyes are held open to determine any deviation to one side or the other. Tympanic membranes must intact for this test to be performed. Eye deviation is assessed for one full minute after the instillation of the cold water; if no movement is seen then the reflex is absent. Corneal reflexes, cranial nerves V and VII, are assessed by drawing a wisp of cotton across the eye. The facial grimace, which also assesses cranial nerves V and VII, is tested for by applying supraorbital pressure or deep pressure to the nail bed and evaluating for a grimace. Cough and gag reflexes, cranial nerves IX and X, are tested by bronchial suctioning with a suction catheter and stimulating the posterior pharynx with a tongue blade. When all cranial nerve reflexes are absent then an apnea test is performed to establish the clinical diagnosis of brain death (Hickey, 2002). During the apnea test, the patient is removed from the ventilator to assess respiratory drive. The patient is preoxygenated with 100% oxygen and a baseline arterial blood gas (ABG) is drawn. After removing the patient from the ventilator, oxygen is supplied by inserting a tube into the endotracheal tube that will deliver oxygen at the level of the carina. The endpoint of the apnea test is an arterial blood gas with a carbon dioxide (CO_2) level of 60 mmHg or a delta of 20 points from the patient's baseline CO_2 level. The patient who is not sedated or receiving analgesics and does not initiate a spontaneous breath indicates there is no hypoxic respiratory drive; the examination is consistent with brain death. This may take as long as 15 minutes to have the CO_2 level rise, during this time the patient may become hemodynamically unstable or desaturated, indicating a need to send the ABG and terminate the apnea test. The CO_2 level at this point may not be high enough to complete the apnea test, then it may be necessary to perform ancillary testing to confirm the diagnosis of brain death (Bhardwaj et al., 2004).

Ancillary Tests. Ancillary tests that measure brain perfusion are the only accepted tests for confirmation of the clinical diagnosis of brain death. A confirmatory test is not mandatory but may be helpful in patients in whom parts of the clinical examination cannot be reliably performed. The gold standard is the four-vessel cerebral angiogram. This is an invasive procedure that requires continuous monitoring of the patient's vital signs, as the patient may be hemodynamically unstable because of loss of the autoregulatory system. Presence of blood flow is determined by injecting contrast material and looking for intracerebral filling at the level of the carotid bifurcation or circle of Willis for at least 1 minute after injection (Young, Shemie, Doing, & Teitelbaum, 2006). Other confirmatory tests that are recognized by the American Academy of Neurology are EEG, TCDs, technetium-99m hexamethylpropleneamineoxime brain scan, and somatosensory evoked potentials ("Practice parameters," 1995).

Summary

Brain death is a clinical diagnosis that is made by a physician, acute care nurse practitioners can participate in the care of the patient but are not able to make the diagnosis of brain death. The number of physicians required to perform the brain death examination and the timing of the two brain death examinations differ from state to state (Wijdicks, 2007).

The American Academy of Neurology suggests that 6 hours be allowed to elapse between the two examinations. Documentation of the etiology and irreversibility of the patient's condition including imaging consistent with an acute central nervous system catastrophe, absence of brainstem reflexes, absence of motor response to pain, and absence of respiratory effort with an arterial CO_2 level of >60 mmHg is required to pronounce the patient brain dead (American Academy of Neurology, 1995). Throughout the process of diagnosis of brain death, the family should be included in the process and the issue of organ donation introduced. Following pronouncement of death, there should be a timely discussion regarding the opportunity to participate in organ donation. The exact procedure for organ donation differs from state to state (Bhardwaj et al., 2004).

References

Adams, H., del Zoppo, G., & von Kummer, R. (2006). *Management of stroke: A practical guide for the prevention, evaluation and treatment of acute stroke* (3rd ed.). USA: Professional Communications Incorporated.

Adams, H., del Zoppo, G., Alberts, M., Bhatt, D., Brass, L., Furlan, A. Grubb, R., Higashida, R., Jauch, E., Kidwell, C., Lyden, P., Morgenstren, L., Qureshi, A., Rosenwasser, R., Scott, P., & Wijdicks, E. (2007). Guidelines for the early management of adults with ischemic stroke. *Stroke, 38,* 1655–1711.

Aggarwal, M., & Khan, I. (2006). Hypertensive crisis: Hypertensive emergencies and urgencies. *Cardiology Clinics, 24,* 135–146.

Allen, M., Kopp, B. and Ersted, B. (2004). Stress ulcer prophylaxis in the postoperative period. *American Journal of Health Systems Pharmacy, 61,* 588–596.

Al-Shahi, R., White, P., Davenport, R., & Lindsay, K. (2006). Subarachnoid haemorrhage. *British Medical Journal, 333,* 235–240.

American Heart Association (2005). 2005 American Heart Association guidelines for cardiopulmonary resuscitation and emergency cardiovascular care [Supplement]. *Circulation, 112 (24).*

American Heart Association Statistics Committee and Stroke Statistics Subcommittee (2006). Heart disease and stroke statistics—2006. *Circulation, 113,* 1–67

American Spinal Cord Injury Association (2006). Standard neurological classification of spinal cord injury. Retrieved January 3, 2008 from http://www.asia-spinalinjury.org/publications/2006_Classif_worksheet.pdf

Aminoff, M., Greenberg, D., & Simon, R. (2005). *Clinical neurology* (6th ed.). Columbus: McGraw-Hill.

Arbour, R. (2004). Intracranial hypertension: Monitoring and nursing assessment. *Critical CareNurse, 24 (5),* 19–34.

Aronen, H. J., Laakso, M., Moser., M., & Perkiö, J. (2007). Diffusion and perfusion-weighted magnetic resonance imaging techniques in stroke recovery. *European Journal of Physical and Rehabilitation Medicine, 43*(2), 271–284.

Bandera, E., Botteri, M, Minelli, C., Sutton, A., Abrams, K., & Latroncio, N. (2006). Cerebral blood flow threshold of ischemic penumbra and infaract core in acute ischemic stroke. *Stroke, 37,* 1334–1339.

Barker, F. G.(2007). Efficacy of prophylactic antibiotics against meningitis after craniotomy: A meta-analysis. *Neurosurgery, 60*(5), 887–894.

Beers, M., Porter, R., Jones, T., Kaplan, J., & Berkwits, M. (Eds.). (2006). *The merck manual of diagnosis and therapy* (18th ed.). Whitehouse Station: Merck Research Laboratories.

Bennet, M. & Haynes, D. (2007). Surgical approaches in the removal of vestibular schwannomas. *Otolaryngologic Clinics of North America, 40,* 589–609.

Bhardwaj, A., Mirski, M., & Ulatowski, J. (2004). *The handbook of neuro-critical care.* Totowa: Humana Press.

Bloch, K. (2006). Infectious diseases. In S. McPhee & W. Ganong (Eds.), *Pathophysiology of disease: an introduction to clinical medicine* (5th ed.). Columbus: McGraw-Hill.

Boakye, M., Patil, C. G., Santarelli, J., Ho, C., Tian, W., & Lad, S. P. (2007). Cervical spondylotic myelopathy: Complications and outcomes after spinal fusion. *Neurosurgery, 62 (2),* 455–462.

Branco F, Cardenas D. D., & Svircev J. N. (2007). Spinal cord injury: a comprehensive review. *Physical Medicine Rehabilitation Clinics of North America 18*(4),651–79.

Brantigan, J. W., Steffee, A., Lewis, M., Quinn, L., & Persenaire J. M. (2000). Lumbar interbody fusion using the Bratigan I/F cage for posterior lumbar interbody fusion and the variable pedicle screw placement system: two-year results from a Food and Drug Administration investigational device exemption clinical trial. *Spine, 25,* 1437–1446.

Bratton, S., Chestnut R., Ghajar, J., Hammond, M., Harris, O., Hartl, R., et al. (2007) . The guidelines for the management of severe traumatic brain injury. *Journal of Neurotrauma 24,* S-1.

Bratzler, D., & Houck, P. M. (2005). Antimicrobial prophylaxis for surgery: An advisory statement from the National Surgical Infection Prevention Project. *The American Journal of Surgery, 189,* 395–404.

Brell, M., Ibáñez, J., Caral, L., & Ferrer, E. (2000). Factors influencing surgical complications of intra-axial brain tumors. *Acta Neurochirurga, 142,* 739–750.

Brkaric, M., Baker, K., Israel, R., Harding, T., Montgomery, D. M., & Herkowitz, H. (2007). Early failure of bioabsorbable anterior cervical fusion plates: Case report and failure. *Journal of Spinal Disorders and Technique, 20*(3), 248–254.

Broderick, J., Connolly, S., Feldmann, E., Hanley, D., Kase, C., Krieger, D., Mayberg, M., Morgenstern, L., Ogilvy, C., Vespa, P., & Zuccarello, M. (2007). Guidelines for the management of spontaneous intracerebral hemorrhage in adults: 2007 update: a guideline from the American Heart Association/American Stroke Association Stroke Council, High Blood Pressure Research Council, and the Quality of Care and Outcomes in Research Interdisciplinary Working Group. *Stroke, 38,* 2001–2023.

Brown, G., & Carley, S. (2004). Does nimodipine reduce mortality and secondary ischaemic events after subarachnoid haemorrhage? *Journal of Emergency Medicine, 21,* 333.

Browne, T. R., & Holmes, G. L. (2001). Epilepsy. *The New England Journal of Medicine, 344*(15), 1145–1151.

Bullock, M. R., Chestnut, R. M., Ghajar, J., Gordon, D., Hartl, R., Newell, D. W., Servadei, F., Walters, B. C., Wilberger, J. E. (2006). Guidelines for the surgical management of traumatic brain injury, *Journal of Neurosurgery, 58 (3),* Supplement, S2-1–S2-111.

Caselli, R. (2003). Current issues in the diagnosis and management of dementia. *Seminars in Neurology, 23,* 231–235.

Castillo, M. (2006). Neuroradiology *Companion: Methods, guidelines, and imaging fundamentals.* Philadelphia: Lipincott, Williams and Wilkins.

Chestnut, R. M., Ghajar, J., Maas, A. I. R., Marion, D. W., Servadei, F., Teasdale, G. M., Unterberg, A., von Holst, H., Walters, B. C. (2007). Early indicators of prognosis in severe traumatic brain injury, *Journal of Neurotrauma, 24,* supplement, S157–S207.

Claassen, J., Hirsch, L. J., Emerson, R. G., & Mayer, S. A. (2002). Treatment of refractory status epilepticus with pentobarbital, propofol, or midazolam: a systematic review. *Epilepsia, 43*(2), 146–153.

Commission on Classification and Terminology of the International League Against Epilepsy (1982). Proposal for a revised clinical and electroencephalographic classification of epileptic seizures. *Epilepsia, 22,* 489–501.

Conti-Fine, B., Milani, M., & Kamanski, H. (2006). Myasthenia gravis: past, present, and future. *The Journal of Clinical Investigation, 116,* 2843–2854.

Cosi, V., & Versino, M. (2006).Guillain-Barré syndrome. *Neurological Sciences, 27,* S47–S51.

Dalakas, M. (2004). Intravenous immunoglobin in autoimmune neuromuscular diseases. *Journal of American Medical Association, 291*(19), 2367–2375.

Davis, A. E., & Briones, T. E.(1998). Intracranial Disorders. In M. R. Kinney, S. B. Dunbar, J. Brooks-Dun, N. Molter, J. M. Vitello-Ciccu (Eds.), *AACN clinical reference for critical care nursing* (4th ed.) (pp. 685–709). St. Louis: Mosby.

de Gans, J., & van de Beek, D. (2002). Dexamethasone in adults with bacterial meningitis. *New England Journal of Medicine, 347,* 1549–1556.

Dehdashti, A., Rilliet, B., Rufenacht, D., & de Tribolet, N. (2004). Shunt-dependent hydrocephalus after rupture of intracranial aneurysms: a prospective study of the influence of treatment modality. *Journal of Neurosurgery, 101,* 402.

Devereaux M. W. (2007). Anatomy and examination of the spine. *Neurologic Clinics, 25(2),* 331–51.

Ditunno, J., Little, J., Tessler, A. & Burns A. S. (2004). Spinal shock revisited: a four-phase model. *Spinal Cord, 42,* 383–395.

Dodson, W. E., DeLorenzo, R. J., Pedley, T. A., et al. (1993).The Treatment of Convulsive status epilepticus: Recommendations of Epilepsy Foundation of America's Working Group of Status Epilepticus. *The Journal of the American Medical Association, 270,* 854–859.

Drappatz, J., Schiff, D., Kesari, S., Norden, A., & Wen, P. (2007). Medical management of brain tumor patients. *Neurology Clinics, 25,* 1035–1071.

Feigin, V., & Findlay, M. (2006). Advances in subarachnoid hemorrhage. *Stroke, 37,* 305–308.

Feigin, V., Rinkel, G., Lawes, C., Algra, A., Bennett, D., van Gijn, J., & Anderson, C. (2005). Risk factors for subarachnoid hemorrhage an updated systematic review of epidemiological studies. *Stroke, 36,* 2773–2780.

Fitch, M., Abrahamian F. M., Moran G. J.,& Talan D. A. (2008). Emergency department management of meningitis and encephalitis. *Infectious Disease Clinics of North America, 22*(1), 33–52.

Frakes, M. A., Lord, W., Kociszewski, C., & Wedel, S. (2006). Efficacy of fentanyl analgesia for trauma in critical care transport. *The American Journal of Emergency Medicine, 24,* 286–289.

Geertz, W., Pineo, G., Heit, J., Bergqvist, D., Lassen, M., Colwell, C., & Ray, J. (2004). Prevention of venous thromboembolism: the Seventh ACCP conference on Antithrombotic and Thrombolytic therapy. *Chest, 126,* 338s–400s.

Gelb, D. (2000). *Introduction to clinical neurology.* Woodburn: Butterworth Heinemann.

Glantz, M. J., Cole, B. F., Forsyth, P. A., Recht, L., Wen, P. Y., Chamberlain, M. C., et al. (2000). Practice parameter: Anticonvulsant prophylaxis in patients with newly diagnosed brain tumors. *Neurology, (54),* 1886–1893.

Goetz, C. (2007). *Textbook of clinical neurology* (3rd ed.). Philadelphia: Saunders.

Goldberg, S. (2007). *Clinical neuroanatomy made ridiculously simple* (3rd ed.). Miami: Medmaster.

Gomes, J., Stevens, R., Lewin, J., Mirski, M., & Bhardwaj, A. (2005). Glucocorticoid therapy in neurocritical care. *Critical Care Medicine, 33,* 1214–1224.

Graham, D. I. & Gennareli, T. A. (2000). Pathology of brain damage after head injury. In P. Cooper, & G. Golfinols (Eds.), *Head Injury* (4th ed.). New York: Morgan.

Grainger, M. B., Allison, D. J. & Dixon, A. (2008). *Grainger & Allison's diagnostic radiology: a textbook of medical imaging* (5th ed.). Philadelphia: Elsevier.

Gunderman, R. (2006). *Essential radiology: clinical presentation, pathophysiology, imaging* (2nd ed.) New York: Thieme.

Hadley, M., Walters B. C., Grabb P. A., Oyesiku N. M., Przybylski G. J., Resnick D. K., et al. (2002). Guidelines for the management of acute cervical spine and spinal cord injuries. *Clinical Neurosurgery, 49,* 407–498.

Hall J. B., Schmidt, G, & Wood, L. (2005). *Principles of critical care* (3rd ed.). New York: McGraw-Hill Companies

Harris, J. H. (2000). Skull & Contents. Retrieved March 25, 2008 from http://www.uth.tmc.edu/radiology/test/er_primer/skull_brain/skull.html

Hassan, E. (2007). Hyperglycemia management in the hospital setting. *American Journal of Health Systems Pharmacy, 64,* s9–s14.

Heegaard, W., & Biros, M. (2007). Traumatic brain injury. *Emergency Medical Clinics of North America, 25,* 655–678.

Hickey, J. (2002). *The clinical practice of neurological and neurosurgical nursing* (5th ed.). Philadelphia: Lipincott, Williams and Wilkins.

Hill, M., Demchuk, A., Tomsick, T., Palesch, Y., & Broderick, J. (2006). Using the baseline CT scan to select acute stroke patients for IV-IA therapy. *American Journal of Neuroradiology, 27,* 1612–1616.

Holmes, G. L. (1997). Classification of Seizures and epilepsies. In S. C, Schachter., & D. L., Schomer (Eds.). *The Comprehensive evaluation and treatment of epilepsy.* San Diego, CA: Academic Press, (pp 1–36). [Electronic version] Retrieved February 1, 2008, from http://professionals.epilepsy.com/page/seizclass_factors.html

Huff, S. (2004). Altered mental status and coma. In J. Tintinalli, G. Kelen, S. Stapczynski, O. Ma & D. Cline (Eds.), *Tintinalli's emergency medicine: a comprehensive study guide* (6th ed.). Columbus: McGraw-Hill.

Hughes, R. A., & Cornblath, D. R. (2005). Guillain-Barré syndrome. *The Lancet, 366,* 1653–1654.

Hutchinson, P., Timofeev, I., & Kirkpatrick, P. (2007). Surgery for brain edema. *Neurosurgical Focus, 22,* 1–9.

Jackson, A. (2000). Overview of spinal cord injury, anatomy and physiology. Retrieved March 25, 2008, from http://www.spinalcord.uab.edu/show.asp?durki=32105.

Jensen, M., and St. Louis, E. (2005). Management of acute cerebellar stroke. *Archives of Neurology, 62,* 537–544.

Kassab, M., Majid, A., Farooq, M., Azhary, H., Hershey, L., Bednarczyk, E., et al. (2007). Transcranial Doppler: an introduction for primary care physicians. *Journal of American Board of Family Medicine, 20,* 65–71.

Kleiter, I., Steinbrecher A., Bogdahn U., & Schulte-Mattler, W. (2006). Autonomic involvement in tick-borne encephalitis (TBE): report of five cases. *European Journal of Medical Research,* 11 (6), 261–2655.

Koehler, P. J. (1995). Use of corticosteroids in neuro-oncology. *Anti-Cancer Drugs,* 6, 19–33.

Kothari, M. (2004). Myasthenia gravis. *Journal of the American Osteopathic Association, 104 (9),* 377–384.

Krumholz, A., Wiebe, S., Gronseth, G., Shinnar, S., Levisohn, P., Ting, T., et al. (2007). Practice parameter: Evaluating an apparent unprovoked first seizure in adults (an evidenced based review). *Neurology, 69,* 1996–2007.

Kupila, L., Vuorien, T., Vainionpaa, R., Hukkanen, V., Marttila, R., & Kotilainen, P. (2006). Etiology of aseptic meningitis and encephalitis in an adult population. *Neurology, 66*(1), 75–80.

Lehmann, H., Hartung, P., Hetzel, G., Stuve, O., & Kieseir, B. (2006). Plasma exchange in neuroimmunological disorders. Part I: Rationale and treatment of inflammatory central nervous system disorders. *Archives of Neurology, 63,* 930–935.

Lehmann, H., Hartung, P., Hetzel, G., Stuve, O., & Kieseir, B. (2006). Plasma exchange in neuroimmunological disorders. Part II: Treatment of neuromuscular disorders. *Archives of Neurology, 63,* 1066–1071.

Lerner, A. J. (1995). *The little black book of neurology* (3rd ed.). St. Louis: Mosby.

Liebenberg, W., Worth, R., Firth, G., Olney, J., & Norris, J. (2005). Aneurysmal subarachnoid haemorrhage: guidance in making the correct diagnosis. *Postgraduate Medical Journal, 81,* 470–473.

Logroscino, G., Hesdorffer, D. C., Cascino, G. D., et al. (2002). Long-term mortality after a first episode of status epilepticus. *Neurology, 58,* 537–541.

Loh J., & Verbalis J. (2008). Disorders of water and salt metabolism associated with pituitary disease; *Endocrinology and Metabolism Clinics, 37 (1),* 213–234.

Lowenstein, D. H. & Alldredge, B. K. (1998). Status Epilepticus. *The New England Journal of Medicine, 338, 14,* 970–976.

Lowenstein, D. H. (2006). The management of refractory status epilepticus: an update. *Epilepsia, 47 (S1),* 35–40.

Lowenstein, D. H., Bleck, T., Macdonald, R. L. (1999). It's time to revise the definition of status epilepticus. *Epilepsia, 40,1,* 120–122.

Lower, J. (2002). Facing neuro assessment fearlessly. *Nursing, 32, (2):* 58–65.

Manno, E. M. (2003). New management strategies in the treatment of status epilepticus. *Mayo Clinical Proceedings, 78,* 508–518.

Marik, P. E., & Varon, J. (2007). Hypertensive crises challenges and management. *Chest, 131,* 1949–1962.

Marik, P. E., & Varon, M. D. (2004). The management of status epilepticus. *Chest, 126* (2), 582–591.

Marmarou, A. (2007). A review of progress in understanding the pathophysiology and treatment of brain edema. *Neurosurgical Focus, 22,* 1–10.

Mayer, S. A., Coplin, W. M., & Raps, E. C. (1999) Cerebral edema, intracranial pressure, and herniation syndromes. *Journal of Stroke and Cerebrovascular Disease, 8*(3), 183–191.

McAvay, G., Van Ness, P., Bogardus, S., Zhang, Y, Leslie, D., Leo-Summers, L. et al. (2006). Older adults discharged from the hospital with delirium: 1 year outcomes. *The Journal of the America Geriatric Society, 54*(8), 1245–1250.

McNamara, J. O. (2001). Drugs effective in the therapy of the epilepsies. In J. G. Hardman, L. E. Limbird, A. G. Gilman. (Eds.), *Goodman & Gilman's The Pharmacologic Basis of Therapeutics* (10th ed.) (pp. 521–547). New York, McGraw-Hill.

McQuillan, K., Truter Von Ruden, K., Hartsock, R., Flynn, M, & Whalen, E. (2002). *Trauma nursing: from resuscitation through rehabilitation.* Philadelphia: Saunders.

Mehta, S. (2006). Neuromuscular disease causing acute respiratory failure. *Respiratory Care, 51*(9), 1016–1023.

Meriggioli, M., & Sanders, D. (2004). Myasthenia gravis: diagnosis. *Seminars in Neurology, 24,* 31.

Morgan, G., Mikhail, & Murray, M. (2006). *Clinical anesthesiology* (4th ed.). New York: McGraw-Hill.

Nair, D. (2003). *The Cleveland Clinic Disease Management Project: Epilepsy.* Retrieved February 1, 2008, from http: //www.clevelandclinicmeded .com/medicalpubs/diseasemanagment/neurology/epilepsy

Nandhagopal, R. (2006). Generalised convulsive status epilepticus: an overview. *Postgraduate Medicine Journal, 82,*723–732.

National Spinal Cord Injury Statistical Center (2006). Retrieved March 15, 2008, from http://www.spinalcord.uab.edu/show.asp

Naval, N., Stevens, R., Mirski, M., & Bhardwaj, A. (2006). Controversies in the management of subarachnoid hemorrhage. *Critical Care Medicine, 34*(2), 511–524.

Newswanger, D. L., & Warren, C. R. (2004). Guillain-Barré syndrome. *American Family Physician, 69*(10), 2405–2410.

New Zealand's Guideline's Group (2006). *Traumatic brain injury: Diagnosis, acute management and rehabilitation.* Retrieved April 13, 2008 from National Guideline Clearinghouse http://www.guideline.gov/ summary/summary.aspx?doc_id=10281&nbr=005397&string=New+ AND+Zealand+AND=group

Nitahara, J., Valencia, M., & Bronstein, M. A. (1998). Medical case management after laminectomy or craniotomy: Do all patients benefit from admission to the intensive care unit? *Neurosurgical Focus, 5*(2), e4.

Noe, K. H., & Manno, E. M. (2005). Mechanisms underlying status epilepticus. *Drugs Today, 41,* 257–266.

Ohira, T., Shahar, E., Chambless, L., Rosamond, W., Mosley, T., & Folsom, A. (2006). Risk factors for ischemic stroke subtypes. *Stroke, 37,* 2493–2498.

Ornstein, E., & Berko, R. (2006). Anesthesia techniques in complex spine surgery. *Neurosurgical Clinics of North America, 17,* 191–203.

Ortiz-Cardona, J., & Bendo, A. (2007). Perioperative pain management in the neurosurgical patient. *Anesthesiology Clinics, 25 (3),* 655–674.

Peters, C. (2008). Infections caused by arthropod and rodent borne viruses. In A. Fauci, E. Braunwald, D. Kaspar, S. Hauser, D. Longo, L. Jameson, & J Loscaizo (Eds.), *Harrison's principles of internal medicine* (17th ed.). Columbus: McGraw-Hill.

Petrozza, P. H. (2002). Major spine surgery. *Anesthesiology Clinics of North America, 20,* 405–415.

Praline, J., Grujic, J., Corcia, P., Lucas, B., Hommet, C., Autret, A., & Toffol, B. (2007). Emergent EEG in clinical practice. *Clinical Neurophysiology, 118,* 2149–2155.

Quality Standards Subcommittee of the American Academy of Neurology, (1995). Practice parameters for determining brain death in adults: Summary statement. *Neurology, 45,* 1012–1014.

Quereshi, A. L., & Suarez, J. I. (2000). Use of hypertonic saline in brain injury. *Critical Care Medicine, 28,* 3301–3313.

Rangel-Castillo, L., & Robertson, C. S. (2007). Management of intracranial hypertension. *Critical Care Clinics, 22,* 713–732.

Raslan, A., & Bhardwaj, A. (2007). Medical management of cerebral edema. *Neurosurgical Focus, 22*(5) 1–12.

Roper, A., & Brown, R. (2005). *Adams and Victor's principles of neurology* (8th ed.). Columbus: McGraw-Hill.

Rosen, D., & MacDonald, R. (2005). Subarachnoid hemorrhage grading scales: a systematic review. *Neurocritical Care, 2,* 110.

Segun, T. D. (2007). *Traumatic brain injury: Definition, epidemiology, pathophysiology*. Retrieved March 27, 2008 from http://www.emedicine.com/pmr/topic212.htm

Seidel, H., Ball, J., Dains, J. and Benedict, G. (2006). *Mosby's physical examination handbook*. St. Louis: Mosby.

Sekhon, L., & Fehlings, M. (2001). Epidemiology, demographics and pathophysiology of acute spinal cord injury. *Spine, 26,* S2– S12. *Spinal Cord 42,* 383–395.

Seneviratne, U. (2000). Guillain-Barré syndrome. *Postgraduate Medicine Journal, 76,* 774–782.

Springborg, J., Frederickson, H., Eskessen, V., & Olsen, N. (2004). Trends in monitoring patients with aneurysmal subarachnoid haemorrhage. *British Journal of Anaesthesia, 94 (3),* 259–270.

Stevens, R. D., Bhardwaj, A., Kirsch, J. R., & Mirski, M. A. (2003). Critical care and perioperative management in traumatic spinal cord injury. *Journal of Neurosurgical Anesthesiology,15(3),* 215–229.

Stone, K., & Humphries, R. (2008). Current Diagnosis & Treatment: Emergency Medicine (6th ed.). East Norwalk: McGraw-Hill.

Thanvi, B., & Lo, T. (2004). Update on myasthenia gravis. *Postgraduate Medical Journal, 80,* 690–700.

Tintanelli, J., Kelen,G., Stapczynski, S., Ma, O., and Cline, D. (Eds.) (2004), *Tintanelli's emergency medicine: a comprehensive study guide* (6th ed.). Columbus: McGraw- Hill.

Towne, A. R., Waterhouse, E. J., Boggs, J. G., Garnett L. K., Brown A. J., Smith J. R. Jr., et al. (2000). Prevalence of non-convulsive status epilepticus in comatose patients. *Neurology, 54,* 340–345.

Toyama, Y., Kobayashi, T., Nishiyama, R. Satoh, K., Ohkawa, M., & Seki, K. (2005). CT for acute stage of closed head injury. *Radiation Medicine, 23 (5),* 309–316.

Tunkel, A., Hartman, B., Kaplan, S., Kaufman, B., Roos, K., & Scheld, W. (2004). Practice guidelines for the management of bacterial meningitis. *Clinical Infectious Diseases, 39,* 1267–1284.

Ullrich, P. (2007). Pain following spinal cord injury. *Physical Medicine and Rehabilitation Clinics of North America, 18*(2), 217–233.

Uniform Law Commissioners in cooperation with the American Medical Association, the American Bar Association and the President's Commission on Medical Ethics. (1980). Retrieved April 12, 2008, from http:/www.nccusl.org/nccusl/uniformact_factsheets/uniformacts-fs-udda.asp.

Unterberg, A. W., Stover, J., Kress, B., & Kiening, K. L. (2004). Edema and brain trauma. *Neuroscience, 129,* 1021–1029.

van de Beek, D., de Gans, J., Spanjaard, L., Weisfelt, M., Reitsma, J., & Vermeulen, M. (2004). Clinica features and prognostic factors in adults with bacterial meningitis. *The New England Journal of Medicine, 351*(18) 1849–1859.

Van de Berghe, Wouters, P., Weekers, F., Verwaest, C., Bruyninckk, F., Schetz, M., et al. (2001). Intensive insulin therapy in critically ill patients. *The New England Journal of Medicine, 345* (19), 1359–1367.

Varelas, P. N., & Mirski, M. A. (2001). Seizures in the adult intensive care unit. *Journal of Neurosurgical Anesthesiology,13(2),* 163–175.

Vinas, F. C. & Pilitsis, J. (2006). *Penetrating head trauma.* Retrieved April 13, 2008 from http://www.emedicine.com/MED/topic2888.htm.

Warrell, D., Cox, T., Firth, J., & Benz, D. (2003). *Oxford Textbook of Medicine* (4th ed.). New York: Oxford University Press.

Weintraub, M. (2006). Thrombolysis (tissue plasminogen activator) in stroke a medicolegal quadmire. *Stroke, 37,* 1917–1922.

Whitley, R. J. (1990). Viral encephalitis. *New England Journal of Medicine, 323,* 242–256.

Wig, J., Chandrashekharappa, K. N., Yaddanapudi, L. N., Nakra, D., & Mukherjee, M. (2007). Effect of prophylactic ondansetron on postoperative nausea and vomiting in patients on preoperative steroids undergoing craniotomy for supratentorial tumors. *Journal of Neurosurgical Anesthesia, 19*(4), 230–242.

Wijdicks, E. (2007). 10 questions about the clinical determination of brain death. *Neurologist, 13 (6),* 380–381.

Young, G., Shemie, S., Doig, C., & Teitelbaum, J. (2006). Brief review: the role of ancillary tests in the neurological determination of death. *Canadian Journal of Anesthesia, 53(6),* 620–627.

Zak, P. (2003). Surgical management of spinal stenosis. *Physical Medicine and Rehabilitation Clinics of North America, 14,* 143–155.

Ziai, W., & Lewin, J. (2006). Advances in the management of central nervous system infections in the ICU. *Critical Care Clinics, 22*(4), 661–694.

Ziai, W. C., Toung, T. J., & Bhardwaj, A. (2007). Hypertonic saline: Firstline therapy for cerebral edema? *Journal of the Neurological Sciences, 261,* 157–166.

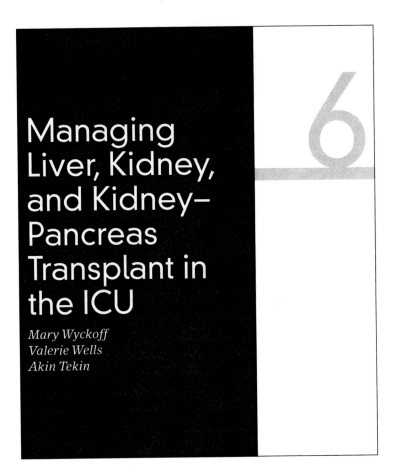

Managing Liver, Kidney, and Kidney–Pancreas Transplant in the ICU

Mary Wyckoff
Valerie Wells
Akin Tekin

Introduction

Managing liver, kidney, and pancreas transplants in the intensive care unit (ICU) are now a major concern of caregivers. Currently, more than 17,000 individuals in the United States are waiting for a liver transplant. From 1988 through January 2008, over 88,600 liver transplants have occurred throughout the U.S. (Organ Procurement and Transplant Network [OPTN]). The United Network for Organ Sharing (UNOS) classifies who meets the criteria to receive a liver transplant by utilizing the Model for End-Stage Liver Disease (MELD) scoring system, which calculates the severity of the disease in each individual. Status 1 is the defined classification for patients with acute severe liver disease or recent development of the disease, or critically ill in an ICU setting with <7 days of life without a liver transplant. The MELD score is based on the probability of death within 3 months and is calculated based on variables of laboratory data including creatinine, bilirubin, international normalized ratio, with the score ranging from 6–40 (Kamath et al., 2001).

Available liver donors are first offered locally to status 1 patients and then accordingly to patients with the highest MELD score. When there are no local recipients available, the liver is then offered regionally and nationally as indicated. Individuals who would not qualify for transplant include those with active alcohol or substance abuse, metastatic cancer, advanced heart and lung disease, severe infections, and massive liver failure with associated brain injury.

Unfortunately, the average waiting time for kidney transplantation is >2 years because of the large waiting list and relatively small pool of organ donors (Kaufman, 2007). As of April 2008, for example, there were 75,514 patients on the UNOS list awaiting cadaver renal transplant, 1,627 awaiting pancreas transplants, and 2,273 awaiting combined renal and pancreas transplant (UNOS, 2008).

Pathophysiology

The liver, weighing approximately 1500 grams has multiple functions within the body and is the largest solid organ. The liver is a unique powerhouse organ managing the carbohydrates, fats, and proteins as the building blocks for growth and vitamins. A functioning liver regulates the blood clotting factors within the body and regulates the bile production. The liver also has functions such as clearance of toxins and host defense.

Indications for Transplant

Cirrhosis accounts for >80% of transplants performed in adults, with hepatitis C and alcoholism being the two most common diagnoses. Other indications include cholestatic liver disease, such as primary biliary cirrhosis (PBC), biliary atresia, primary sclerosing colangitis (PSC), chronic hepatitis (autoimmune hepatitis, hepatitis B), metabolic disease such as hemochromatosis or Wilson disease, nonalcoholic steatohepatitis (NASH), primary hepatocelluler carcinoma, Budd–Chiari syndrome, and fulminant hepatic failure (FHF) (Luu, Van Gelder, & Conrad, 2006). Ascites, hepatic encephalopathy, and hepatorenal syndrome are common symptoms of decompensated liver disease. Spontaneous bacterial peritonitis (SBP) may also occur secondary to bacteria within the ascites. Scarring or fibrosis secondary to liver disease may cause portal hypertension and splenomegaly, which will subsequently destroy red blood cells and trap thrombocytes, which will cause thrombocytopenia. Esophageal varices may also occur and may require intervention such as endoscopic banding and embolization (Guillen, Black, & Grace, 2005). Major pediatric indications for liver transplant include biliary atresia and metabolic liver disease.

Patients who require pre–liver transplant have an enhanced risk of bleeding from the gastrointestinal tract secondary to portal hypertension that requires beta blockade to decrease the portal pressure. Lactulose is also generally indicated to facilitate the clearance of toxins when the liver is not functioning (Guillen et al., 2005). Metronidazole may be considered to decrease the gastrointenstinal bacterial load. Liver failure presents as acute, chronic, and fulminant, usually encompassing multiorgan failure. Patients may present with hepatic encephalopathy (HE) that subsequently entails cerebral edema and intracranial hypertension. These alterations in cerebral metabolism are of major sequelae, because the brain uses glucose as an energy source only under normal physiological conditions. Hyperammonemia is consistent with liver failure and correlates with alterations in brain metabolism (Strauss, Moller, Larsen, Kondrup, & Knudsen, 2003).

The pretransplant evaluation is a complex workup that includes multiple specialists such as a transplant surgeon, anesthesiologist, hepatologist, cardiologist, nephrologist, and, if necessary, psychiatrist and social worker. The pretransplant evaluations include laboratory evaluation of the liver function tests, hematological studies, electrolytes and kidney function tests, tumor markers, hepatitis serology, viral serology, blood type, tuberculosis testing, computerized testing of the liver, and ultrasound.

Contraindications

Contraindications to liver transplant are center specific. Many centers have a multidisciplinary meeting that discusses and evaluates whether patients are candidates for transplant. Some of the diagnosis that are questioned include cholangiocarcinoma, exceedingly large hepatoma, active substance abuse, including an inability to stop alcohol abuse, extrahepatic malignancy, advanced cardiac or pulmonary disease, and absence of ability to maintain care of the organ (Bufton, Emmett, & Byerly, 2008). Some examples include psychological inability to cope, absence of family or social network, and homelessness. These diagnoses and situations are discussed, and the ability to rectify the situations is generally evaluated. Should the underlying conditions be complicated by need of a coronary artery bypass, lung or heart transplant, or kidney failure, these patients may be scheduled prior to, or during the liver transplant. Some patients have received heart, lung, and kidney transplant (Bufton et al., 2008). The health care society is in rapid growth, and it continues to move forward with unique advancements to extend and prolong life depending on the underlying well health of the individual.

Transplantation

Intraoperative Techniques

There are multiple types of liver transplant including a whole liver, reduced liver, or a partial segment. The orthotopic liver transplantation generally involves a disruption of portal and inferior vena caval blood flow that occasionally might require venovenous bypass, which is indicated to divert the blood to the superior vena cava during the anhepatic phase of the liver transplant. The inferior vena cava, portal vein, hepatic artery, and the biliary duct are anastomosed. A Roux-en-Y choledochojejunostomy connects the bile duct to the bowel and may be indicated when a duct-to-duct anastomosis is not feasible (Bufton et al., 2008). The surgical incision is in the shape of a chevron opening both on lower chest and abdomen, which may cause patients postoperative difficulties in mobility. Pain management is significant in promoting mobility, respiratory survivability, extubation, and early ambulation.

Postoperative Management

Detailed acute postoperative management is key to survival and prevention of infections. Operative blood loss, hypotension, or cardiac problems before, during, or after reperfusion, and use of venovenous bypass are the important information that needs to be known for early management of patients. Fluid management is used to stabilize blood pressure and urine output, which is crucial to the resuscitation of patients. Patients who had hepatorenal syndrome and significant hemodynamic instability during the operation will continue to have renal insufficiency postoperatively and might require temporary dialysis. Most patients with hepatorenal syndrome with a functioning liver graft will recover from renal insufficiency in the immediate postoperative period.

Patients who have critical chronic liver disease may be hyperdynamic postoperatively, exhibiting a low systemic vascular resistance (SVR), high cardiac output (CO), and cardiac index (CI). Considering the chronicity of this patient population, it is important to keep in mind that these hyperdynamic numbers might reflect sepsis secondary to infection, which was not recognized prior to the transplantation.

Management may incorporate fluid resuscitation but with limitations and inotropic support. Maintaining adequate fluid balance facilitates the perfusion of the liver and the hepatic artery to prevent cellular death, which is vital to the organs (Bufton et al., 2008). Patients' post–liver transplant evaluation and follow up must be done systematically. During the first few hours and days after the transplant, patients' general clinical condition, even without any laboratory workup, provides significant information about the function of the transplanted liver graft. Maintaining normotension is specifically imperative based on thrombocytopenia. Hypertension with systolic blood pressures >140 mmHg may precipitate an intracranial hemorrhage, specifically those with thrombocytopenia. Medications indicated to maintain normotension include, but are not limited to, continuous infusions of labetalol based on heart rate, and nicardipine may be another consideration once the pain has been managed. An awake patient with good urine output most likely has functioning graft including self-correction of lactic acidosis and coagulopathy, which reflects good synthetic function of the liver. Also, the fibrinogen levels >100 are the main prognostic indicator of a functioning liver. Daily follow up of liver function tests and liver duplex ultrasound to check vascular anastomotic patency are routine in the postoperative period of liver transplant patient. Daily levels for calcineurin inhibitors, which facilitate dose adjustment, are significantly important in the early postoperative period to prevent rejection. Patients must be aggressively mobilized and, if possible, be weaned to extubation if not extubated in the operating arena.

Evaluation of medications, pain management, and monitoring of antirejection medication levels while preventing hospital-acquired infection facilitates a rapid ICU discharge and home environment. Arranging discharge planning, social work involvement, and physical and occupational therapy will further enhance the recovery period. Family and patient education with clear communication facilitates long-term outcomes.

Fluid and Electrolyte Management

Management of fluids and electrolytes is important in the initial postoperative period. The primary focus is to maintain patients normovolemia. Whether patients are volume overloaded or volume under loaded is always the challenging factor. This may be based on the actual surgical procedure and the resuscitative effort indicated to maintain stability. The goal is to keep patients slightly hypervolemic in the initial postoperative period. Blood pressure, CVP, and pulmonary artery (PA) catheter information will assist in determining volume status and in determining when fluid boluses are required. Monitoring serum chemistries for electrolyte status will improve outcomes. Magnesium and potassium are generally the electrolytes that need the most replacements.

Blood Glucose Management

A continuous infusion of regular insulin is often required post–liver transplant. Steroids such as methylprednisolone are administered preoperatively and postoperatively, causing the blood glucose to require close attention. Insulin sliding scales facilitate the management of blood sugar and enhance the healing process.

Respiratory Management

Patients who required transplant are extubated once pain management is controlled. The chest radiograph, intake and output, breath sounds, oxygen saturation, and patients' clinical appearance must be monitored based on preoperative conditions and urine output. As with all postoperative patients, aggressive pulmonary therapy and early ambulation are encouraged.

Gastrointestinal Prophylaxis

Prevention of stress- and steroid-induced peptic ulcer disease is essential postoperatively especially in patients with preexisting esophageal varices. Patients are routinely placed on proton pump inhibitors, H2 receptor blockers, antacids, or sucralfate, with the preference being proton pump inhibitors. Upon return of bowel function, the nasogastric tube is removed, and patients are placed on a progressive diet; ulcer prophylaxis may be continued, particularly if the immunosuppressive regimen includes corticosteroids.

Immunosupression

Graft survival is paramount and is accomplished through immunosuppression following the transplant. Immunosuppression therapy includes a combination of corticosteroids, a calcineurin inhibitor such as cyclosporine or tacrolimus, and an antiproliferative agent. During the immediate postoperative period and at the time of induction, high-dose corticosteroids and an antithymocyte globulin or a monoclonal antibody, such as alemtuzumab (Campath), is administered. The monoclonal antibody binds to CD52 surface antigen of multiple cell types, which results in lysis.

Postoperatively, immunosuppression is maintained with tacrolimus and weaning doses of corticosteroids. Tacrolimus known as FK–506 is a macrolide antibiotic produced by streptomyces tsukubaensis. Tacrolimus inhibits calcineurin recruitment, decreases IL-2 production, and suppresses humoral immunity through the inhibition of B-lymphyocyte activation. Tacrolimus is metabolized in the liver through the cytochrome P450 system. The oral dose in liver transplant recipients is 0.1–0.15 mg/kg per dose. Tacrolimus may also be given as a continuous intravenous therapy when absorption is questionable. Daily levels are monitored, and there is a lower incidence of hypertension and hyperlipidemia, but a higher rate of diabetes and neurotoxicity (Luu et al., 2006; Bufton et al., 2008).

Corticosteroids are administered in a high dose with a daily weaning scale following transplantation. They inhibit cytokine gene transcription and prevent recruitment and activation of T cells. The initial dosing is IV methylprednisolone and then changed to oral form. Acute rejection should be treated with high dose IV methylprednisolone. The secondary effects of steroids include hypertension, cushingoid appearance, personality changes, weight gain, dyslipidemia, osteoporosis, hyperglycemia, diabetes, cataracts, and increased risk of infection (Luu et al., 2006).

Primary Nonfunction

Once reperfusion occurs graft function is viable, but primary nonfunction may occur secondary to preservation injury, which leads to multiorgan failure. Some of the causative factors include donor age, prolonged donor hospitalization, and prolonged cold ischemic time. The risk of primary nonfunction is approximately 2% to 5%, and retransplantation is indicated or patients will die (Bufton et al., 2008).

Maintaining optimal fluid balance also decreases the potential for early hepatic artery thrombosis. The initial signs are deterioration including an elevated alanine aminotransferase (AST), aspartate aminotransferase (ALT), and/or fever. Even though the prothrombin time may be as high as 19 or 20 seconds, careful observation and follow up will be acceptable, unless there are signs of bleeding. Platelet transfusion also might not be necessary, unless the level goes below 20,000/L. There is a concern of thrombosis of hepatic artery occurring by overcorrecting the coagulopathy. There is no clear cause for this occurrence, but it may be secondary to a kink or narrowing in the artery and must be ruled out if primary nonfunction occurs (Bufton et al., 2008).

Acute Rejection

Acute rejection generally occurs within 7–14 days postoperative in approximately 20% to 70% of patients. Clinically, these patients present with hyperbilirubinemia, a rise in alkaline phosphatase, and an elevation in ALT and AST. The clinical symptomology includes fever, liver tenderness, general malaise, and symptoms of infection. Acute rejection is treated with high-doses steroids, generally methylprednisolone 1 gram for 3 days or alternatively with monoclonal therapy such as OKT3. These treatment regimines are effective in 65% to 80% of patients (Luu et al., 2006).

Chronic Rejection

Liver transplant patients may also present with general malaise, jaundice, pruritius, elevated serum alkaline phosphatase, and bilirubin. This is generally a chronic graft rejection that occurs in approximately 5% of postoperative liver transplant patients. This diagnosis is made by liver biopsy, because loss of liver synthetic function does not occur until later in the course.

Infection is another primary problem in postoperative liver transplant patients secondary to immunosuppression. Patients may present with fever, abdominal pain, and hyperthermia or hypothermia. This population is generally so immunosuppressed that they usually cannot mount a white blood cell count (WBC) or a fever. A complete septic evaluation would include a complete blood count, a full chemistry panel, liver function profile, coagulation studies, urinalysis, urine culture, and blood culture including viral studies. Other tests would generally include a liver duplex ultrasound, computerized tomography with contrast, kidney function test, evaluation for abscess, and a liver biopsy.

Infections are primarily hospital acquired, such as *Acinetobacter baumanii, Pseudomonas aerigonsa, Enterococci, Staphylococcus aureus, Klebsiella pneumonae,* and *Candida* species, which are 75% of the infections. Patients presenting with fevers, malaise, arthralgias, atypical lymphocytes, thrombocytopenia, and elevated transaminase levels may be harboring a cytomegalovirus (CMV), which infects 25% to 85% of patients who require liver transplant during their 1st and 3rd postoperative months. This viral infection may be fatal if it becomes disseminated. CMV pneumonitis is demonstrated on a chest radiograph as bilateral infiltrates. The treatment regimine for CMV is intravenous ganciclovir for 2–4 weeks. *Pneumocystis carinii* pneumonia (PCP) can be a complicating factor with CMV infection, and transplant recipients are placed on PCP prophylaxis with trimethoprim sulfamethoxazole 1 gram single strength 3 times per week to potentially prevent these sequelae.

Liver transplant patients presenting with rejection symptoms, who are placed on increased immunosupression therapy, are exposed to other opportunistic pathogens such as *Candida* species, herpes zoster, toxoplasmosis, or hepatitis C reccurrence, which occurs in 50% to 80% of postoperative patients. Hepatitis B is less common and only reoccurs in 10% of patients. The second leading cause of late death in liver transplant recipients is lymphomas, squamous cell carcinoma, and posttransplant lymphoproliferative disorder (PTLD), which is the adverse effect of immunosupression.

Outcomes

The survival rates vary from center to center, but overall, the 1-year survival rate after liver transplantation is approximately 90% for those who come to the hospital to receive their transplant. Patients in the ICU preoperatively and at the time of transplant, are critically ill, generally have a much lower rate of survival, approximately 60%. In 5 years, the survival rate in compliant patients is 80% (Luu et al., 2006).

Kidney Transplantation

Kidney transplant is the treatment of choice for patients with chronic end-stage renal disease, which is defined as an irreversible glomerular filtration rate of <20 ml/min (Lipshutz & Wilkinson, 2007; Klingensmith, Amos, Green, Halpin, & Hunt, 2005). Kidney transplant affords prolonged survival rates and improved quality of life compared with the alternative therapy, dialysis. Renal transplant recipients have a higher success rate of becoming productive, active members of the community posttransplantation (Johnston, 2007; Matas, 2003).

Pancreas Transplantation

Whole vascularized pancreas transplant is the treatment of choice for type 1 diabetes mellitus, an autoimmune disease that results in destruction of the insulin-producing islets of Langerhans within the pancreas (Lipshutz & Wilkinson,

2007). In addition, pancreas transplant rates are increasing for patients with complicated type 2 diabetes (Hummel, Langer, Wolters, Senninger, & Brockmann, 2008). Diabetes is a chronic illness that causes devastation to end organs and leads to complications such as blindness, cardiovascular disease, cerebrovascular disease, loss of limbs, and dyslipidemia within 10–20 years of diagnosis (Lipshutz & Wilkinson, 2007).

Pancreas transplantation normalizes blood glucose levels more effectively than any other treatment currently available. A successful graft results in freedom from insulin administration, frequent blood sugar measurements, prevention or improvement of secondary complications, a halt to the progression of end-organ failure, a lack of dietary restrictions, and an improved quality life (Kaufman, 2007; Lipshutz & Wilkinson, 2007). Pancreas transplant yields the best results in patients whose disease has not yet caused severe target-organ damage (Bindi et al., 2005). Approximately 34% of patients with diabetes develop renal failure within 15 years; therefore, it is not surprising that >90% of the pancreas transplants are performed simultaneously with kidney transplants (Lipshutz & Wilkinson, Wikipedia, 2008).

Indications for Kidney Transplant

Most kidney transplants are performed secondary to end-stage renal failure (ESRF) (Johnston, 2007). Most renal transplant recipients are surviving because of hemodialysis, hemofiltration, or peritoneal dialysis. Those who have a living donor available may choose to receive a transplanted kidney prior to the initiation of dialysis, because this has been shown to have improved outcomes.

Renal failure, secondary to diabetes mellitus, comprises approximately 25% to 31% of the cases in the United States and is now the most common disease requiring kidney transplant. Other common diseases leading to ESRF are previous graft rejection, hypertension, chronic glomerulonephritis, polycystic kidney disease, lupus, scleroderma, chronic pyelonephritis, interstitial nephritis, nephrotic syndrome, hypertensive nephrosclerosis, obstructive uropathy, amyloidosis, and traumatic causes, such as vascular occlusion or parenchymal destruction (Kaufman, 2007; Organ Procurement and Transplantation Network [OPTN], 2006).

Indications for Pancreas Transplant and Combined Kidney Pancreas Transplant

Indications for pancreas transplant include type 1 diabetes or type 2 diabetes with significant secondary sequelae. Individuals with diabetes, in addition to end-stage renal disease, which is usually >90% of pancreas transplants, generally will receive a simultaneous pancreas and kidney transplant (SKP) from a cadaver donor. This is considered the intervention of choice, minimizing patients' risk by performing one surgical intervention and limiting the recipient exposure to one donor human leukocyte antigen (HLA). This will further minimize the potential for rejection. An individual with severe metabolic complications of type 1 diabetes and maintains a creatinine clearance of 60–70 ml/min or greater will receive a pancreas transplant alone (PTA). Patients with diabetes and renal failure may receive a kidney transplant only when the pancreas is not available and then receive a pancreas transplant after the kidney when the organ is available (PAK), which is the common surgical intervention (Hummel et al., 2008; Kaufman, 2007; Lipshutz & Wilkinson, 2007).

Contraindications

Contraindications to kidney and pancreas transplant are center specific and often relative contraindications. Some commonly accepted contraindications to kidney and pancreas transplant are substance abuse, HIV, and AIDS. Relative contraindications include systemic infections, sepsis, multisystem organ failure, severe cardiopulmonary insufficiency, recent cancer within the past 2–5 years, and history of noncompliance (Johnston, 2007). Most centers have variations of age criteria and are based on individual functionality. Some centers, such as Jackson Health System in Miami, Florida, have performed kidney transplantation on patients older than 85 years, patients who are HIV positive, and in some circumstances within 2 days after heart transplantation, utilizing the same donor with the kidney maintained on a pump in a preservation solution. Therefore, end-stage cardiac failure is not an absolute contraindication to kidney transplant. Similarly, patients who are HIV positive with well-maintained cluster of differentiation 4 (CD4) counts may be candidates for transplantation at some centers.

Intraoperative Techniques

Kidney Transplant Operative Technique

Although alternate techniques may be employed, the most common operative technique for kidney transplantation is retroperitoneal placement in the right iliac fossa as opposed to intra-abdominal placement. Patients who may be candidates for pancreas transplant at a later time should have the kidney placed in the left iliac fossa, with the right side reserved for the pancreas. The donor renal artery is anastomosed to the external iliac artery of the recipient, and the renal vein is anastomosed to the external iliac vein (Matas, 2003; Klingensmith et al., 2005). The donor ureter is implanted in the recipient's bladder, with the creation of an extravesicular ureteroneocystostomy known as Lich–Gregoir reimplantation to prevent obstruction and posttransplant reflux pyelonephritis (Johnston, 2007; Klingensmith et al., 2005; Matas, 2003).

Alternatively, intravesical ureterocystostomy may be done when necessary. During this technique, the bladder is incised, which is known as a Leadbetter–Politano reimplantation, and a urethral catheter is placed to drain the bladder. This catheter is left in place for 3–7 days postoperatively (Klingensmith et al., 2005). Prophylactic ureteral stents are commonly used to reduce complications such as urine leaks and ureteral stenosis and are retrieved within a few weeks postoperatively via cystoscopy (Johnston, 2007; Wilson, Bhatti, Rix, & Manas, 2005). Sometimes, ureteral stents are tied to a foley catheter intraoperatively and are removed with the foley.

The native kidneys are usually left in place. A native nephrectomy may be performed prior to transplantation in necessary circumstances, such as in cases of chronic parenchymal infection, unmanageable proteinuria, polycystic kidney disease, intractable hypertension, infected stones, or acquired renal cystic disease (Klingensmith, et al., 2005).

Pancreas Transplant Operative Technique

The donor pancreas may be placed retroperitoneally in the right iliac fossa, or may be placed intraperitoneally. Typically, the arterial anastomosis is achieved by using the donor splenic and superior mesenteric artery anastomosed to the

Y-graft formed from the donor iliac artery prior to implantation and attaching it to the recipient's common or external iliac artery. Connection of the venous system entails the donor's portal vein being anastomosed to the recipient's common or external iliac vein. The recipient retains the native pancreatic exocrine function to aid in digestion, and exocrine secretions of the graft must be managed to minimize complications. Management of the pancreatic fluid produced by the graft is accomplished by enteric drainage or bladder drainage.

Enteric drainage necessitates an intra-abdominal operation and carries the risk of development of an enteric leak. Drainage of the pancreas into the bladder avoids these risks and permits measurement of urine amylase and lipase as a measure of pancreatic graft function. This is a less physiologic process, and it results in higher incidence of urinary tract infections, dehydration, and metabolic derangements secondary to loss of high amounts of bicarbonate (Lipshutz & Wilkinson, 2007; Matas, 2003; Rainer & Sutherland, 2004).

Early Postoperative Management

In many centers, patients with uncomplicated renal transplant may recover in the postanesthesia recovery unit (PACU) and then be transported to a regular floor or transplant floor that utilizes nurses who are trained in the care of postoperative transplant patients. Adequate staffing is essential to accommodate the demanding needs of post-transplant patients specifically in monitoring of intake and output to prevent graft failure. Patients with simultaneous pancreas and kidney transplants, or those with significant comorbidities, may be best served by admission directly from the operating room to the surgical intensive care unit (SICU). Immediate postoperative care includes management of hemodynamic status, acid–base balance, fluid and electrolyte status, blood glucose, respiratory management, gastrointestinal prophylaxis, assessment of graft function, monitoring of immunosuppression, and patient education. Research by Bindi et al., (2005) identified the mean ICU stay as 4.7 days for isolated pancreas transplants as well as simultaneous kidney–pancreas transplant recipients.

Hemodynamic Status

Postoperative transplant patients generally arrive in the ICU with a central venous catheter and an arterial catheter, although blood pressure may be frequently assessed with the use of noninvasive monitoring alone. Although not necessary for most kidney–pancreas recipients, patients with significant cardiac risk factors may be monitored with the use of a PA catheter to achieve optimum cardiac function monitoring. Kidney and kidney–pancreas transplants experience rapid fluid changes and generally are managed on milliliter of urine output per milliliter of fluid replacement. The goal of intense monitoring is to prevent pulmonary edema, volume overload, or dehydration during this initial postoperative period of rapid changes in fluid status.

Hypotension must be avoided because decreased perfusion pressures increase the risk of acute tubular necrosis or graft thrombosis; hypertension increases the risk of postoperative bleeding and stroke (Matas, 2003). Most of renal and pancreas transplant recipients have a past medical history of hypertension, while perioperative use of corticosteroids further causes sodium and fluid retention that contributes to postoperative hypertension. Typical goal parameters in the immediate postoperative period for systolic blood pressure are 120–150 mmHg or mean arterial pressure of 90–105 mmHg (Klingensmith et al., 2005). Central venous pressure (CVP) monitoring is useful in guiding the ACNP's choice of interventions in the face of low urine output, specifically because CVP trends are more useful than absolute numbers. A decreasing urine output with a decreasing CVP and blood pressure indicate the need for a fluid challenge, whereas low urine output with an elevated CVP and elevated blood pressures usually indicates the need for a diuretic. Furosemide drips may be initiated ranging from 5–20 mg/hr. Dopamine administered at a dose of 2–5 $\mu g \cdot kg^{-1} \cdot min^{-1}$ intravenously is used to elevate a low blood pressure and promote urine output once preload (intravascular fluid volume status) has been optimized (Klingensmith et al., 2005). Pharmacologic agents, such as intravenous beta-blockers (labetalol, lopressor, esmolol), calcium channel blockers (nicardipine), or vasodilators (hydralazine) are frequently used to control postoperative hypertension.

Tachycardia is to be avoided, especially in patients with cardiovascular disease or risk factors such as diabetes, hypertension, or dyslipidemia. Pain as a cause of tachycardia should be assessed, and intravenous morphine or other narcotics are appropriate for postoperative pain management. Tachycardia may be an indication of inadequate perfusion, although blood pressure appears relatively normal. Decreasing bicarbonate levels and worsening base deficit on the arterial blood gas, as well as elevated lactic acid level may provide clues that tachycardia is a result of inadequate perfusion and impending cellular death. These laboratory values combined with a decreasing CVP indicate the need for increasing intravenous fluids. Once pain and hypoperfusion has been assessed and managed, if tachycardia remains unresolved, administration of beta-blockers may be effective in controlling heart rate and minimizing associated increased myocardial oxygen demand. During cases of suspected myocardial stress, the ACNP should evaluate patients for potential myocardial ischemia or infarction by electrocardiogram and appropriate laboratory tests such as cardiac enzymes and troponin level as adjusted for creatinine levels.

The posttransplant patient must be monitored for signs of hemorrhage, including continuous monitoring of the surgical drains for sanquinous output, hematuria that progresses to a continuous sanguineous urine, falling hematocrit, decrease in blood pressure that responds to fluid boluses initially, persistent tachycardia, and worsening metabolic acidosis indicating the possibility of bleeding. Replacement with packed red cells and correction of any coagulopathy is the initial treatment, and the surgical team is notified to evaluate the need for exploration. Frequently, the bleeding tamponades, and immediate surgical intervention is not necessary; however, evacuation of the hematoma may be indicated at a later time (Matas, 2003).

Acid Base Balance

Renal Transplant Recipients. Until the transplanted kidney is functioning well, the postoperative patient will continue to have a renal tubular acidosis (RTA). After ruling out hypoperfusion as a cause of metabolic acidosis, bicarbonate administration may be necessary to normalize serum pH. Generally, a good functioning kidney helps to correct the acidosis, minimizing the need for bicarbonate administration.

Pancreas Transplant Recipients. When pancreas grafts are surgically placed to drain into the duodenum, bicarbonate can be reabsorbed. However, when there is 800–1,000 ml/day of exocrine pancreatic fluid drained into the bladder, the loss of bicarbonate may result in a metabolic acidosis. Bicarbonate replacement may be necessary (Kaufman, 2007).

Fluid and Electrolyte Management

Management of fluids and electrolytes is challenging in the postoperative kidney transplant patient. Initially, the goal is to keep patients slightly hypervolemic. Urine output is measured hourly and replaced with 0.45 normal saline milliliter for milliliter, and a maintenance intravenous fluid to replace insensible losses infuses at 30–60 ml/hr (Klingensmith, 2005). Half-normal saline is used as a replacement fluid to prevent a high chloride load that could cause acidosis secondary to the high volume urine output. Blood pressure and CVP can assist with determining volume status and need for fluid boluses. Patients who receive a marginal graft may be oliguric or even aneuric and may only require maintenance intravenous fluids without replacement. Communication with the surgical transplant team is necessary to determine postoperative expectations of the transplanted kidney. Information regarding patients' native renal function and preoperative urine production are useful in determining the amount of urine production by the transplanted kidney. A sudden cessation of urine output may indicate an obstruction in the urinary catheter that requires gentle irrigation.

Monitoring of serum chemistries for electrolyte status is imperative. Potassium levels must be monitored, because hypokalemia may develop with posttransplant diuresis and fluid replacement. Potassium is replaced cautiously and conservatively in the absence of dysrhythmias. Hyperkalemic patients with poor initial graft function may require aggressive treatment and may ultimately become an indication for posttransplant dialysis.

Blood Glucose Management

A continuous infusion of regular insulin is often required post–kidney transplant as well as post–pancreas transplantation. When steroids such as methylprednisolone have been administered perioperatively, blood glucose control requires close attention. During the immediate postoperative period, blood sugars are monitored hourly, and some centers use continuous infusions of 50% dextrose and regular insulin simultaneously for patients receiving pancreas transplants.

Respiratory Management

The post–renal and post–pancreas transplant patients are normally extubated prior to admission to the ICU, or rapidly weaned and extubated shortly after arrival. Some indications for prolonged mechanical ventilation are hemodynamic instability and pulmonary edema due to aggressive intraoperative fluid resuscitation (Matas, 2003). The transplant team may decide to maintain an endotracheal airway until the first dose of the muromonab (OKT3), an immunosuppressive, is given, as the most concerning drug reaction related to monoclonal antibody is pulmonary edema. This is an unusual condition, because most immunosuppressive induction and maintenance regimens do not include OKT3 currently. The chest radiograph, intake and output, breath sounds, oxygen saturation, and patients' clinical appearance must be monitored as urine output is rapidly replaced post–renal transplant. As with all postoperative patients, aggressive pulmonary toilet and early ambulation are encouraged.

Gastrointestinal Prophylaxis

Prevention of stress and steroid-induced peptic ulcer disease is essential postoperatively. Patients are routinely placed on proton pump inhibitors, Histamine 2-receptor agonists, antacids, sucralfate, or a combination thereof (Matos, 2003). Upon return of bowel function, the nasogastric tube is removed, and patients are placed on a progressive diet. The ulcer prophylaxis may be continued, particularly if the immunosuppressive regimen includes corticosteroids.

Assessment of Graft Function

Renal Graft Assessment. Hourly urine output is assessed upon arrival to the SICU, and while urine production may be adequate, the function of the kidney is further assessed by monitoring blood urea nitrogen (BUN) and creatinine. Serum pH, bicarbonate, and base excess should begin to normalize as the kidney reabsorbs bicarbonate.

Initial renal graft function can be categorized into three groups including immediate graft function (IGF), slow graft function (SGF), or delayed graft function (DGF). IGF is evident in recipients when the creatinine falls rapidly, and diuresis occurs immediately postoperative. Most living renal donor and half of cadaveric renal donor grafts display immediate function. Recipients have fewer episodes of rejection and better long-term results than those with delayed graft function. SGF recipients are oliguric with a slowly decreasing creatinine, and do not require dialysis. DGF recipients have very poor initial graft function, are mostly anuric, and require dialysis. DGF is usually attributed to prolonged ischemic time but may occur as a result of marginal donor quality or high panel reactive antibodies, and usually manifests as acute tubular necrosis (ATN). DGF is not a result of other complications that may impact graft function such as urine leaks, graft thrombosis, or accelerated acute rejection. Graft function improves slowly over days to weeks, and is linked to a higher risk for acute rejection as wells as decreased graft survival (Johnston, 2007; Kaufman, 2007; Matos, 2003).

When renal graft function suddenly declines, renal artery or vein graft thrombosis should be suspected. These complications most frequently occur within the first 2–3 days after transplantation (Klingensmith, 2005). Some centers routinely perform regular renal scans and duplex ultrasound of the graft on the first postoperative day to identify graft and artery complications.

Pancreatic Graft Assessment. Postoperative blood glucose levels normalized with minimal use of exogenous insulin demonstrate good pancreatic graft function. Recipients who have bladder drainage of pancreatic enzymes require urine measurements of amylase and lipase, which can identify intact endocrine function as an indication of a healthy graft, and a biopsy, if indicated, may be achieved via cystoscopy. Pancreatic graft anastomosis, connecting to the duodenum of the recipient as a means of exocrine drainage allows for visualization of the graft via gastroscopy (Hummel, 2008). Pancreatic graft Doppler ultrasonography is important in the postoperative period to follow venous thrombosis and, if identified, immediate action including anticoagulation and possible surgical intervention should be taken.

Immunosuppression

Prescribing immunosuppressive therapy prevents the recipient's immune system from destroying the transplanted graft(s). The surgical transplant team implements its center-specific protocols and actively monitors immunological markers and drug levels to adjust drug therapy daily. The ACNP needs to have an understanding of the intended action of common immunosuppressive medications prescribed and the side effects of these agents. The various forms of rejection are discussed below.

Rejection. *Hyperacute rejection* occurs within hours of transplantation, when preformed HLA antibodies attack the graft and result in vessel thombosis quickly progressing to necrosis of the graft. The graft is unsalvageable and must be immediately removed.

Accelerated acute rejection occurs from 12 hours to 1 week after transplantation. Immediate therapy with antilymphocyte globulin and pulse corticosteroids results in frequent recovery of graft function.

Acute rejection occurs 1–3 months posttransplant, and is T-lymphocyte mediated. Diagnosis is confirmed with biopsy. Treatment is with corticosteroids alone or in conjunction with anti-T cell antibodies.

Chronic rejection can occur weeks to years after transplant and involves progressive irreversible destruction to the graft and its vessels (Kaufman, 2007; Klingensmith, 2005).

Induction Therapy. Anti-T cell antibodies that block or inhibit T-cell response to the graft(s) are used for induction therapy immediately after transplant or for treatment of episodes of acute rejection. Examples of these agents are antithymocyte globulin, muromonab-CD3, daclizumab, and alemtuzumab. Use of these powerful agents increases the recipient's risk of infection. Alemtuzumab has been associated with rash, thrombocytopenia, bronchospasm, and hypotension. Monitoring concerns with muromonab-CD3 include cytokine release syndrome, fever, chills, risk of pulmonary edema, neurotoxicity, and nephrotoxicity. Attention to fluid status prior to administration is essential. Premedication with an acetaminophen, an antihistamine, and corticosteroid can minimize these adverse events.

Corticosteroid therapy can also be used to treat episodes of acute rejection. Methylprednisolone is the drug of choice; secondary sequelae include complicated blood glucose management, gastrointestinal ulceration, extreme mood swings, psychosis, delayed wound healing, elevated blood pressure because of sodium and water retention, and a sudden elevation in WBC count.

Maintenance Therapy. A combination of immunosuppressive agents is used for prevention of graft rejection. A calcineurin inhibitor such as tacrolimus or cyclosporine is commonly prescribed. Patient management involves the careful assessment of drug interactions, because these immunosuppressive drug levels may elevate or decrease with concomitant use of various pharmacologic agents involving the cytochrome P450 system, which is routinely used in the ICU. Tacrolimus and cyclosporine have dose-related nephrotoxicity, and care is taken to monitor levels of these immunosuppressives while avoiding coinciding use of other nephrotoxic agents whenever possible. The adverse effects of tacrolimus and cyclosporine are dose dependent and are difficult to compare without stating the relative dose used. Renal toxicity may be reversible secondary to renal vasoconstriction, and irreversible nephron loss may occur with atrophy and fibrosis secondary to the vascular damage. Calcineurin inhibitors, specifically tacrolimus, have neurotoxic effects and may cause seizures and in addition to a calcineurin inhibitor, mycophenolate or azathioprine may be used. Renal function must be monitored closely. Mycophenolate inhibits proliferation of B cells and T cells selectively; nausea and diarrhea are the primary side effect. Azathioprine inhibits lymphocyte cell division and can lead to severe leukopenia. Sirolimus is an agent useful in limiting the dose of calcineurin inhibitor required, thereby minimizing toxic effects of cyclosporine or tacrolimus; however, marked thrombocytopenia may occur, and therapy may be complicated by multiple drug interactions (Johnston, 2007; Kaufman, 2007).

Corticosteroids usually have a role in initial maintenance therapy, but with the advances in current immunosuppression protocols, steroids have been avoided or minimized to avoid long-term side effects such as hypertension, ulcer disease, osteoporosis, infection, obesity, hypercholesterolemia, and glucose intolerance (Johnston, 2007).

Outcomes

Prognosis after transplantation is excellent; the 1-year graft survival is 95% for kidney and 80% to 85% for pancreas (Johnston, 2007). Discharge teaching is a high priority for success of the graft and should begin while patients demonstrate readiness to learn, and can begin gradually in the immediate postoperative period. Posttransplant education is focused toward understanding early postoperative monitoring and treatment, understanding new medications and related effects of these medications, lifestyle modifications, and the importance of compliance (Kaufman, 2007).

Summary

Although management of patients who have undergone liver transplant, kidney transplant, and pancreas transplant requires close monitoring, frequent interventions, and an elaborate medication regime, the benefits to the recipients are well described. Collaboration between the ACNP and surgical transplant teams is essential in the immediate postoperative period to quickly identify and prevent complications and ensure optimal graft function.

References

Bindi, M. L., Biancofiore G., Pasquini C., Lugli D., Amorese G., Bellissima G., et al. (2005). Pancreas transplantation: problems and prospects in intensive care units. *Minerva Anestesiologica, 71(5)*, 207–221.

Bufton, S., Emmett, K., Byerly, A., (2008). Liver transplant. In L. Ohler & S. Cupples. *Core curriculum for transplant nurses* (pp. 423–452). St. Louis: Mosby Elsevier.

Guillen, S., Black, M., & Grace, T., (2005). *Liver Transplant.* Retrieved April, 2008, from http://www.emedicinehealth.com/liver_transplant/article_em.htm

Hummel, R., Langer, M., Wolters, H. H., Senninger, N., & Brockmann, J. G. (2008). Exocrine drainage into the duodenum: a novel technique for pancreas transplantation. *Transplant International, 21(2)*, 178–181.

Johnston, T. D. (2007). Renal transplantation (urology). *eMedicine.* Retrieved September, 2008 from http://www.emedicine.com/med/topic3406.htm

Kamath, P. S., Wiesner, R. H., Malinchoc, M., Kremers, W., Therneau, T. M., Kosberg, C. L., et al. (2001). A model to predict survival in patients with end-stage liver disease. *Hepatology 33(2)*: 464–70. Retrieved September, 2008 from doi:10.1053/jhep.2001.22172. PMID 11172350.

Kaufman, D. B. (2007). Pancreas transplantation. *eMedicine.* Retrieved September, 2008 from http://www.emedicine.com/med/topic2605.htm

Kaufman, D. B. (2007). Renal transplantation (medical). *eMedicine*. Retrieved September, 2008 from http://www.emedicine.com/med/topic2604.htm

Kidney transplantation. (2008). In *Wikipedia, the free encyclopedia*. Retrieved November, 2008 from http://en.wikipedia.org/wiki/kidney_transplant

Klingensmith, M. E., Amos, K. D., Green, D. W., Halpin, V. J., & Hunt, S. R. (Eds.). (2005). *Washington Manual of Surgery, 4th Edition,* pp. 469–476.

Lipshutz, G. S., & Wilkinson, A. H. (2007). Pancreas–kidney and pancreas transplantation for the treatment of diabetes mellitus. *Endocrinology and Metabolism Clinics, 36(4),* 1015–1038.

Luu, L., Van Gelder, C. M., & Conrad, S. A. (2006). *Transplants, Liver*. Retrieved February 6, 2008, from http://www.emedicine.com/emerg/topic605.htm

Matas, A. (Ed.). (2003). *Manual of Kidney Transplant Medical Care*. Minneapolis, MN: Fairview Publications.

Organ procurement and transplantation network. Retrieved May, 2008, from http://www.optn.org/latestData/rptData.asp

Organ procurement and transplantation network. (2006). http://www.optn.org/organdatasource/about.asp?display=kidney

Pancreas transplantation. (2008). *Wikipedia*. http://en.wikipedia.org/wiki/Pancreas_transplantation

Rainer, W. G., & Sutherland, D. E. (Eds.). (2004). *Transplantation of the pancreas*. New York: Springer.

Strauss, G. I., Moller, K., Larsen, F. S., Kondrup, J., & Knudsen, G. M. (2003). Cerebral glucose and oxygen metabolism in patients with fulminant hepatic failure. *Liver Transplant 9(12),* 1244–1252.

United Network for Organ Sharing. (2008). http://www.unos.org/data/default.asp?displaytype=usdata

Wilson, C. H., Bhatti, A. A., Rix, D. A., & Manas, D. M. (2005). Routine intraoperative ureteric stenting for kidney transplant recipients. *Transplantation, 80(7),* 877–882.

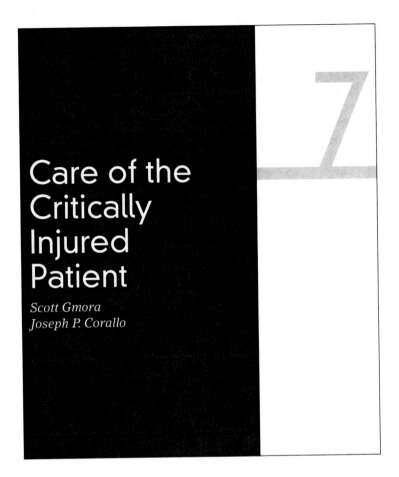

Care of the Critically Injured Patient

Scott Gmora
Joseph P. Corallo

Introduction

In the United States, trauma is the leading cause of death among children, adolescents, and adults under the age of 35 years. In 2003, the Centers for Disease Control (CDC) estimated that more than 400 U.S. residents died each day from injury. Motor vehicle and transportation-related injuries accounted for most of these deaths (29%), followed by firearm injuries (18%), and falls (11%). A recent study that examined the economic impact of trauma in the Unites States found that the total lifetime costs associated with medically treated injuries was over $400 billion annually. The greatest financial and often psychological burden associated with trauma is the extensive disability that may result from injuries, often in young persons in the early part of their work career (Corso, Finkelstein, Miller, Fiebelkorn, & Zaloshnja, 2006). The epidemic of trauma-related deaths is a global health crisis with a staggering 1 in 10 deaths worldwide resulting from injury (Mackenzie & Fowler, 2008).

Governments have responded in part to this public health crisis by creating trauma systems to manage and coordinate the care of individuals who have been significantly injured. These systems are organized using several identified phases of trauma care that include prehospital care, acute inpatient care, and rehabilitation. The primary goal of these systems is to coordinate health care from the initial injury through the rehabilitation phase so that outcomes are optimized, and patients can regain maximal functionality. The critical care nurse practitioner is typically involved in only a part of this long sequence of events to recovery.

In this chapter, we will focus on the acute care management of trauma patients. A discussion of the initial assessment of the injured patient and the approach to managing shock states and resuscitation will be discussed. An overview of commonly encountered injuries will be provided with an emphasis on thoracic, intra-abdominal, and musculoskeletal injuries.

Initial Assessment of the Injured Patient

The primary survey and subsequent management of critically injured patients remains a daunting task even for the most experienced practitioner. The forces sustained during a major trauma are formidable and can result in a diverse array of seemingly unrelated injuries that involve multiple regions of the body. The most important element of the initial trauma assessment is to maintain an orderly sequence of evaluations regardless of the distracting nature of presenting injuries. This orderly sequence of evaluations is referred to as the *primary survey* and can be recalled using a modification of the commonly taught mnemonic ABCDE.

1. *Airway:* Confirm and maintain airway patency with cervical spine immobilization.
2. *Breathing:* Establish the presence of spontaneous respirations and exclude life-threatening impairments to normal ventilation (e.g., tension pneumothorax, neurological injury, influence of drugs and/or alcohol).

3. *Circulation:* Ensure the presence of effective circulation and exclude exsanguinating hemorrhage. Establish intravenous access.
4. *Disability:* Perform a gross neurological assessment to rule out significant intracranial injury and determine the patient's level of consciousness using the Glasgow Coma Scale (GCS).
5. *Exposure:* Remove all clothing and scan the patient head-to-toe to rule out significant life-threatening injury. Ensure appropriate measures to prevent hypothermia.

Most critically injured patients have sustained a sufficient force of injury to warrant the initial presumption of cervical spine injury, so their cervical spine should be immobilized before beginning any assessment. This includes the application of a hard cervical collar and maintenance of inline spine immobilization. In certain situations, the trauma team leader may elect to forgo immobilization if the mechanism of injury is clearly incompatible with cervical spine injury (e.g., penetrating injury to the extremities).

The highest priority in any resuscitation is determining whether the patient's airway is patent. Injured patients often demonstrate diminished levels of consciousness (e.g., brain injury, intoxication, shock, etc.) that may prevent them from protecting their own airway. Traumatic injuries to the face can also result in significant nasopharyngeal bleeding, leading to airway obstruction. If the patient is conscious, the simple act of responding to questions is often sufficient to preclude any obstruction. Signs of airway obstruction include stridorous and labored breathing. Any evidence of obstruction requires immediate intervention via oropharyngeal suctioning, inserting a nasopharyngeal airway, or endotracheal intubation.

After the airway has been deemed patent, the presence of spontaneous breathing needs to be established. Patients who are not breathing spontaneously require supported forms of ventilation. A rapid and focused respiratory examination should also be conducted to exclude significant thoracic injury. Inspection of the chest wall for signs of external trauma (contusion, deformity, laceration) often provides the first indication that there is an underlying lung injury. The presence of subcutaneous emphysema on palpation may also signify serious pulmonary trauma. Auscultation is performed to establish that there is normal and equal air entry bilaterally. Diminished air entry may signify an underlying hemothorax and/or pneumothorax. Patients with hemodynamic instability and clinical evidence of a pneumothorax require immediate decompression of their pleural space with needle and tube thoracostomy. Supplemental oxygen is administered, and oxygen-saturation monitoring is established.

The patient's pulse and blood pressure are quickly assessed at this point to ensure adequate circulatory function. A rapid visual scan of the patient's body should also be conducted to exclude significant external hemorrhage. Intravenous (IV) access is critical and is established early with 2 large-bore peripheral IVs (14 or 16G) or via central venous catheterization. Crystalloid fluids and blood products are administered as indicated.

A cursory neurological examination should be subsequently performed to rule out significant intracranial trauma. The patient's pupils are assessed for size and reactivity. A fixed and dilated pupil suggests a significant underlying brain injury and necessitates intervention to decrease intracranial pressure. The patient's level of consciousness should be assessed using the GCS (Table 7.1). A GCS score below 9 indicates severe brain injury requiring immediate neurosurgical consultation (see Chapter 5).

The patient's clothing should be completely removed. It is critical that all bandages applied in the prehospital setting eventually be removed and be carefully inspected by the trauma team. It is not uncommon to miss subtle findings in the field setting that would dramatically affect management. A small laceration, for example, may actually represent a small tear from an underlying open fracture. "Arterial pumpers" observed in the field may represent inconsequential bleeding from subcutaneous tissues or might indeed be a major vascular injury. It is important to rely only on what you or your team has personally visualized and not on the assessment of prehospital personnel or transferring physicians. Hypothermia is also a serious concern in trauma patients, particularly when there is evidence of hemorrhagic shock. Strategies employed to minimize lowering of the patient's core body temperature include the use of warmed resuscitation fluids and warming blankets, as well as increasing the ambient room temperature when feasible.

7.1 Glasgow Coma Scale (GCS)

	Score
Eyes	
Opens eyes spontaneously	4
Opens eyes in response to voice	3
Opens eyes in response to painful stimuli	2
Does not open eyes	1
Verbal	
Oriented, converses normally	5
Confused or disoriented	4
Inapropriate words	3
Incomprehensible sounds	2
Makes no sounds	1
Motor	
Obeys commands	6
Localizes painful stimuli	5
Withdraws (normal flexion) to painful stimuli	4
Abnormal flexion to painful stimuli (decorticate response)	3
Extension to painful stimuli (decerebrate response)	2
Makes no movements	1

GCS ≤ 8 = Severe; GCS 9–12 = Moderate; GCS ≥ 13 = Mild

Investigations and Monitoring Adjuncts to the Primary Survey

Once the primary survey has been completed, several adjuncts are employed to monitor patients' physiologic status. If the primary survey has not already been done, patients should be attached to a pulse oximetry device to ensure adequate oxygenation and have electrocardiographic (ECG) monitoring leads attached. Catheterization of the bladder is performed early to allow for monitoring of volume status and organ perfusion and to prevent bladder distention. Urethral catheterization is absolutely contraindicated in patients with a suspected urethral injury. The presence of blood at the urethral meatus or a "high-riding" prostate on digital rectal examination should alert the clinician to the possibility of such an injury. In this situation, catheterization should be deferred until definitive imaging of the distal genitourinary tract has been performed.

An orogastric (OG) or nasogastric (NG) tube is commonly inserted to decompress the stomach contents and minimize the risk of aspiration. Trauma patients are at increased risk for aspiration, because they are physically immobilized on spine boards and often have a diminished capacity to protect their airway. Insertion of an NG tube is absolutely contraindicated in patients with a suspected basal skull fracture, because there have been rare case reports of NG tubes inadvertently being passed through a fractured cribiform plate into the cranial vault. In these cases, gastric decompression via oral intubation is preferred.

Laboratory studies should be drawn from patients during this phase of resuscitation. Although protocols vary across hospitals, commonly ordered studies include a complete blood count (CBC), a chemistry panel, coagulation parameters, and arterial blood gases. All patients are screened for blood type and crossmatch when blood transfusion is required.

Radiological imaging is an important component of the initial assessment, and arrangements should be made to have the appropriate personnel and equipment available. A plain anterior–posterior (AP) chest and AP pelvic film are mandatory in all polytrauma patients. For patients who are not undergoing brain imaging with computed tomography (CT), plain films of the cervical spine should be obtained, including AP, lateral, and odontoid views.

Shock and the Trauma Patient

Shock plays a central role in the assessment and management of critically injured patients. The initial goal of all trauma resuscitations is to recognize the possible presence of shock and to identify and treat the condition(s) responsible for its occurrence. *Shock* is an umbrella term used to describe a life-threatening physiological state in which there is marked impairment in blood flow and oxygen delivery to vital organs.

It occurs when the cardiovascular and/or pulmonary system malfunction to such an extent that vital organs no longer receive sufficient oxygen and nutrient delivery to perform their baseline functions. This impaired delivery of blood together with the accumulation of cellular waste products results in severe cellular derangements, organ dysfunction, and eventually death.

Approach to the Patient in Traumatic Shock

One of the most significant obstacles in managing patients in shock is recognizing its presence in the first place. Because shock exists along a continuum rather than as an all-or-none phenomenon, its manifestations can be quite subtle, especially in the early phases and among young healthy patients with significant physiological reserve. There have been countless attempts of researchers to identify a single laboratory test or physical examination finding that can reliably establish the presence of shock. To date, no such parameter has been found.

To diagnose shock, clinicians must rely on the integration of various different clinical findings and biochemical tests that, when combined, highly suggest a state of hypoperfusion (see Table 7.2). Clinicians cannot depend on any single finding to reliably establish or rule out the presence of shock. Consequently, a high degree of suspicion is required when dealing with all critically injured patients.

Clinical Findings. Because shock refers to impaired blood flow and oxygen delivery to vital organs, the body's initial response is to compensate by increasing its heart rate in an attempt to improve tissue perfusion. In adults, a heart rate above 100 beats/min should raise the clinical suspicion of circulatory shock. It is important to recognize, however, that the absence of tachycardia does not exclude the possibility of shock. Elderly patients, for example, often have a blunting of their cardiac response to adrenergic stimulation and may be incapable of mounting a tachycardic response to hypovolemia, or a consideration of baseline beta-blockers may cause inhibition. Patients with neurogenic shock may also be incapable of compensating with a tachycardic response resulting from loss of sympathetic tone. Another early manifestation of shock is cutaneous vasoconstriction as the body increases vascular tone. Accordingly, trauma patients who are cool and

7.2 Shock Classification Table

Classification	Description	Differential Diagnosis	Intervention
Hemorrhagic	— An inadequate circulating volume of blood resulting from loss of whole blood leading to impaired tissue perfusion — By far, the most common form of shock in trauma patients	Bleeding	— Fluid administration with crystalloids +/− blood — Surgical hemostasis as indicated
Nonhemorrhagic Cardiogenic	— Inadequate tissue perfusion resulting from primary cardiac dysfunction	Myocardial infarction Arrythmias Blunt cardiac injury	— ACLS protocol (see Chapter 4) — Cardiac telemetry
Distributive	— A hemodynamic state caused by loss of sympathetic tone resulting in arteriolar and venular dilatation	Sepsis Anaphylaxis Neurogenic Shock	— Infectious source control — Antibiotics — +/− inotropic support — Epinephrine — +/− steroids — Fluids — Vasoactive medications if refractory
Obstructive (extracardiac)	— Mechanical obstruction of the great vessels of the heart, leading to diminished blood flow through the cardiopulmonary circuit	Cardiac tamponade Tension pneumothorax	— Pericardiocentesis/ pericardotomy — Surgical repair of cardiac injury — Decompressive needle thoracostomy — Chest tube insertion

tachycardic must be presumed to be in a state of shock until proven otherwise (American College of Surgeons Committe on Trauma, 2004).

When the degree of organ perfusion worsens, additional clinical findings begin to emerge. The kidney is exquisitely sensitive to decreases in blood delivery and responds by decreasing the amount of urine produced. Clinicians tend to rely heavily on the trend of urine output to identify patients in shock and monitor the degree of end-organ perfusion. A normal urinary output is approximately 0.5–1.0 $ml·kg^{-1}·hr^{-1}$.

Alterations in mental status should also alert the clinician to the possibility of shock. In the early phases of shock, these changes can be quite subtle. Patients initially exhibit varying degrees of anxiety that eventually progresses to confusion, lethargy, and coma while cerebral perfusion diminishes.

The sine qua non of profound circulatory collapse, however, is hypotension. When compensatory mechanisms become inadequate to maintain perfusion, a significant fall in systolic blood pressure ensues (typically <90 mmHg). It is important to note that up to 30% blood volume loss is needed before hypotension begins to manifest. Given this delay in presentation, clinicians cannot rely solely on hypotension as an indicator of shock. The presence of any degree of hypotension should be interpreted as representing a profound degree of circulatory collapse and requires immediate attention and intervention.

Identify and Correct the Underlying Cause

Restore Tissue Perfusion. In the acute phase of management, the overwhelming majority of trauma patients who exhibit signs of shock are bleeding and are consequently hypovolemic. These patients require aggressive fluid resuscitation beginning with warmed isotonic crystalloids or colloid solutions and progressing to blood products as necessary. The American College of Surgeons Committee on Trauma recommends an initial bolus of 1–2 L to expand the intravascular space and replenish interstitial and intracellular losses (American College of Surgeons Committee on Trauma, 2004). Patients in hypovolemic shock who fail to respond fully to this fluid challenge, or respond only transiently, should have blood products transfused to restore the oxygen-carrying capacity of their intravascular volume.

An interesting paradigm shift is currently emerging in the resuscitation of patients with penetrating injuries. There is increasing, albeit not yet conclusive, evidence to suggest that patients with penetrating injuries may benefit from a more limited approach to fluid resuscitation. This strategy, known as *permissive hypotension*, operates on the assumption that aggressive fluid resuscitation may be detrimental to patients with penetrating injuries, because even normal systolic blood pressures may be sufficiently high to dislodge clots that have formed on bleeding blood vessels. Thus, in selected cases, trauma physicians may elect to limit the amount of fluid administered and maintain lower systolic blood pressures as means for bridging patients to definitive operative repair.

Although the administration of fluids and blood products may temporize the effects of hypovolemic shock, trauma patients often have significant underlying bleeding that will continue unabated unless surgically corrected. Accordingly, the presence of shock in an injured patient demands that a surgeon be immediately involved to assess the need for operative intervention.

Common Injuries in the Critically Injured Trauma Patient

Rib Fractures, Flail Chest, and Pulmonary Contusion

Rib fractures are the most common injury sustained following blunt chest trauma. It has been estimated that 10% of all trauma admissions have fractured ribs, although the incidence is likely higher, because chest x-rays fail to detect up to 50% of such injuries. Although simple rib fractures are rarely life-threatening, they can carry significant morbidity because of pain, atelectasis, and underlying lung injury. This increased morbidity and mortality is particularly apparent in the elderly population. Bulger, Alnerson, Mock, and Jurkovich (2000) found that elderly patients with blunt chest trauma and rib fractures have twice the mortality of younger patients. Moreover, each additional rib fracture in the elderly results in a 19% increase in mortality.

When three or more consecutive ribs are fractured in two or more places, a situation is created where the injured segment of thoracic wall becomes detached from the remaining chest wall. This condition is known as a *flail chest,* and results in an island of chest wall that moves independently from the remaining thoracic cage. That is, the flail segment moves inward while the rest of the chest moves out and vice versa. Although this instability of the chest wall may independently result in significant respiratory impairment, the primary clinical concern is the pulmonary contusion that invariably accompanies this injury.

A pulmonary contusion is an injury to lung parenchyma that is characterized by interstitial and alveolar edema, hemorrhage, and loss of normal lung structure and function. It is a "bruising" of the lung that occurs when a significant amount of kinetic energy is transferred to the chest, such as when an unrestrained driver strikes the steering column or when an overlying rib fracture lacerates the pulmonary parenchyma. Hypoxemia and respiratory distress develop over the course of 24–48 hours, with some patients progressing to an acute respiratory distress syndrome (ARDS). The diagnosis of pulmonary contusion is confirmed with radiographic imaging on plain chest x-ray or CT that demonstrates nonanatomic, infiltrative lesions and associated rib fractures.

The management of simple rib fractures, flail chests, and pulmonary contusions is largely supportive. Pain relief is an important component of therapy to minimize restriction of patient's respiratory effort (splinting), which leads to atelectasis and pneumonia. For severe chest wall injuries, continuous epidural infusion is an excellent form of analgesia and should be strongly considered. The addition of nonsteroidal anti-inflammatory drugs are also extremely effective but should be used with caution in patients with high bleeding risks. In patients with pulmonary contusions, excessive fluid administration should be avoided to minimize increasing the edema within the contused lung. Aggressive pulmonary toilet should also be provided. Large pulmonary contusions may significantly affect gas exchange, particularly within the first 24–48 hours after injury and may require endotracheal intubation. Endotracheal intubation should not be performed in an attempt to "treat" the contusion and prevent subsequent respiratory decompensation; it should only be performed in response to subjective and objective clinical signs of respiratory distress in patients. The use of nonin-vasive ventilation in this setting is usually quite effective in maintaining oxygenation, and clinicians are encouraged to consider the use of this respiratory adjunct in the hemody-namically stable patient who is significantly hypoxemic after a pulmonary contusion.

Simple Pneumothorax or Hemothorax

Normal respiratory function is predicated on the ability to move air into and out of the lungs. Humans have evolved an ingenuous mechanism for enabling this process to occur. The pleural sac surrounding each lung acts as a natural adhesive that closely approximates each lung to the chest wall. During inspiration, humans employ several muscle groups to expand their chest wall, causing the adherent lung to expand in tandem. This expansion creates a negative pressure gradient drawing air into the lung.

A traumatic pneumothorax (or "collapsed lung") occurs when air is inadvertently allowed to enter the pleural space. This could result from blunt trauma (e.g., a fractured rib that lacerates the lung causing air to escape into the pleural space) or penetrating lung trauma (e.g., stab wound). Regardless of the cause, the accumulation of air in the pleural space inter-feres with the ability of the lung to remain adherent to the chest wall. This causes the lung to collapse away from the chest wall, thereby impeding the normal indrawing of air when the thoracic cage expands.

The clinical manifestations of this condition depend largely on the degree of collapse. On one end of the spectrum, patients with small pneumothoraces often remain entirely asymptomatic. Patients with large pneumothoraces, however, typically present with shortness of breath or pleuritic chest pain. Auscultation classically reveals diminished air entry on the affected side. Definitive diagnosis is made with plain radiographs that demonstrate a displacement of the pleura away from the chest wall and accumulation of intrapleural air on the affected side.

The management of this condition consists of placing a thoracostomy tube into the pleural space. The tube is connected to a suction device to allow for removal of the misplaced air and permit re-expansion and adherence of the lung to the chest wall. The tube is typically left in place for

48–72 hours, until there is evidence of lung re-expansion on x-ray and an absence of air leakage on the suction device. Occasionally, a second tube may need to be inserted for large pneumothoraces.

A *hemothorax* occurs when blood is allowed to enter the pleural space. This blood can originate from injury to the soft tissue and muscles of the chest wall, intercostal vessels, or laceration of the lung parenchyma. Managing of hemothorax is usually limited to placement of a thoracostomy tube to allow for drainage of the blood. In cases of excessive ongoing blood loss, surgical exploration to arrest the bleeding may be required. Meticulous documentation of the nature and amount of output by the nursing staff is critical in managing injured trauma patients. It is also important that all of the blood be completely evacuated from the pleural space.

Even small amounts of residual blood can lead to fibrothorax, a condition in which a thick fibrin peel forms over the pleural surfaces. This peel restricts normal lung movement during the respiratory cycle that results in impaired lung function. This condition often requires surgical exploration to remove the peel, which can carry a significant morbidity (Meyer, 2007).

Tension Pneumothorax. A tension pneumothorax is a life-threatening condition that occurs when air progressively accumulates under pressure in the pleural space. It is an extreme form of a simple pneumothorax that is thought to occur when the lung and adjacent pleura are injured in such a way that a one-way valve is created. This valve opens during inspiration, allowing air to accumulate in the pleural space, but closes during expiration. This effectively prevents escape of the accumulated air. The accumulation of air progresses unabated until there is complete lung collapse, impairment of venous return to the heart, and mechanical compression of the heart. The precise point at which a simple pneumothorax becomes a tension pneumothorax is not always clear. Most clinicians, however, consider a pneumothorax to be under tension when it results in significant cardiorespiratory compromise that reverses on decompression of the pleural space (Leigh–Smith & Harris, 2005).

A tension pneumothorax must be considered in trauma patients who experience a sudden deterioration in their cardiorespiratory status. Given the importance of timely intervention to prevent complete cardiorespiratory collapse, the diagnosis is strictly clinical and should not be based on radiological findings. Patients typically present with shortness of breath, pleuritic chest pain, and decreased air entry on the affected side. The defining features of this condition, however, are hypoxemia, tachycardia, and hypotension. Occasionally, these patients present with tracheal deviation and distended neck veins; however, the presence of these findings is inconsistent.

A high index of suspicion is required so that definitive therapy can be instituted prior to complete cardiovascular collapse. Given the importance of minimizing delay in intervention, needle decompression followed by tube thoracostomy is considered the treatment of choice. It is vital to appreciate that a tension pneumothorax is a clinical diagnosis and should not be made based on radiographic findings. Needle decompression involves insertion of a large bore cannula or needle through the pectoralis muscles at the second intercostal space in the midclavicular line. A rush of air is often heard when air escapes under pressure and is accompanied by immediate amelioration of the patient's clinical status. This maneuver is not diagnostic. A tension pneumothorax cannot be definitively excluded, simply because no air escapes on needle decompression. Placement of a tube thoracostomy is mandatory after a therapeutic needle decompression.

Cardiac Tamponade

The heart is enclosed within a fibrous sac, called the *pericardial sac* (or pericardium), that permits only a limited amount of elasticity. Traumatic cardiac tamponade refers to a life-threatening condition in which blood accumulates within the pericardial sac causing acute compression of the cardiac chambers. In the trauma patient, cardiac tamponade occurs most commonly as a result of a penetrating injury to the heart. With each contraction of the myocardium, more and more blood extravasates into the pericardial space leading to further compression of the cardiac chambers, decreased diastolic compliance, and eventually obstruction of venous inflow. It has been estimated that as little as 100 ml of blood is sufficient to cause a tamponade effect (Spodick, 2003).

Cardiac tamponade reflects a spectrum of physiological compromise as blood continues to accumulate within the pericardial sac. Although the compromise in cardiac filling ultimately leads to profound cardiovascular collapse, the initial physical findings can be difficult to detect. The classical findings are referred to as Beck's triad and include (a) hypotension, (b) jugular venous distention, and (c) muffled heart sounds. Another key diagnostic finding is pulsus paradoxus, defined as a cyclical fall in systolic blood pressure of 10 mmHg or more with each inspiration. Ultrasonography is highly accurate in detecting the presence of hemopericardium and is the diagnostic modality of choice in most trauma situations. In stable patients with equivocal findings, echocardiography can be employed for definitive diagnosis.

The presence of a traumatic cardiac tamponade is a surgical emergency requiring immediate pericardial decompression. Because all trauma patients with blood in the pericardial sac are presumed to have a concomitant injury to the heart, open surgical decompression with exploration and repair of the heart is the decompression technique of choice. Although needle decompression (pericardiocentesis) is highly effective for nontraumatic causes of cardiac tamponade (e.g., fluid, pus), it tends to be less effective at aspirating clotted blood and obviously does not address any underlying injury. The use of pericardiocentesis in trauma is increasingly limited to situations in which a patient has become unstable from cardiac tamponade and there is no surgeon available for open decompression.

Abdominal Trauma

Abdominal trauma is a leading cause of morbidity and mortality among trauma patients, and it accounts for a significant percentage of allocated critical care resources. Although we usually think that the abdomen is comprised only of that part of the torso extending from costal margins to the groin, it is important to recognize that significant intra-abdominal injury can result from injuries to the lower chest, back, and flank regions. The abdominal cavity is typically divided into four anatomic zones, namely; intraperitoneal, retroperitoneal, thoracoabdominal, and pelvic. Within these anatomical confines, there are solid organs (liver, spleen, pancreas, and kidneys), hollow viscous organs (distal esophagus, stomach, small intestine, colon, and rectum), and numerous vascular structures.

The abdominal assessment is a notoriously difficult component of the initial evaluation of an injured patient. Unlike the chest and musculoskeletal regions of the body, injuries within the abdomen are typically not apparent without the aid of advanced imaging technologies (e.g., CT) or surgical exploration. Clinicians are often forced to rely only on indirect findings of injury (e.g., tenderness, hemodynamic

7.3 Abdominal Trauma

| Organ(s) | Diagnosis | | Management Options | |
	Clinical Findings	Diagnostic Modality	Hemodynamically stable	Hemodynamically unstable
Spleen	— Left-sided rib fractures — Left upper quadrant (LUQ) contusion/ tenderness — Referred pain to left shoulder	1. FAST 2. CT scan	— Close observation if no other indication for surgery and stable hematocrit	— Splenectomy — Splenic repair (less common)
Liver	— Right-sided rib fractures — RUQ contusion/ tenderness	1. FAST 2. CT scan	— Close observation if no other indication for surgery and stable hematocrit	— Surgical exploration and repair of liver injury — Angio-embolization (less common)
Stomach/ Duodenum	— Epigastric contusion/ tenderness — Diffuse peritonitis	1. Chest radiograph (CXR): Free air (poor sensitivity) 2. CT scan	— Surgical exploration and repair of injury mandatory.	

instability, free fluid on ultrasound) when formulating their treatment plan. Given the "black box" nature of abdominal injuries, the key when initially assessing trauma patients is often not to accurately diagnose the type of injury, but rather to recognize that there is an injury.

Assessment of the Abdomen

Trauma surgeons rely heavily on physical examination findings when assessing patients for the possibility of intra-abdominal injury. Although the physical examination technique is similar to that of noninjured patients, the interpretation of these physical findings is tailored to the detection of signs suggesting an underlying injury.

Inspection. Physical examination begins with careful inspection of the abdomen for external evidence of injury. In blunt trauma, contusions of the abdominal wall suggest that a significant force was applied to the abdominal cavity and that a high degree of suspicion for injury needs to be maintained. Bruising in the shape of a seat belt ("seat belt sign") has been shown to be associated with underlying pancreatic injury, intestinal perforation, and fracture of the lumbar vertebrae. In patients who present with penetrating injuries, it is critical that the patient be completely exposed and that a meticulous search for penetrating wounds is conducted. This includes hidden areas such as the axilla and gluteal clefts, and logrolling the patient to examine the back. Finally, clinicians should note the shape of the abdomen, because a distended abdomen may indicate internal bleeding.

Percussion. In patients with a protuberant abdomen, dullness on percussion suggests a fluid-filled cavity, (i.e., intra-abdominal bleeding) and tympany suggests gastric distention or, less commonly, pneumoperitoneum from a perforated viscous. However, percussion provides a means of identifying patients with peritonitis. Patients with peritoneal inflammation often demonstrate exquisite tenderness when their abdominal wall is percussed. This tenderness is a highly abnormal finding and should alert the clinician of the possibility of underlying injury.

Palpation. The primary purpose of abdominal palpation is to elicit signs suggestive of peritoneal irritation. Signs that indicate peritonitis include tenderness to palpation, increased abdominal wall rigidity, voluntary and/or involuntary guarding, and pain with movement. It is important to determine whether these findings are present diffusely throughout the entire abdominal wall or remain localized to particular quadrants. When localized, the point of maximal tenderness will often provide a clue to which organ is injured. For example, splenic injuries typically present with left upper quadrant tenderness, whereas renal injuries may present with flank pain. The presence of diffuse peritonitis is an indication for surgical exploration of the abdomen.

Digital Rectal Examination. Digital rectal examination (DRE) is typically performed when the patient is logrolled to assess the posterior torso and spine. The presence of gross blood on digital examination suggests the possibility of colorectal injury. The presence of rectal bleeding and palpable bony fragments within the rectum indicates the presence of an open pelvic fracture. In men, a high-riding or difficult-to-palpate prostate gland may indicate the presence of an underlying urethral injury. Finally, anal sphincter tone and sensation should be assessed for possible spinal cord injury.

Adjunct Diagnostic Tests and Procedures

In the past decade, abdominal ultrasound has assumed a prominent role in the management of severely injured trauma patients. Once the sole domain of radiologists, the ultrasound has now become a critical tool in the trauma physician's armamentarium to identify the presence of internal hemorrhage. The technique known as *focused assessment with sonography for trauma* (FAST) evaluates several discrete regions within the peritoneal cavity and pericardium to determine whether free fluid (i.e., blood) is present. The use of ultrasound is particularly helpful for patients who are hemodynamically unstable; because in this context, the finding of free fluid is an indication for emergent surgical exploration. Patients who are hemodynamically unstable require immediate transport to the operating room so that internal bleeding can be surgically arrested. Although there are certain limitations inherent to this diagnostic modality, the FAST examination is inexpensive, readily obtainable, and quite sensitive in the appropriate setting for identifying even small quantities of blood.

Diagnostic peritoneal lavage (DPL) is another technique used to detect intra-abdominal injury. This technique involves placing a catheter into the peritoneal cavity and instilling 1L of fluid (normal saline or Ringer's lactate). The fluid is then drained under gravity from the peritoneal cavity and sent for laboratory analysis. It is analyzed macroscopically and microscopically to quantify the amount of red blood cells, white blood cells, and amylase present. Numerous studies have established that a certain concentration of each of these indices can reliably predict the presence of intraperitoneal bleeding and/or bowel injury.

In recent years, this test has been largely overshadowed by newer diagnostic modalities (i.e., ultrasound). Currently, DPL is primarily employed in situations where a patient is hemodynamically unstable, and trauma ultrasonography is not readily available or remains indeterminate. It is also occasionally employed when there is a suspicion of bowel injury on CT but no evidence of peritonitis on physical examination.

CT has assumed a central role in the modern management of trauma patients. Technological advances have made CT scans extremely sensitive and accurate in the detection of most types of body injury. CT scans have become readily accessible, with dedicated machines located near most resuscitation bays. Injuries that had previously gone undiagnosed are now identified early in the assessment process so that appropriate treatment can be provided. Interestingly, however, many now argue that CT scans are becoming overutilized in trauma patients and should be limited to situations where there is a high probability of injury or when a reliable clinical examination cannot be obtained (e.g., severe traumatic brain injury, intoxication, distracting injuries).

Musculoskeletal Injuries

Musculoskeletal injuries are exceedingly common in patients who have sustained blunt trauma. It is estimated that orthopedic surgeries for skeletal trauma outnumber all other trauma operations by 5:1 (Harkess, Ramsey, & Harkess, 1991). These injuries range in severity from minor to life and limb threatening. This section addresses the clinical examination of the musculoskeletal system and outlines an approach to fracture management.

Assessment

Although musculoskeletal injuries are sometimes dramatic in their appearance, it is critical that the primary survey take precedence in the evaluation of all trauma patients. With the exception of exsanguinating external hemorrhage (e.g., amputation or mangled extremity), the assessment and management of all extremity injuries should begin only after a properly conducted primary survey.

Once the primary survey has been completed, a head-to-toe examination of the patient is performed to exclude additional injuries—a process referred to as the *secondary survey*. The musculoskeletal system forms an integral part of the secondary survey and involves evaluation of both the axial and appendicular structures for possible injury.

Assessment of musculoskeletal trauma begins by asking patients to localize any bone pain. The bone structure is then inspected for deformity, swelling, and bruising. It is important to inspect the overlying skin for small tears that might indicate the possibility of an open fracture. The extremity is palpated for tenderness; and a neuromotor examination is performed with attention to sensory function, range of motion, and muscle strength. A focused evaluation of the peripheral vascular system is also mandatory. Distal pulses are palpated, and capillary refill of the digits and toes are assessed. A Doppler probe is frequently employed to supplement this assessment. All pulse points should be compared with the contralateral extremity for symmetry.

Finally, any abnormal clinical examination findings (e.g., pain and deformity) should be followed up with appropriate x-ray imaging to confirm and define the nature of the injury.

Principles of Fracture Management

The primary goal of fracture management is to have the broken bone segments heal in a position that will produce optimal functional recovery and to prevent fracture and soft-tissue complications. The initial approach to managing skeletal fractures consists of realigning the broken segments and then immobilizing the limb.

Once a fracture has been identified, clinicians must determine whether realignment (i.e., reduction) is necessary. Most significantly displaced, shortened, or angulated fractures will require some form of reduction to reappose the fractured segments. This can usually be accomplished using a closed technique by applying manual traction along the long axis of the injured limb in a direction opposite the mechanism of injury. Operative intervention to reduce the fracture (i.e., open reduction) may be necessary if closed reduction fails, the fracture is unstable, or there is intra-articular displacement.

Once the injured segments have been successfully reduced, it is necessary to immobilize the limb to prevent further soft tissue and neurovascular injury. Immobilization also provides a degree of symptomatic relief for most patients. Immobilization is most commonly accomplished using a splint or cast; however, external fixation is occasionally required. A neurovascular examination should be performed before and after reduction and immobilization to ensure that patient's neurovascular status remains intact.

Finally, orthopedic consultation should be obtained to plan definitive care and to ensure appropriate follow-up and rehabilitation.

Cervical Spine

An overwhelming majority of trauma patients undergo spinal immobilization to prevent additional spinal cord injury in the event of vertebral fracture. Prior to the removal of spinal immobilization precautions, it is necessary to exclude bone and ligament injury. For decades, the standard of care for excluding body spine fracture was plain radiograph. This has included three views of the cervical spine (lateral, anterior–posterior, and odontoid) and imaging of the thoracolumbar spine. Recently, it has been demonstrated that plain x-rays may miss more than one third of all clinically significant fractures (Barrett, Mower, Zucker, & Hoffman, 2006; Richards, 2005). This has prompted many traumatologists to move to CT imaging, particularly in patients in whom there is a high degree of suspicion for injury. Because these patients often have head-associated injuries, a CT scan from the skull base to the top of the thoracic spine is often obtained concurrently with brain imaging.

However, not all trauma patients require radiologic imaging. Clinical clearance of the spine can be carried out in the following circumstances (Hoffman, Mower, Wolfson, Todd, & Zucker, 2000; Richards, 2005; Stiell et al., 2001):

1. the patient is alert and oriented
2. absence of tenderness on palpation of the cervical spine
3. absence of focal neurological deficits
4. no significant distracting injuries
5. low risk mechanism of injury
6. age <65 years

Once bone injury has been excluded radiographically, the patient should be reassessed for tenderness of the cervical spine and pain with active range of motion. If there is no pain, the hard cervical collar can be removed. However, if pain is elicited with either of these maneuvers, the patient should be maintained in a cervical collar and imaged further for the possibility of ligament injury (e.g., cervical spine MRI or flexion–extension radiographs).

Because it is not possible to clinically clear the cervical spine of patients with diminished levels of consciousness (e.g., coma), two general approaches have been adopted. The first approach is to maintain the patient in cervical spine immobilization until they are sufficiently alert to permit clinical clearance. The second approach is to rule out ligamentous injury using MRI. Published literature is not definitive regarding which approach is better, because the sensitivity of MRI for ligament injuries is still a matter of debate (Richards, 2005; Stassen, Williams, Gestring, Cheng, & Bankey, 2006).

Pelvic Fractures

The pelvis is a ring-like bone structure located at the base of the spine. In addition to its role as a supportive structure, the pelvis also serves to protect the lower abdominal viscera and vessels from injury. This protective role can be a double-edged sword because pelvic fractures also have the potential to cause significant internal injury. Pelvic fractures are most commonly associated with urogenital (bladder and urethra), gastrointestinal (rectal), and vascular injuries. The latter group poses a significant problem for trauma physicians, because they can cause a significant amount of bleeding that is difficult to control. Unlike vessels in the extremity, bleeding pelvic veins and arteries are typically covered by bone and are not amenable to external compression. Moreover, even in the operating room, pelvic vessels are extraordinarily difficult to expose and control.

The initial assessment of pelvic fractures is similar to that of other skeletal structures. The pelvic bones are inspected and palpated for tenderness and deformity. The perineum and urogenitalia are also examined for possible injury. A digital rectal examination is mandatory to rule out an open pelvic fracture and to assess for a high-riding prostate in men. A thorough vascular examination is conducted with special attention to femoral and lower extremity pulses. The diagnosis is confirmed with a standard anterior–posterior plain x-ray.

In the face of hemodynamic instability, treatment begins with the primary survey and institution of appropriate resuscitative measures. Because pelvic fractures are ubiquitous in the bluntly injured patient, a search for alternate sources of bleeding is critical. Thoracic and abdominal bleeding is excluded with careful clinical examination and radiologic imaging, including chest x-ray and trauma ultrasound or DPL. Long-bone fractures are another source of ongoing bleeding that need to be ruled out. As previously discussed, patients with hemodynamic instability and intraperitoneal fluid on ultrasound generally require an exploratory laparotomy for definitive surgical hemostasis.

Certain types of pelvic fractures are amenable to external reduction for control of venous bleeding. In particular, anterior–posterior compression injuries tend to result in disruption of the pubic symphysis and/or sacroiliac joints and can cause an opening of the pelvic ring or "open-book" fracture. As the pelvic ring opens and the bone volume increases, bridging vessels are at significant risk of being torn. Fortunately, reclosing the pelvic ring and reducing the bony volume can often arrest this form of bleeding. This can be accomplished using various commercially available pelvic binders or simply tightening a bed sheet around the patient's waist and upper thighs. If blood loss continues despite the use of a pelvic binder and there is no evidence of intraperitoneal bleeding, patients should undergo angioembolization in the interventional suite to stop possible arterial bleeding. In select circumstances, surgeons may elect to proceed to the operating room to tamponade the bleeding with extraperitoneal packing. A definitive stabilization procedure, if needed, will be conducted after the patient is resuscitated and medically stable for the procedure.

Summary

The management of trauma patients who have serious illness requires knowledge of current evidence-based standards of care, sound practitioner judgment, and a careful and thorough approach to initial patient assessment. Identification and subsequent treatment of injuries should follow established clinical algorithms, in order of priority, as described above. Completeness of the primary and secondary surveys are vitally important to fully understand the patient's injuries and to ensure their prompt treatment. Prompt identification and early resuscitation of shock states is crucial in achieving optimal patient outcomes and in minimizing organ dysfunction during and after the acute phase of patient care.

Online Resources

http://www.facs.org/trauma/index.html (American College of Surgeons-Trauma Programs)

http://www.amtrauma.org (American Trauma Society)

http://www.cdc.gov/ncipc (National Center for Injury Control and Prevention)

http://www.trauma.org (non-profit educational organization)

http://www.aast.org (American Association for the Surgery of Trauma)

References

American College of Surgeons Committee on Trauma. (2004). *Advanced Trauma Life Support* (7th ed.). Chicago, Illinois: ACS.

Barrett, T., Mower, W., Zucker, M., & Hoffman, J. (2006). Injuries missed by limited computed tomographic imaging of patients with cervical spine injuries. *Annals of Emergency Medicine, 47*(2), 129–133.

Bulger, E., Arneson, M., Mock, C., & Jurkovich, G. (2000). Rib fractures in the elderly. *Journal of Trauma, 48*(6), 1040–1046; discussion 1046–1047.

Corso, P., Finkelstein, E., Miller, T., Fiebelkorn, I., & Zaloshnja, E. (2006). Incidence and lifetime costs of injuries in the United States. *Injury Prevention: Journal of the International Society for Child and Adolescent Injury Prevention, 12*(4), 212–218.

Harkess, J. W., Ramsey, C. W., & Harkess, J. W. (1991). Biomechanics of fractures. In D. P. Green & R. W. Bucholz (Eds.), *Fractures in adults*. New York: Lippincott.

Hoffman, J., Mower, W., Wolfson, A., Todd, K., & Zucker, M. (2000). Validity of a set of clinical criteria to rule out injury to the cervical spine in patients with blunt trauma. National Emergency X-Radiography Utilization Study Group. *The New England Journal of Medicine, 343*(2), 94–99.

Leigh–Smith, S., & Harris, T. (2005). Tension pneumothorax—time for a rethink? *Emergency Medicine Journal, 22*(1), 8–16

Mackenzie, E. J., & Fowler, C. J. (2008). Epidemiology. In D. V. Feliciano, K. L. Mattox, & E. E. Moore, *Trauma* (6th ed., pp. 25–40). New York: McGraw Hill.

Meyer, D. (2007). Hemothorax related to trauma. *Thoracic surgery clinics, 17*(1), 47–55.

Richards, P. J. (2005). Cervical spine clearance: A review. *Injury, 36,* 248–269.

Spodick, D. (2003). Acute cardiac tamponade. *The New England Journal of Medicine, 349*(7), 684–690.

Stassen, N., Williams, V., Gestring, M., Cheng, J., & Bankey, P. (2006). Magnetic resonance imaging in combination with helical computed tomography provides a safe and efficient method of cervical spine clearance in the obtunded trauma patient. *Journal of Trauma, 60*(1), 171–177.

Stiell, I., Wells, G., Vandemheen, K., Clement, C., Lesiuk, H., De Maio, V., et al. (2001). The Canadian C-spine rule for radiography in alert and stable trauma patients. *JAMA, 286*(15), 1841–1848.

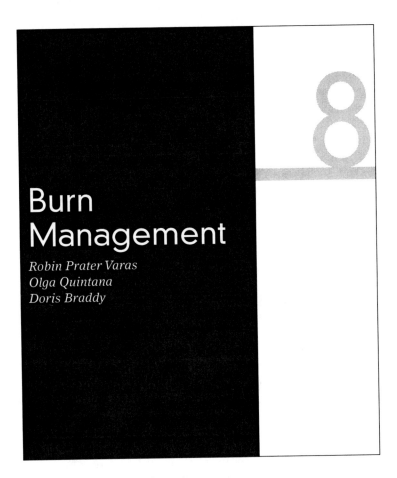

Burn Management

Robin Prater Varas
Olga Quintana
Doris Braddy

Introduction

Approximately 1.25 million people are burned yearly in the United States; 50,000 of these require hospitalization, and 4,500 die annually. Care of the critically burned patient requires a multidisciplinary team approach to provide the comprehensive, coordinated, long-term care required for the best outcome. Major burn injuries should be cared for in a burn center (U.S. Fire Administration [FEMA], 2008; Centers for Disease Control [CDC]; Pruit, Wolf, & Madison, 2007).

The Acute Care Nurse Practitioner (ACNP) is in a prime position to orchestrate this care to ensure consistency and continuity of care and to facilitate communication among all team members. The principles of Advanced Trauma Life Support (ATLS) apply to all burn patients. Initial care of the burn patient is similar to that of critically ill patients with other diseases or multiple trauma. Burn patients are considered trauma patients first until proven otherwise. The extent or appearance of the burn injury should not distract from the ABC's of the primary survey. Initial attention is focused on hemodynamic stability, including fluid and electrolyte balance, respiratory support and ventilation, surveillance of infections with appropriate culture-directed antibiotic coverage, release of pressure in compartments influenced by restrictive eschar, early nutritional support, and monitoring for adrenal insufficiency.

The integumentary system is the largest organ system in the body. It is the body's first line of defense against infection, body fluid loss, and thermal regulation. When the integrity of the skin is breached because of severe burn injury, the entire body is affected. The magnitude of the physiologic response is dependent on the depth, extent, and the cause of the burn.

The outermost layer of the skin is the epidermis. The epidermis has five stratified layers containing diversified cell types. These include keratinocytes, which provide strength, flexibility, and waterproofing by producing the protein keratin. Merkel cells are sensory cells for touch reception. Melanocytes produce the melanin that pigments the skin and helps to protect against ultraviolet rays. Langerhans cells in the epidermis help regulate the immune response to external antigens. Burns involving only the epidermis are considered first degree. First-degree burns are erythematous and locally painful. There are no blisters, and the skin retains its ability to prevent invasion of microorganisms and retain the protection from fluid and electrolyte losses. For this reason, first-degree burns have little physiologic impact on the body and are not included when calculating the extent of burn (Patal & Hartman, 2005).

The second layer of the skin is the dermis. The dermis is the living layer that consists of fibroelastic connective tissues. The layer just below the epidermis is the papillary layer, which contains Meissner corpuscles. These layers are sensory touch receptors and are the microcirculation that delivers nutrition to the epidermis.

The deeper reticular layer of the dermis contains most of the fibroblasts that produce the protein collagen, reticular fibers, and elastin, that combine with nonfibrous substances such as glucosaminoglycans to form the extracellular matrix, which provides strength, structure, and elasticity to the skin. Also located in the reticular layer of the dermis are the sensory receptors for pain and deep touch called the Pacinian corpuscles and lymph vessels.

Skin appendages, including sebaceous glands, apocrine and eccrine sweat glands, and hair follicles originate within the dermis or just below the dermal subcutaneous junction. The region of the hair follicle known as the *follicular bulge* is the area responsible for regeneration of skin cells and sebaceous glands following injury (Bessy, 2007). The smooth muscles located in the dermis aid in temperature regulation. Burns that destroy the entire epidermis and extend into the dermis are considered second-degree or partial-thickness burns. Superficial partial-thickness injury extends into the superficial papillary layer and is characterized by fluid-filled blisters. These wounds are very moist and painful but usually heal in 2–4 weeks.

Deep partial-thickness burns involve the entire dermis, both the papillary and reticular layer, but the skin appendages are spared. They are characterized by formation of dead and devitalized tissue called *eschar*. The eschar is dry, inelastic, and may be yellow or brown in color. Deep partial-thickness wounds take several weeks for the epidermis to regenerate depending on the number of surviving hair follicles. Wounds that extend into the reticular dermis and heal secondarily take 3 or more weeks to heal and have a greater potential for hypertrophic scarring (Bessy, 2007).

The third layer of the skin is the subcutaneous layer. The adipose tissue insulates and pads the body and gives the body form. The subcutaneous tissue contains blood vessels and lymph vessels. Burns into the subcutaneous layer are considered third-degree or full-thickness burns. The wound will have a thick, dry, leathery eschar that is lacking in elasticity because the entire extracellular matrix has been destroyed. Full-thickness injuries are insensate because of the loss of the nerves that are located in the dermal layer (Standring, 2005; Revis & Seagle, 2006).

Pathophysiology

When the skin comes in contact with a heat source, a burn injury occurs. In 1953, Jackson described three zones of tissue injury that results following a thermal injury. The zone of coagulation is the area that has the most contact with the heat source. This consists of dead and dying cells as a result of coagulation necrosis and is devoid of blood supply. The wound may appear white or charred. Adjacent to the zone of coagulation is an area characterized by capillary vasoconstriction and ischemia called the zone of stasis. The tissues in this area contain a combination of nonviable, damaged, and viable cells. These potentially viable cells could convert to a zone of coagulation as a result of edema, decreased perfusion, or infection. The cells in the zone of stasis appear deep red and may have petechial hemorrhages. The third zone, the zone of hyperemia, is more distant from the heat source. Inflammatory mediators incite vasodilatation. The cells in this area will typically remain viable (Pham, Gibran, & Heimbach).

A major goal of wound management is to protect the viability of the zone of stasis to promote wound healing with desirable cosmetic and functional outcomes. Several factors have been attributed to the progressive demise of cells in the zone of stasis. Thromboxane A_2 is produced by platelets in the wound, causing vasoconstriction and increasing the ischemia beneath the wound. The release of prostaglandin derivatives and oxygen free radicals, such as xanthine oxidase, in the burn wounds contribute to vasodilatation and the formation of burn edema, decreased tissue perfusion, and can increase the depth of the burn wound from partial to full thickness.

Adults with thermal injury extending over 20% of their body surface area experience both a local and systemic response to the tissue injury that begins immediately postburn. The major physiologic effects that occur in the first 24–48 hours postburn are concentrated around fluid losses caused by an increased capillary permeability, an increased intravascular hydrostatic pressure, and a negative pressure in the interstitial tissues at the site of the injury (Shirani, Vaughhan, Mason, & Pruitt, 1996).

At the time of injury, the thermally injured cells release histamine from their mast cells, causing immediate increase in capillary permeability. Macrophages and neutrophils infiltrate the wound, releasing prostaglandins into the general circulation. The prostaglandins promote vasodilatation and increased capillary permeability. As the capillaries become more permeable, plasma proteins are permitted to enter the interstitial space, exerting colloid osmotic pressure, causing rapid and sometimes massive edema to form. Because of the massive leak of fluids and resultant edema, patients experience intravascular hypovolemia.

The resultant decrease in perfusion and oxygen delivery to the tissues leads to further cellular damage and ischemia. Ischemia stimulates a release of catecholamines, vasopressin, and angiotensin that cause peripheral and splanchnic bed vasoconstriction, affecting all of the major organ systems including the heart. Myocardial contractility may be reduced because of the circulating inflammatory cytokines, tumor necrosis factor-α, and oxygen free radicals (Horton, White, Maass, & Sanders, 2004). The reduced cardiac contractility exacerbates the ischemic problem by shunting blood away from the liver, kidneys, and gut. Burn injury also causes changes at the cellular membrane level. In a major burn, this occurs systemically and is not isolated to the thermally injured cells. The cellular transmembrane potential is decreased, resulting in an alteration of the sodium–potassium pump, thus increasing cellular edema (Morris, 2006).

A cycle is established of inflammatory mediator-induced capillary permeability causing increasing edema, hypovolemia, and hyperviscosity, which in turn leads to tissue ischemia, acidosis, reduced cardiac function, and multiorgan dysfunction. The ensuing acidosis and reduced oxygenation of the tissues leads to further cellular destruction, releasing more vasoactive mediators. Burn shock results from the massive fluid leak, changes in hydrostatic pressures, and cardiac and multiorgan system failure. The cycle will continue in a downward spiral without aggressive intervention. The goal of fluid resuscitation is to deliver an adequate supply of oxygen to the cells by providing adequate tissue perfusion (Cartotto, Choi, Gomez, & Cooper, 2003).

Compartment Syndrome

The elastic properties of the skin are lost in deep partial-thickness or full-thickness wounds. When the burn edema develops beneath the nonelastic eschar, the skin is unable to expand to accommodate the increased fluid mass. If the wound is circumferential, the result is increased pressure in the compartments of the extremities. Initially, the increased pressure occludes the venous outflow, causing pressure to build up rapidly until the pressure increases enough to halt arterial capillary inflow. When the pressure exceeds the capillary filling pressure, the blood supply is cut off from the extremity, resulting in death of the muscle. Muscular infarction produces release of myoglobin, edema, and acidosis. If the pressure is not released, death of the extremity will ensue (American Burn Association, 2001).

Metabolic Response

As with other forms of major trauma, the stress response is triggered in response to burn injury. The stress response in patients with burns over 40% of their total body surface area (TBSA) causes increased metabolic rates up to twice the normal increased oxygen consumption, accelerated fat breakdown, and erosion of body mass. The hypermetabolic, hypercatabolic state peaks within the first 1–2 weeks and progressively returns to normal in the months following wound closure. Increased protein consumption associated with the hypermetabolic state hinders the immune response and slows wound healing (Norbury & Henderson, 2007).

Postburn Anemia

Postburn anemia occurs in patient with thermal injuries over 10% of their body surface area. Initially, there is a trapping of red blood cells in thrombosed capillaries as well as destruction of the erythrocytes from the heat. The inflammatory mediators that are released following thermal injury work to decrease the life span of the erythrocyte from their normal 80–120 days. Production of new red blood cells is slowed because of bone marrow suppression. These factors, added to the loss of blood during dressing changes, excision of wounds, and phlebotomy, lead to significant anemia in patients with major burns (Kwan, Gomez, & Cartotto, 2006).

Inhalation Injury

Respiratory pathophysiology in a burn patient results directly from thermal injury to the upper airway, inhalation of smoke and the by-products of combustion, and indirectly from the pulmonary response to the inflammatory mediators. Thermal injury to the airways is rare. Usually, this occurs secondary to the exposure to superheated steam, inhalation of scalding liquids, or flammable gases under pressure. Thermal injury of the airway is usually limited to the upper airway, because the larynx closes as a reflex to the superheated air. Resultant edema of the structures in the upper airway may cause obstruction of the airway. When the fluid resuscitation progresses and the edema expands, progressive worsening of the airway obstruction is to be anticipated (McCall & Cahill, 2005).

Inhalation injuries that occur below the glottis are usually chemical in nature as a result of the noxious chemicals that are released during a fire. In the course of a fire, organic carbon containing substances burn, and carbon monoxide is formed as a by-product of incomplete combustion. Carbon monoxide combines to the body's hemoglobin molecules, creating carboxyhemoglobin. The carbon monoxide has an affinity for hemoglobin that is 200 times greater than that of oxygen. Oxygen delivery to the cells is decreased as a result of the decreased oxygen-carrying capacity of the hemoglobin, as well as the fact that greater affinity blocks the release of the oxygen to the tissues (McCall & Cahill, 2005). Normal blood concentration of carboxyhemoglobin is <1%. Smokers and people who are exposed to heavy traffic have a carboxyhemoglobin around 5% to 10%. Although 15% to 40% of the hemoglobin is bound to carbon monoxide, the victim may experience various symptoms of cerebral hypoxia, including impaired judgment and confusion. Carboxyhemoglobin levels of 40% to 60% causes patients to become obtunded and may cause subsequent loss of consciousness. Levels above 60% lead to unconsciousness, respiratory failure, and death (American Burn Association, 2001).

When plastics and synthetic materials are consumed by fire, hydrogen cyanide is released. Hydrogen cyanide causes inhibition of the cytochrome oxidase system by binding with the ferric iron atom, rendering the cells incapable of using any available oxygen. The cells convert to anaerobic production of ATP, and lactic acid is produced. The result is increased hypoxia and metabolic acidosis (Schraga & Pennardt, 2008). When both carbon monoxide and hydrogen cyanide is present, there is a synergistic effect that increases tissue hypoxia and acidosis and further decreases cerebral oxygen consumption (Traber, Herndon, Enkhbaatar, Maybauer, & Maybauer, 2007).

Noxious chemicals such as aldehydes, sulfur oxides, and phosgenes are released and carried on the surface of the smoke particles. When they come in contact with the epithelium of the airways, the ciliary activity is impaired, reducing the body's ability to clear the noxious agents. The inflammatory process is initiated including hypersecretion, edema formation, increased blood flow, and ulceration of the mucosa. The timing of the onset of symptoms of an inhalation injury is unpredictable and depends in part on the volume of smoke inhaled. The bronchi and the bronchioles may go into severe spasm with higher doses of smoke inhalation. Wheezing and respiratory distress will occur immediately in patients with prolonged exposure to a smoke-filled environment. The edema formation and inflammatory response may not be evident initially but will increase with fluid resuscitation. Mucosal sloughing may occur as late as 4–5 days postinjury, so patients with history that suggests a high suspicion of inhalation injury need to be observed closely (American Burn Association, 2001).

Clinical Manifestations/Symptoms

Criteria for admission of a burn victim into the intensive care unit include the following:

- Adults with burns >20% TBSA
- Pediatrics with burns >10%–15% TBSA
- Inhalation injury
- High voltage electrical injury
- Patients with premorbid diseases such as diabetes, cardiac, or renal disease
- Full-thickness injuries
- Associated trauma
- Extremes of age

Neurological. Burn victims are generally awake, alert, and oriented on admission, if not, look for associated trauma. Changes in level of consciousness occur with hypovolemia, medications, and smoke inhalation. Patients may be fearful, distraught, agitated, anxious, and in pain as a result of the events surrounding the accident. Suspected hypoxia or hypovolemia must be ruled out immediately. Obtaining the patient's medical and social history, including the details of the accident, is a priority if the patient is stabilized. A proxy or health care surrogate should be named, and advanced directives should be initiated prior to intubation or sedation when possible.

Pulmonary. Pulmonary dysfunction is a major cause of death in burn victims. Patients with inhalation injury may present with or without cutaneous burns. A history of being in an enclosed space during a fire should raise an index of suspicion for inhalation injury. Signs and symptoms of inhalation injury include singed nasal or facial hair, facial burns, hoarseness, agitation, and carbonaceous sputum. Presence of symptoms does not necessitate immediate intubation but does require 24-hour observation for signs of airway compromise. Signs and symptoms of inhalation injury may not be present until 18–36 hours post injury. Chest radiograph and arterial blood gases may have normal results in the first 24 hours. Direct laryngoscopy can be used to visualize the upper airway if there is a suspicion of injury. Visualization of erythema, edema, ulceration, and soot deposits makes bronchoscopy useful in evaluating the extent of injury to the tracheobronchial tree (Serebrisky, Nazarian, & Connolly, 2008). The presence of carbonaceous material, edema, erythema, or lesions below the vocal cords confirms the diagnosis of inhalation injury.

Initial and ongoing assessment includes monitoring for the actual or potential loss of the airway. Extensive face or neck burns, hoarseness, or stridor may necessitate early intubation. Tracheal intubation should be considered early before progressive edema, exacerbated by fluid resuscitation, begins to compromise the airway in patients with extensive burns of the face and neck. The head of the bed should be elevated 30–45 degrees to help decrease facial edema. Supplemental humidified oxygen is initiated on all burn patients and patients with suspected inhalation injury.

Serial blood gases will reveal metabolic acidosis and abnormal carboxyhemoglobin levels. Carbon monoxide decreases the blood oxygen content and hinders the release of oxygen from hemoglobin to the tissues. Pulse oximetry values may be normal, because it monitors saturation and makes no distinction between carbon monoxide and oxygen.

Treatment for carbon monoxide poisoning is supplemental oxygen at 100%. The supplemental oxygen hastens the dissociation of carbon monoxide from hemoglobin in direct relation to the partial pressure of oxygen. Treatment continues until values are normal.

Treatment for smoke inhalation injury is supportive.

- Auscultate breath sounds.
- Monitor chest excursion and need for escharotomies.
- Observe depth and rate of respirations.
- Observe need for suctioning.
- Note the color, consistency, and amount of the sputum.
- Continually reassess the patient for the need for intubation and ventilatory support.

Ongoing fluid resuscitation may compromise the airway by edema formation that necessitates continual reassessment for the need of intubation and ventilatory support. Use of the high-frequency percussive ventilator has been shown to reduce mortality in inhalation injury with further human trials ongoing. (Sanford & Herndon, 2001).

Circumferential full-thickness burns of the torso may impede respiratory excursion, making it difficult to ventilate the patient because of the inelasticity of burn eschar. Increased peak inspiratory pressures (PIPs), decreased tidal volumes, or inability to adequately ventilate the patient with a bag valve mask may indicate the need for escharotomies of the torso. Tracheostomy may be indicated in special situations. Indications include prolonged intubation, emergent airway access, facial trauma, and deep partial-thickness or full-thickness wounds of the face or neck with significant edema.

Cardiovascular. Major burn injuries cause a dramatic increase in catecholamine release, resulting in tachycardia and increased myocardial work. Burn shock follows the same pathway as other forms of hypovolemic shock including decreased venous return, ventricular filling pressures, stroke volume and cardiac output with resultant hypotension, increased peripheral vascular resistance, and decreased tissue perfusion. Decreased tissue perfusion can increase the depth of the burn wound from partial to full thickness.

Monitor adequate circulation by palpating peripheral pulses and checking capillary refill. Monitor for signs of compartment syndrome in circumferentially burned extremities and torso. Circumferentially burned extremities should be elevated continually above heart level to help decrease edema formation. Monitor hourly intake and output, vital signs, and heart rhythm. Fluid requirements exceeding calculated resuscitation amounts after 24 hours suggest an inhalation component to the injury.

Patients with electrical injuries may have sustained ventricular fibrillation at the scene and may have received CPR. Sinus tachycardia and nonspecific ST-T segment changes remain the most common cardiac findings. Most arrhythmias seen on admission spontaneously resolve in a few hours. Patients who present in the emergency room without evidence of cardiac arrhythmia rarely develop them later.

Progressive anemia because of loss of cell mass and decrease in the half-life of the red blood cell leads to low hematocrit, so monitor trends. Transfuse the patient only if the patient is symptomatic, has a cardiac history, or has poor oxygenation. Blood transfusion increases the infection and mortality rates in critically ill burn patients. The accepted trigger point for transfusion is 7g/dl and 21%. (Palmieri, Caruso, Foster, Cairns, Peck, Gamelli et al., 2006).

Fluid Management. Massive fluid shifts occur in the first 24 hours after a major burn injury, which leads to hypovolemic shock and death if interventions are not initiated. Two large-bore IVs are inserted for initial fluid resuscitation. Intravenous catheters can be placed through burn eschar if access is difficult. Increased capillary permeability leads to loss of fluid and plasma proteins into the interstitial space. Burn edema occurs in burned tissue and in unburned tissue, causing sodium to be translocated into skeletal muscle and other tissues through the leaky capillaries. Large amounts of fluid are required to maintain hemodynamic stability, and often patients are under-resuscitated because of fear of volume overload.

There are various burn fluid resuscitation formulas. The American Burn Association's consensus formula is commonly used to guide the resuscitation. The formula is as follows: ringers lactate 2–4 ml/kg of body weight per percent of TBSA burned (4 ml × kg × % burn). First-degree burns are not included in the TBSA. One half of the calculated volume is given in the first 8 hours post burn and the second half is given over the next 16 hours.

For example, a 70-kg man with a 50% TBSA burn would require 4 ml × 70 kg × 50% = 14,000 ml over 24 hr. Therefore, 7,000 ml would be infused over the first 8 hours at 875 ml/hr and 7,000 ml over the next 16 hours at a rate of 438 ml/hr.

Glucose is not initially used because of glucose intolerance and potential for glycosuria that could lead to an osmotic diuresis, thereby eliminating the urine output as an accurate monitoring tool for fluid management. In addition to the calculated fluid resuscitation, a vitamin C drip may be administered at a rate of 66 mg·kg^{-1}·hr^{-1} for the first 24 hours. Vitamin C has been shown to decrease the required resuscitation volume and decrease the number of ventilator days (Tanaka et al., 2000).

The 24-hour timeframe for initiating fluid resuscitation begins at the time of injury, not at the time of arrival to the hospital. The formulas are guidelines and are based on individual patient response. The rate of resuscitation fluid is based on hourly urine output via a Foley catheter. The urine is monitored hourly and should be 0.5 ml·kg^{-1}·hr^{-1} or 30–50 ml/hr (American Burn Association, 2001). The exception is electrical injuries, where an increased urine output is warranted and should be >100 cc/hr to avoid the accumulation of hemachromagens in the renal tubules. Sodium bicarbonate may be given to alkalinize the urine to avoid clumping of the hemachromagens, which occurs in an acid environment and may block the renal tubules. If the urine output requirements are greater or less than the calculated resuscitation amounts, increase or decrease the intravenous rate by 25%. Fluid boluses result in an increase in intravascular hydrostatic pressure and are therefore lost in the tissues. If the fluid required exceeds the calculated amounts by 2–3 times at the end of the 24-hour period, this is indicative of an inhalation component to the burn injury. The resuscitation formulas do not take into account fluid loss from the leaky pulmonary capillaries. Practitioners who are inexperienced in the care of burn patients often underresuscitate patients because of the enormous volume of fluids that patients require to maintain hemodynamic stability.

Hematocrits initially can be in the 50–60 g/dl range because of hemoconcentration. The hematocrit will begin to trend down with adequate fluid replacement. Capillary leak begins to resolve in 24 hours, preventing the leak of fluids into the interstitium. Colloids are started after the first 24 hours of resuscitation to assist mobilization of fluid into the intra-vascular space where it is excreted. Loss of plasma proteins contributes to the loss of intravascular fluid. Colloids, such as salt-poor albumin in drip form, will help replace the proteins once the capillary leak has been resolved.

The use of central lines and pulmonary artery catheters has limited use during the initial resuscitation period. The central venous pressure (CVP) and the pulmonary artery occlusion pressures (PAO) will read below normal because of the fluid shifts from the intravascular space. There is a risk of overloading patients with fluid during the resuscitation because normal CVP and PAO pressures will be elusive until the capillary leak resolves in 18–24 hours.

Renal

Renal failure is rare in appropriately resuscitated patients in the early phase of care. Decreased urine output, decreased cardiac output, accumulation of hemachroma-gens in the renal tubules, and underresuscitation can lead to acute tubular necrosis. The use of diuretics during the primary resuscitation phase is contraindicated except in rare instances.

Infection Control

The first line of defense against the invasion of microorgan-isms is breached with loss of the skin. Infection remains the number one cause of death in the burn patients. Central lines are guidewired every 3 days and sent for culture until the burn wounds close. According to CDC recommenda-tions, routine guidewire exchange of central venous cath-eters (CVC) should not be done after burn wounds close, and timing of replacement of CVCs is a matter of some debate. Positive catheter segment culture (>15 cfu) war-rant the removal of the line (King, Schulman, Pepe et al., 2007). Prophylactic antibiotics are not routinely given in burn patients. Surveillance for infection is constant, and administration of antibiotics is culture driven. Empiric anti-biotics are initiated when signs of sepsis appear without a documented source while awaiting culture results. Broad-spectrum antibiotics are initiated and should be guided by unit or hospital-specific antibiograms until speciation of the bacteria is identified.

Temperature Regulation

Heat loss through an open burn wound can be excessive; therefore, keeping the environment warm with radiant heating devices is imperative. The temperature in the operating room is usually 80–90° F. Use of warming catheters has been useful in maintaining patients' core temperature during long operative procedures. Warm blankets, warm fluids, and covering the patient's head aid in heat conservation.

Temperature regulation of the hypothalamus is reset after a major burn injury. Burn patients are hypermetabolic and suffer the effects of the systemic inflammatory response. Unless there is a change in mental status or vital signs, patients do not need to have cultures ordered secondary to fever in the first 4–5 days post injury.

Drug pharmacokinetics can be altered in patients with major burn because of altered capillary permeability, loss of plasma proteins from the intravascular space, and edema that increase the volume of distribution (Weinbren, 1999). For this reason, systemic antibiotics are frequently given at higher than normal doses to burn patients. Antibiotic serum concentrations are monitored for proper dosing.

Burn Wound Management

Calculation of TBSA is required because fluid resuscitation formulas are based on this percentage. The Lund–Browder burn sheets are used to accurately estimate the percent of the body burned. The percentages take into consideration the body parts that change with age such as the head, thighs, and lower legs. For example, a burn wound of a 2-year old whose entire head is burned would calculate to be 13%, compared with the adult head, which would be 7%. The palm and fingers of the patient's hand equals approximately 1% and can be used to calculate the percent of burn. This method is useful for wounds that are scattered over the body in a splatter-type pattern, which occur when an agent like tar or grease spill onto a body part. The burn wound is the source of the systemic response seen clinically when the body reacts to the dead and dying tissue.

In electrical injuries, the appearance of the outer cutaneous burn wound is not reflective of the extent of damage below the burned or nonburned skin. This type of wound is described as the "tip of the iceberg." Electrical current that enters and exits the body produces the most damage where current meets the most resistance. Bone creates the most resistance and, therefore, the most heat damage. These types of injuries usually result in some form of amputation. Technetium-99 pyrophosphate scanning of an extremity can aid in deciding whether to amputate and/or attempt to save the limb when the degree of injury is not obvious by direct observation.

The goal of wound management is to prevent infection, expedite wound closure, and prevent conversion of the wound to a deeper level. Infection or desiccation of the burn can cause conversion of the wound from a partial-thickness injury to a full-thickness injury. Burn wounds at the extremes of age are deceptive in the first 24–48 hours because of the thinness of the skin. In the elderly and young children, viewing the wounds initially may provide a false sense of the burn wound depth, because it may appear superficial. After 24 hours, what was thought to be a nonoperative, superficial wound, often results in a deep wound requiring excision and/or grafting for wound closure.

The depth of the wound is determined by skin structures and layers that have been damaged or destroyed. When describing the burn wounds, it is important not to fixate on correctly naming or classifying the wounds according to the depth. The best way to document the appearance of the wound is to describe what is observed or assessed. For example, description of the wound may include, color, absence or presence of hair follicles, absence or presence of pain, and whether there is blanching of the wound with applied pressure. A wound that is pink, clean, moist, and painful to touch with intact hair follicles usually indicates a partial-thickness injury. Eschar is a dead devitalized tissue and is often confused with the protein exudates or pseudoeschar that accompanies partial-thickness wounds. Eschar that is dry, leathery, nonblanching with pressure, and anesthetic to pain is indicative of a full-thickness injury. Deep circumferential burns of the extremities or thorax can cause a tourniquet-like effect because of the inelasticity of the eschar. This can be exacerbated by the edema formation that occurs with the fluid resuscitation.

In circumferentially burned extremities, it is important to perform hourly neurovascular checks to assess the compartments. Checking capillary refill, palpating the compartments for tightness and measuring compartment pressures are effective tools for evaluating compromise. Patients who are responsive may be able to describe tingling and numbness in the extremities, which may be the first sign of compromise.

Removal of eschar can be done through surgical, enzymatic, or biomedical debridement (maggots). Wounds are cleansed with soap and tap water, and then covered with an antimicrobial topical cream such as silver sulfadiazine. Ionic silver has antimicrobial properties, and there are various commercially available dressings that contain ionic silver that can be used to cover the wound. The dressings can be left in place and provide antimicrobial coverage for 4–7 days depending on the product. This avoids the painful twice-daily dressings that include removal of the antimicrobial topical agent, which have been the mainstay of burn care. The occlusive dressings protect the nerve endings, decrease evaporative losses, decrease pain, decrease nursing time, and decrease the amount of pain medications used for dressing changes.

The natural contraction of wounds that are healing secondarily puts patients at risk for contractures. The position of comfort is the position of deformity for burn patients. Occupational and physical therapists follow their patients on a daily basis for passive or active range of motion exercises involving joints and foot drop, such as splinting of extremities to avoid contracture formation. The therapists assist in developing a positioning program to counteract the contractile forces of wound healing. Applying the splints and adjunctive equipment as ordered by the therapist facilitate optimization of function.

Burn patients requiring wound care may be uncooperative, restless, and confused. Hypoxia and hypovolemia must be assessed and evaluated, before assuming that it is pain or anxiety. Once these have been ruled out, patients may be medicated with intravenous opioids and anxiolytics in small increments after resuscitation fluids are infusing. Medications are given intravenously; no intramuscular medications (except for tetanus prophylaxis) are given during the resuscitation period. Medications given intramuscularly will become sequestered in the muscle. Once the capillary leak subsides, remobilization of fluid back into the general circulation can cause an overdose of the medication.

Burn wounds are the source of the most unimaginable pain one can experience. Burn wound pain increases as the wounds progress toward healing because of the exposure of nerve endings to the environment once the eschar or protein layer is removed and the edema resolved. Pain management revolves around three types of pain, namely, background pain, procedural pain, and breakthrough pain. Intubated burn patients in the intensive care unit may be placed on fentanyl- and propofol-continuous infusions. Additional medications are given prior to dressing changes and physical or occupational therapy.

Nutrition

Major burn injuries cause a dramatic alteration in metabolism, leading to hypermetabolism and hypercatabolism. Metabolic rates of burn patients can exceed 2–3 times normal and can cause tremendous wasting of lean body mass within a few weeks of injury. The hyperdynamic state and hypermetabolism require increased nutritional requirements. On admission, small silastic feeding tubes are inserted, and enteral feeds are started to avoid malnutrition. Various formulas are available in calculating individualized caloric requirement, which should include 100:1 or 150:1 kilocalories (kcal) to nitrogen.

Gastric and duodenal ulceration has long been recognized as a complication of burn injury. (McAlhany, Colmic Czaja, & Pruitt, 1976) Mucosal ulceration prophylaxis is accomplished by early administration of enteral feedings. H2 blocker or proton pump inhibitors in combination with antacids should be added to maintain a gastric pH above 5 (Mozingo & Mason, 2007). Monitoring of nutrition laboratories and following the trends can be useful in guiding caloric intake. When possible, patients should be weighed weekly. The administration of oxandrolone, an anabolic steroid, has been shown to limit muscle wasting in patients with large burn injuries, with less androgenic effects. Oxandrolone can be given orally. Patients on regular diets with poor appetites also benefit from the addition of appetite stimulants such as dronabinol. Nutritional requirements in patients with major burn injuries exceed 2–3 times the normal daily caloric intake and may increase with associated injuries.

Maintaining high ambient temperature and relative humidity can reduce caloric requirements by up to 20%. Antibiotics and routine early burn wound excision have reduced infection and modulated hypermetabolism. In addition, covering burn wounds with autograft, allograft, or synthetic substitutes shortens the duration of hypermetabolism. Mechanical ventilation and chemical sedation or paralysis reduce energy requirements.

Several formulas for calculating nutritional requirements are available The major energy source for burn patients should be carbohydrates. Glucose is the preferred fuel for healing wounds (Saffle & Graves, 2007). Protein catabolism can exceed 150 g/day; as burn size increases progressively, more protein is required for positive nitrogen balance (Matsuda, Kagan, Hanumadass, & Jonasson, 1983). Current recommendations require 1.5–2.0 g of protein/kg of body weight per day. Enteral nutrition and high protein intake are important; expenditure needs fluctuate throughout hospitalization and need to be reevaluated frequently.

Prognosis and Outcome

The chance of survival from a burn injury has increased over the past several decades. Several risk factors identified by Ryan et al., (1998) continue to be the strongest predictors of death in the burn patient. These risk factors are age >60 years, a burn >40% of the body surface area, and the presence of inhalation injury. In the presence of no risk factors, patients' chance of mortality is 0.3%; patients with one risk factor have a 3% chance of mortality; patients with two risk factors have a 33% chance of mortality, and all patients with three risk factors have approximately a 90% chance of mortality. Other factors have also been identified as determining factors in the survival of the burn patient. In a study conducted on a national sample of over 31,000 burn patients the presence of preexisting medical conditions at admission increased the risk of mortality and required a longer hospital stay than patients of similar age, sex, and burn injury characteristics, but with less comorbidity (Thombs, Singh, &

Haloren, 2007). Predicting mortality for a burn patient is not the priority issue. The new challenge has become to facilitate an improved quality of life for patients who are surviving these injuries

Even after survival, patients will most likely encounter extended surgical, medical, psychological, and rehabilitation interventions for years. An expert in multidisciplinary burn care team to guide and support patients increases the probability of patients to obtain a desirable quality of life, because no longer is survival the sole goal and desired outcome; a successful outcome is determined by the ability of the burn survivor to be integrated back into the community with an acceptable quality of life as determined by the survivor. With no predetermined notion of what patients' definition of quality of life may be, this presents a challenge.

Recent studies have demonstrated that most burn survivors appear to have adjusted satisfactory to their limitations over time (Sheridan et al., 2000). The first year is usually plagued with physical difficulties and discomforts that are transient. Psychological adaptation continues over several years and should be periodically assessed by experts in the field. Massively burned individuals cannot be returned to their preinjury appearance and function, but the combination of expert acute care with supportive multidisciplinary rehabilitative care can produce satisfying long-term outcome.

References

American Burn Association. (2001). *Advanced burn life support provider's manual*. (A. A. Committee, Ed.) Chicago: American Burn Association.

Bessy, P. Q. (2007). Wound care. In D. N. Herndon, *Total burn care* (3rd ed., pp. 127–134). Philadelphia, PA: Saunders Elsevier.

Cartotto, R., Choi, J., Gomez, M., & Cooper, A. (2003). A prospective study on the implications of a base deficit during fluid resuscitation. *Journal of Burn Care and Rehabilitation, 24*, 75–84.

Centers for Disease Control and Prevention (CDC). (n.d.). *Fire deaths and injuries: Fact sheet*. Available at http://www.cdc.gov/ncipc/factsheets/fire.htm

Horton, J. W., White, D. J., Maass, D., & Sanders, B. (2004). Left ventricular contractile dysfunction as a complication of thermal injury. *Shock, 22*(6), 495–507.

Jackson, D. M. (1953). The diagnosis of the depth of burning. *British Journal of Surgery, 40*(164), 588–596.

Kramer, G. C., Tjostolv, L., & Beckum, O. K. (2007). Pathophysiology of burn shock. In D. N. Herndon, *Total burn care* (3rd ed., pp. 93–103). Philadelphia, PA: Saunders Elsevier.

Kwan, P., Gomez, M., & Cartotto, R. (2006). Safe and sucessful restriction of transfusion in burn patients. *Journal of Burn Care and Research 27*, 826–834.

King, B., Schulman, C., Pepe, A., et al. Timing of central venous catheter exchange and frequency of bacteremia in burn patients. *Journal of Burn Care and Research, 28*(6), 859–860. November/December 2007.

Matsuda, T., Kagan, R., Hanumadass, M., & Jonasson, O. (1983). The importance of burn wound size in determining the optimal calorie: Nitrogen ration. *Surgery, 94*, 562–568.

McAlhany, J. C. Jr., Colmic, L., Czaja, A. J., Pruitt B. A. Jr. (1976) Antacid control of complication from acute gastroduodenal disease after burns. *Journal of Trauma, 16*(08), 645–649.

McCall, J. E., & Cahill, T. J. (2005). Respiratory care of the burn patient. *Journal of Burn Care and Rehabilitation, 26*(3), 200–206.

Morris, S. E. (2006). Shock, multiple organ sysfunction syndrome, and burns in adults. In K. L. McCance, & S. E. Huether, *Pathophysiology: The biologic basis for disease in adults and children* (5th ed., pp. 1642–1651). Philadelphia, PA: Elsevier Mosby.

Mozingo, D. W., & Mason A. D. Jr. (2007). Hypophosphatemia. In D. N. Herndon (Ed.), *Total burn care* (3rd ed., pp. 392). Philadelphia, PA: Saunders Elsevier.

Norbury, W. B., & Herndon, D. N. (2007). Modulation of the hypermetabolic response after burn injury. In D. N. Herndon, *Total burn care* (pp. 420–421). Philadelphia, PA: Saunders Elsevier.

Palmeri, T. L., Caruso, D. M., Foster, K. N., Cairns, B. A., Peck, M. D., Gamelli, R. L., et al. (2006). Effect of blood transfusion on outcome after major burn injury: a multicenter study. *Critical Care Medicine 34*, 1602–1607.

Patal, N., & Hartman, J. K. (2005). Burn injuries. In L. E. C. Copstead, & J. L. Banasik, *Pathophysiology* (3rd ed., pp. 1338–1361). Philadelphia, PA: Elsevier/Saunders.

Pham, T. M., Gibran, N. S., & Heimbach, D. M. (2007). Evaluation of the burn wound. In D. N. Herndon, *Total burn care* (3rd ed., p. 120). Philadelphia, PA: Saunders Elsevier.

Pruit, B. A., Jr., Wolf, S. E., & Mason, A. D., Jr. (2007). Epidemiological, demographic, and outcome characteristics of burn injury. In D. N. Herndon (Ed.), *Total burn care* (3rd ed., pp. 14–32) Philadelphia: Elsevier Inc.

Revis, D. R., & Seagle, M. B. (2006, February 17). *Skin Anatomy*. Retrieved March 21, 2008, from eMedicine from WebMD available at http://www.emedicine.com/plastic/TOPIC389.htm

Ryan, C. M., Schoenfeld, D. A., Thorpe, W. P., Sheridan, R. L., Cassem, E. H., & Tompkins, R. G. (1998). Objective estimates of the probability of death from burn injuries. *The New England Journal of Medicine, 338*, 362–366

Saffle, J., & Graves, C. Nutritional support of the burned patient. In D. N. Herndon (Ed.), *Total burn care* (3rd ed., p. 402). Philadelphia, PA: Elsevier Inc.

Sanford, A. P., & Herndon D. N. (2001). Current therapy of burns. *Surgical treatment: evidence-based and problem oriented*. W. Zuckschwerd Verlag, München, Bern, Wein, New York, ISBN 3–88603–714–22001.

Schraga, E. D., & Pennardt, A. (2008, March 11). *CBRNE-Cyanides, Hydrogen*. Retrieved April 16, 2008, from eMedicine from WebMD, available at http://www.emedicine.com/EMERG/topic909.htm

Serebrisky, D., Nazarian E. B., Connolly, H. (2008). Inhalation Injury. *eMedicine*. Retrieved from http://emedicine.medscape.com/article/1002413-overview

Sheridan, R. L., Hinson, M. I., Liang, M. H., Nackel, A. F., Schoenfeld, D. A., Ryan, C. M., et al. (2000). Long-term outcome of children surviving massive burns. *Journal of the American Medical Association, 283*, pp. 69–73

Shirani, K. Z., Vaughhan, G. M., Mason, A. J., & Pruitt, B. J. (1996). Updates on current therapeutic approaches in burns. *Shock, 5*(1), 4–16.

Standring S. (2005). Systemic overview: Skin and its appendages. In S. Standring (Ed.), *Gray's Anatomy 39th Edition* (39th ed., pp. 157–170). Spain: Elsevier.

Tanaka, H., Matsuda, T., Miyagantani, Y., Yukioka, T., Matsuda, H., & Shimazaki, S. (2000). Reduction of resuscitation fluid volumes in severely burned patients using ascorbic acid administration. *Archives of Surgery, 135*, 326–331.

Traber, D. L., Herndon, D. N., Enkhbaatar, P., Maybauer, M. O., & Maybauer, D. M. (2007). The pathophysiology of inhalation injury. In D. N. Herndon (Ed.), *Total burn care* (3rd ed., pp. 248–261). Philadelphia: Saunders Elsevier.

Thombs, B. D., Singh, V. A., Haloren, J., Diallo, A., & Milner, S. M. (2007). The effects of preexisting medical comorbidities on mortality and length of hospital stay in acute burn injury: Evidence from a national sample of 31,338 adult patients. *Annals of Surgery, 245*.

U.S. Fire Administration. (n.d.). *Federal Emergency Management Agency (FEMA)*. Last reviewed February 5, 2008, from www.usfa.dhs.gov/statistics/index.shtm

Weinbren, M. J. (1999). Pharmacokinetics of antibiotics in burn patients. *Journal of Antimicrobial Chemotherapy 44*, 319–327.

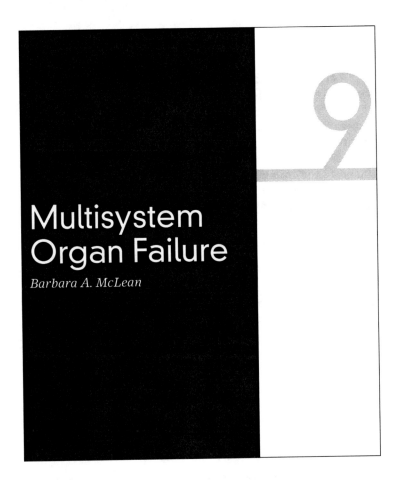

Multisystem Organ Failure

Barbara A. McLean

Introduction

> The problem of organ failure continues to perplex clini-
> cians and scientists, and it contributes to fatal outcomes
> for patients with illnesses, infections, and injuries after
> operations.
>
> *—Dr. Roger Bone, 1992*

Multiple organ dysfunction syndrome (MODS/MOF/
MSOF) is a constellation of acute or acute-on-chronic systemic
disorders that profoundly affect mortality and morbidity. The
continuum of sepsis, severe sepsis, and septic shock are inti-
mately linked to multiorgan dysfunction and may ultimately
result in organ failure and death.

Technological advances in acute care, such as volume resuscitation and blood transfusion, decreased the incidence of renal failure; however, the resulting increased survival rate gave rise to a post resuscitation lung disorder that later became known as acute lung injury and acute respiratory distress syndrome. Understanding the malignant, destructive, uncontrolled inflammatory and coagulation process became the primary focus in the management of patients exhibiting signs and symptoms of severe sepsis and MODS (Figure 9.1).

The American College of Chest Physicians/Society of Critical Care Medicine Consensus Conference offered a specific approach for identification of high-risk patients in 1992 (see Exhibit 9.1 on page 321). This method of evaluating patients was based on their clinical presentation, risk factors and ultimately laboratory diagnosis. The high-risk patient

9.1

The Continuum of SIRS to Septic Shock

SIRS	SEPSIS	SEVERE SEPSIS	SEPTIC SHOCK
SIRS: BE Aware !!!	*Control The Source!!!*	*Stop the Organ Dysfunction!!*	*Maintain the blood pressure*
• Temperature core <38.3° C or <36° C	• As in SIRS + Documented or suspected infection	*Support the Organs!!*	• As in SIRS + SEPSIS + Severe
• Heart Rate >90 bpm or >2 SD above normal for age and context	• Altered Mental Status	• As in SIRS + SEPSIS	• loss of vascular tone refractory to volume requires vaso-pressors
• Respiratory Rate >20 pm or >20 MV	• Significant + fluid balance >20mL/Kg in 24 hours	• simple signs of acute organ dysfunction	^amaldistribution of blood flow
• White Blood Count >than 12,000 cells mm-3 or <4000 cells mm-3 or greater than 10% immature (band) forms	• Blood Glucose >140 mgm in absence of diabetes	• simple signs of tissue hypoperfusion	• inappropriate shunting of oxygenated blood

Exhibit

9.1 Systemic Inflammatory Response Syndrome (SIRS)

1 Temperature >38°C or <36°C
2 Heart rate >90 beats/min
3 Respiratory rate >20 breaths/min or $PaCO_2$ <32 torr
4 WBC >12,000 cells mm-3 or <4,000 cells mm-3 or >10% immature (band) forms

Bone, R. C. et al., (1992).

must present at least two of the specified indicators. The criteria are very sensitive and require the astute practitioner to utilize the identifiers in conjunction with critical intuition and a comprehensive analysis of the patient's history.

Because the terms for identifying systemic inflammatory response syndrome (SIRS) are simplistic, nonspecific, and sensitive, others have suggested additional evaluations beyond the initial presentation (Levy et al., 2003; Cunneen, & Cartwright, 2004) (Exhibit 9.2). These include evaluation of tissue hypoxia and simple organ indicators of dysfunction to promote a strategic identification of the patient's risk and may facilitate a more timely and accurate intervention.

In severe sepsis, the inflammatory response to a nidus of infection (or inflammation) is fulminating and out of control. Stimulated by-products of antigen ingestion, activated neutrophils, and other humoral mediators combine, activate, and potentiate an ongoing endothelial injury with a concomitant proinflammatory, procoagulating, antifibrinolytic responses. Among other mediators, an increased presence of tissue factor persistently stimulates thrombin, which ultimately increases fibrinogen conversion to fibrin and promotes platelet aggregation. In addition to the increased platelet activity, excessive thrombin production and a secondary decrease in endothelial production of plasminogen activator, thrombomodulin, and activated protein C, profoundly increases microcoagulation while limiting fibrinolysis. The endothelial regulation of appropriate blood flow related to a balanced expression of vasodilators (i.e., nitric oxide NO) and vasoconstrictors (e.g., endothelin) becomes uncoupled and nonspecific. The corresponding loss of

Exhibit

9.2 Modification of SIRS and MODS

Clinical Inflammatory Signs

Hyperthermia
Hypothermia
Heart rate >90 bpm or 20 higher
  than normal (persistent)
Hyperventilation: RR > 20 bpm
Altered mental status

Laboratory Measures of Inflammation

Leukocytosis
Leukopenia
Normal WBC count with
  bands >10%
↑ C-reactive protein
↑ procalcitonin
Hyperglycemia >150 mgm
measured × 2 1 hour apart

Tissue Perfusion/Hemodynamics

$SvO_2-ScVO_2 < 70\%$ or >70%
  in the presence of clinical
  compensatory signs
Lactic Acidosius > 4 mMol/dL
Lactate Clearance of <10% / 24 hours
Anion gao > 20

Stroke volume variation >15% in a
  ventilated patient. Measured with
  controlled positive pressure breaths.

Cardiac Index >4.0 L·min·m² or
  <2.5 L·min·m²

Heart rate >90 bpm or 20 higher than
  normal

Organ Dysfunction

Failure of arterial oxygenation
▪ $P/F < 200$ on ≥ 0.40 FiO_2 or
▪ A-a difference >normal
   20 mmHg (corrected for baro-
   metric pressure and FiO_2) or
▪ Oxygenation index >15

Plateau pressure (inspiratory
  hold) >30 cm H_2O in the
  absence of chest wall
  compliance disorders or
  space occupying lesions
  (hemothorax, pneumothorax)
  measured on a ventilated
  patient with a controlled
  breath.

Urine output <0.5 ml/kg
  following fluid resuscitation.
  Cr ↑ >50%

Coagulation abnormalities:
↑ PT, INR, D-Dimers
↓ platelets, fibrinogen

Levy, M. M., Fink, M. P., Marshall, J. C., et al., 2003; Cunneen, J. and Cartwright, M., 2004.

Exhibit

9.3 An Example of the Expression of Unopposed Inflammation

Failure of vascular tone (nitric oxide synthase and induced NO release)
Vasodilatation due to local metabolites
Loss of reactivity of smooth muscle
Consumption of coagulating proteins
Activation of tissue factor, thrombin, fibrinogen
Diminished activation of protein C, tissue plasminogen
Alteration in red blood cell deformability
Hemoconcentration, sludging, intravascular coagulation, occlusion of the capillaries
AV Shunting
Capillary leak and intestitial edema
Inflammatory responders such as cortisol, glucagons, epinephrine promoting insulin resistance and hyperglycemia

vascular tone and maldistribution of blood flow occurs at the both the macrovascular and microvascular level, resulting in a scenario of mixed ischemia and hyperemia at the same surface area Frequently the patient's blood pressure will begin to decrease, signifying a loss of compensatory vasoconstriction. In addition, myocardial depressant factor is released and ultimately may contribute to the loss of the compensatory cardiac output (CO) (Exhibit 9.3).

A patient with sepsis presents with at least two of the previously mentioned SIRS criteria: an abnormal body temperature, elevated heart and respiratory rates, and an altered white blood cell (WBC) count. Sepsis with one or more acute organ dysfunctions is considered severe sepsis. Septic shock is severe sepsis with cardiovascular dysfunction (primary loss of vascular tone) that does not respond to fluid resuscitation, requiring the administration of vasopressors.

Multiple Organ Dysfunction Syndrome (MODS)

Patients with severe sepsis or prolonged tissue hypoxia, the problem is not as simple as a nidus of infection; it is more concisely the inflammatory response that is out of control, wreaking havoc on the endothelium.

The term *MODS* is used to identify the early phase of organ dysfunction and was coined by Marshall as a relative predictor of overt failure (Marshall et al., 1995). The potential for organ failure looms large during this period, and currently the primary therapy is based on the initial identification and suppression of the nidus of inflammation focusing on the management and support of each organ that is dysfunctional as well as supporting blood flow, cardiac output and ultimately vascular tone. Quite simply, rapid diagnosis, constant vigilance, and appropriate and timely therapeutic intervention can significantly reduce the evolution of sepsis to MODS. Under recognized and underresuscitated, severe sepsis (presence of MODS with indicators of sepsis) frequently leads to organ failure and ultimately death.

Deconstructing this complex process into a few simple tools, guidelines, and protocols is nearly impossible. However, if therapy is initiated in an emergent manner, the progression may be arrested, and therefore mortality and morbidity may indeed be decreased. The acute care nurse practitioner (ACNP) evaluates clinical signs and symptoms of SIRS and correlates the assessment with an index of suspicion, patient's history, and complaints of illness, then designs an appropriate evaluation, early treatment, and reevaluation platform. Early treatment involves rapid volume resuscitation of 20 ml/kg over 30–60 minutes or an even shorter time frame, depending on the vital signs, history and age,. Resuscitative fluids will impact tissue perfusion. Following the drawing of blood cultures and other appropriate cultures, a broad-spectrum antibiotic must be administered intravenous (IV), based on unit antibiogram (chapter 11).

Endothelial Dysfunction

Despite numerous clinical trials aimed at supporting or antagonizing humoral mediators and cellular communicators, no single strategic method of control has been identified. Indeed, controlling one cascade often leads to another problem (Figure 9.2).

There is no predictable model for MODS, a complex, nonlinear monolith, affecting inflammation (both pro and anti), apoptosis (a process referred to as cellular suicide or programmed cell death), coagulation, and fibrinolysis referred to as endothelial dysfunction. In the absence of the

9.2

Inflammatory Cascade

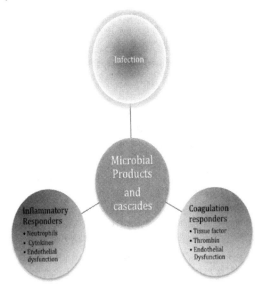

presentation of a specific nidus, the ACNP should consider the patient's condition and where they sit on the continuum of sepsis, making treatment decisions accordingly. Rapidly instituting a therapy driven toward increasing and maintaining blood flow, therefore decreasing the heart rate and respiratory rate (as compensatory measures), increasing the diastolic blood pressure and pulse pressure, and clearing lactic acid, is an important intervention. All of these therapies combined will increase endothelial protection.

Assuming that the focal point of inflammation is infectious, the ACNP should perform blood and appropriate system cultures and should initiate broad-spectrum antibiotics (Chapter 11) within 4 hours after patient identification. If cultures cannot be obtained, antibiotics should be initiated regardless. In the presence of a hypotensive state, rapid diagnosis and administration of antibiotic therapy appears to be essential to reduce mortality (Kumar et al., 2006)

The endothelium was historically considered a passive barrier between tissues and blood. Over the last 2 decades, cell traffic, proinflammation and antiinflammation, coagulation, fibrinolysis, and vascular tonal control have been uncovered as just a few of the many endothelial functions.

The primary stimulation for this endothelial chaos is the systemic and local release of inflammatory mediators (Figure 9.3). The cytokine-based communicators activate the endothelium and attract WBC, which further generates endothelial activation. The heightened activation trips the coagulation component, in a prothrombin and antifibrinolytic cascade. Unopposed, this process may lead to a profound consumptive coagulopathy, diminished distal blood flow as a result of microcoagulation, and activated apoptosis (Aird, 2002). The blood flow necessary to maintain tissue oxygenation and aerobic metabolism, nutrient transfer, and metabolic waste removal is profoundly threatened.

There are two basic types of endothelial cells: the quiet endothelial cells expressing antiadhesive, anticoagulation, and vasodilation mediators, and the activated cells, which perform the opposite functions. There is an intricacy of function and molecular components contributed by the endothelium.

The presence of continuous flowing blood (and the dynamic shear stress generated when blood is ejected), an acidotic pH, the increased presence of thrombin, and cell-to-cell communications of dysfunction significantly impacts the complexity of endothelial function. Heightened apoptosis also significantly impacts the complexity, and dysfunction, of the endothelial properties. Apoptosis is the pogram of cell death. Cells can die in two ways: by damaging their cell membrane

9.3

Endothelial Cascade

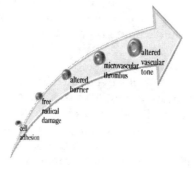

Inflammatory stimulation
1. microbial activation
2. activation of neutrophils
3. cytokine actovation

Consequences
1. Refractory hypotension
2. Consumption of coagulation products
3. Capillary leak

and then undergoing necrosis or by shrinking and blebbing the intact cell membrane. This process is a normal one: all cells have a programmed life and death. There is evidence to suggest that an increase in the apoptotic processes may play a determining role in the outcome to sepsis syndromes. Therapeutic efforts in modulating the apoptotic response, particularly by interfering with cell signaling pathways that lead to early and increased apoptosis, represent an attractive therapeutic target for the patient with sepsis.

The evolution of sepsis to MODS resulting ultimately in organ failure and death initially presents as a form of hypovolemia (distributive shock). To the unsuspecting practitioner, the early signs of arterial underperfusion may be masked by the patient's appearance and relative health history. Sepsis and severe sepsis are equal opportunistic inflammatory states; no age, gender, or requirement of prior health issues are necessary for the process to occur or to render a patient resilient to the process, although there are multiple issues that may place the patient in higher risk category.

The primary mechanism for initial compensation is an acute stress, inflammation, or a hypermetabolic state that increases cardiac output. Attention to the details of inflammation and compensation (Figure 9.1) followed by an immediate intervention may significantly improve survival and prevent the patient's imminent decompensation, significantly reducing the evolution to MODS (see Figure 9.3 on page 326).

Cellular Perfusion

At the bedside, three basic assumptions drive practice.

Assumption One: If everything looks normal, "it is."

Patients will frequently appear "normal" because their cardio–pulmonary–vascular systems compensate for early inflammation and hypermetabolism with hyperventilation and/or increased heart rate or vasoconstriction. The color and temperature of the peripheral extremities is one of the common evaluation tools determining blood flow that might lead the provider astray. An inherent error may occur in the patient who has the microcirculatory deficits of severe sepsis, because their blood flow is essentially maldistributed. The hands and feet may be warm because the patient is infarcting cells and organs that are unseen and unable to be evaluated.

Assumption Two: If blood pressure is normal, blood flow "must" be adequate.

When patients present in the early stages of shock, catecholamines, neuroendocrine responses, and the corresponding cardiac response may profoundly impact the actual blood pressure, maintaining pressure while masking the inadequacy of blood flow. Blood pressure monitoring may not be a sensitive indicator for the patient with compensated shock. Profound reductions is blood pressure is a sign of end-organ decompensation; the goal is to recognize the symptoms prior to this severe decompensation.

Assumption Three: If the pulse oximeter is acceptable, oxygenation "must" also be good

Traditional pulse oximetry, both SpO_2 as well as SaO_2, are not strong indicators of cellular oxygen, although both importantly (indirectly and directly) reflect the alveolar capillary gas exchange. When saturation of hemoglobin (Hgb), arterial oxygen content, and PaO_2 appear to be adequate, the cells may still be profoundly hypoxic.

Contributors to Blood Flow and Tissue Oxygenation

From the time of the early work of Shoemaker et al., (1988) and Kreymann et al., (1993), it has been well established that global tissue hypoxia accompanies *all* forms of shock. Categorically, oxygen delivery in shock (cardiac, hypovolemic, and hemorrhagic) affect the mechanics of oxygen supply and availability, while systemic inflammatory response or severe sepsis with the secondary effects of endothelial dysfunction, vasodilation, inflammatory mediation, and unopposed procoagulation, interferes with the utilization of oxygen at a microcirculatory and cellular level. This persistent hypoxia further exacerbates the systemic response, and if unresolved, it will lead to organ dysfunction and eventually death (Table 9.1).

SIRS can rapidly progress from severe sepsis to septic shock, with tissue hypoxia undetected by traditional measurements. Tissue oxygenation indicators provide a framework of reference that should direct therapy toward a more valid perfusion goal. When the potential for a hypoxic states exists, two primary physiological responses occur to maintain

9.1 Comparing Shock Types

Type/indicator	Heart rate	Cardiac output	Filling pressures	SVR	Pulse pressure	SvO₂
Cardiogenic	↑	↓	↑	↑	↓	↓
Hypovolemic	↑	↓	↓	↑	↓	↓
Hemorrhagic	↑↑	↓	↓↓	↑	↓	↓↓
Neurogenic	↓	↓	↓	↓	↑	↓
Anaphylaxis	↑	↓	↓	↓	↑	↓
Compensated Severe Sepsis	↑	↑	↓	↓	↑	↓↓
Decompensated Severe Sepsis	↑↓	↓	↑	↑	↓	↑

tissue oxygen consumption: increasing the delivery of oxygen (primarily via increased CO) and increasing the release rate of oxygen from Hgb (desaturating Hgb at the capillary level) expressed as a shift to the right of the saturation of hemoglobin (oxyHgb) dissociation curve (Figure 9.4).

9.4

Oxyhemoglobin Dissociation

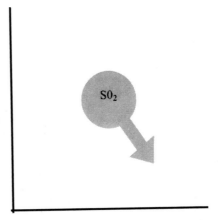

Bound to HgB: SO₂

Reserve: Measured in the venous Compartment

Dissolved in Blood: Usable and Unbound: PO₂

Maintaining Oxygen Consumption

The adequate delivery and consumption of oxygen can be assured only in the face of an adequate CO and appropriate release of bound oxygen, as well as oxygen content (Figure 9.5). CO is the product of heart rate × stroke volume (see Figure 9.6). Although heart rate is easily measured and evaluated, the evaluation of stroke volume must be performed with echocardiography or tissue oxygenation monitors and then leading to increasingly invasive mechanisms including volumetric end tidal CO_2, continuous arterial signal processes, Fick calculations based on arterial and central venous or mixed venous oxygenation measures, and intrapulmonary (thermodilution) or intra arterial techniques. The appropriate release of bound oxygen (traditionally inferred from the mixed venous saturation of Hgb) requires a continuous method of measuring the central or mixed venous Hgb saturations as well as correlating the aerobic/anerobic environment of the tissues (traditionally inferred from the anion gap, lactic acid levels, base deficit, serum CO_2, and calculated bicarbonate). The methodology ultimately depends on the resources available as well as the expertise of the providers. The clinician must be aware of the limitations of any measurement technique that is selected and utilize all measures to create a strong picture of the pathologic process.

9.5

Maintaining Oxygen Balance

Release of Oxygen

Oxygen Delivery

SvO$_2$

Oxygen Consumption

Cardiac Output
Hemoglobin
SaO$_2$

9.6

Maintaining Cardiac Output/Index: Balance of Heart Rate and Stroke Volume

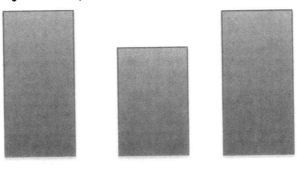

Heart Rate   Cardiac Output/Index   Stroke Volume

Oxygen Content

Content of arterial oxygen (CaO_2) is defined as the amount of bound Hgb (SaO_2) plus the amount of dissociated, dissolved oxygen (PaO_2) found in the arterial blood. The role of the saturated Hgb is to transport and then release oxygen as the blood flows through the capillaries, maintaining a relatively constant partial pressure of oxygen in the dissolved (usable) state. Every Hgb cell that is fully saturated with oxygen, transports approximately 1.34–1.36 ml of oxygen, and is the only reservoir for oxygen that appropriately balances tissue demands (Table 9.2 on page 332). As the red cells deform, flow into the capillaries, and past the cells, a constant dissociation occurs as the partial pressure of dissolved oxygen decreases based on cellular uptake of oxygen. The ability of Hgb to release oxygen when cellular demand is increased is the second most important compensatory mechanism utilized to sustain cellular integrity. In terms of the oxyHgb dissociation curve, this reflects a shift to the right or a release of bound oxygen to the dissolved or usable state (PaO_2). This process occurs at the capillary interface level and therefore cannot be directly measured in the arterial blood. When arterial blood volume is inadequate, ventricular function is poor and/or Hgb levels do not fulfill oxygen-carrying capacity criteria, the second compensatory mechanism, shifting to the right, may save the day.

9.2 Measurements of Oxygen Content

Measures	Hgb	Saturation	PaO$_2$/PvO$_2$	Formula	Normal
Arterial	14 gm	0.95–1.00	80–100 mmHg	SaO$_2$ (Hgb × 1.36) + PaO$_2$ (0.03)	18–20 ml/dl
Mixed Venous (PAC) Oximetry	14 gm	0.60–0.80	40–45 mmHg	SvO$_2$ (Hgb × 1.36) × PaO$_2$ (0.03)	11.5–15 ml/dl
Central Venous (CVP) Oximetry	14 gm	0.65–0.85	40–45 mmHg	ScvO$_2$ (Hgb × 1.36) + PaO$_2$ (0.03)	13–16 ml/dl

Values based on Reinhart, K., et al., (2004) and Reinhart, K., et al., (2006).

Typically, the oxygen delivery (CO × content of oxygen) is in profound excess of the tissue demand (see Table 9.3) representing the normal reserve of saturated Hgb. Normally, tissues consume about 20% to 30% of reserve oxygen, desaturating Hgb to approximately 70%. When oxygen delivery (DaO$_2$) decreases, because the CO has gone down or there is an inadequate oxygen-carrying capacity, the reserve will be tapped at a greater level. However, when tissues cannot use the oxygen delivered to them, the initial compensatory mechanism is to increase the delivery via an increase in CO.

Cardiac Output: Delivering the Oxygen Content

Heart Rate. The first compensatory mechanism that expresses the patient's attempt to increase oxygen delivery is an increase in the intrinsic heart rate. Patients who are unable to manifest increase in heart rate (as a result of beta blockade or acute cervical spinal cord injury) will have a limited ability to compensate. In the appropriate clinical circumstances, persistent tachycardia should be considered as an attempt to increase oxygen delivery compensating for low hemoglobin, high tissue demand or inadequate oxygenation at the cellular level

9.3 Measurements of Oxygen Delivery

Measures	Content	Cardiac Output	Formula	Normal
Arterial	18–20 ml/dl	4–8 L/min	CaO_2 (10) Cardiac output	1000 ml/min
Mixed Venous (PAC) Oximetry	11.5–15 ml/dl	4–8 L/min	CvO_2 (10) Cardiac output	830 ml/min 460–1200
Central Venous (CVP) Oximetry	13–16 ml/dl	4–8 L/min	$CcvO_2$ (10) Cardiac output	920 ml/min 520–1280

Legend Mixed Venous
Lowest 11.5(4)10 = 460
Highest 15 (8(10 = 1200
mean average = 830

Legend Central Venous
Lowest 13(4)10 = 520
Highest 16(8)10 = 1280
mean average = 920

Values based on Reinhart, K., et al., (2004) and Reinhart, K., et al., (2006).

until proven otherwise (diagnosis of exclusion). Optimal management calls for increasing the stroke volume and thereby decreasing the heart rate., as well as utilizing sedation and pain management strategies to reduce tissue demands. The ability to evaluate the stroke volume or CO may significantly impact the treatment measures and patient outcome. The variables that affect the stroke volume include contractile function, preload, and afterload. Invasive and noninvasive methods can be used to indirectly or directly to assess these components (Figure 9.7).

Stroke Volume

Contractility. Contractility is the intrinsic ability of cardiac muscle to develop force for a given muscle length. The ability to develop tension or power is related to the intrinsic myocardial state. The amount of force required (tension or afterload) and the filling volume (preload) are essential factors which impact contractility. However, the contractile function is ultimately an independent one and is independently affected by crossbridges, calcium, mitochondrial function, and oxygen

9.7

When Cardiac Output is Inadequate for the Oxygen Consumption/Demand

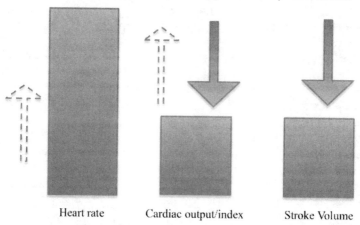

| Heart rate | Cardiac output/index | Stroke Volume |

delivery. There are no known bedside measures that directly monitor the true contractile state of the myocardium.

Preload. Frank and Starling are credited with the seminal observation that peak ventricular ejection increases as the end-diastolic volume (EDV) increases in an intact ventricular model. The integral distendability of the chamber and the volume load it can accept are the basis of the Frank–Starling curve: the more filling, the greater the stretch; the greater the stretch, the better the ejection. Until overdistension is reached the volume load will no longer equal the ejection volume, this volume load is usually estimated from the easily measured pressure in the venous column (measured in the vein or the atria) prior to the ventricle that is being filled. The right and/or left ventricular end-diastolic pressures are therefore indirectly reflected in the central vein or the pulmonary artery respectively.

Preload pressure is a measure or estimate of the ventricular volume load in the chamber at the end of diastole. These two preload pressures are reflective of the EDV as well as the compliance of the ventricular wall (Exhibit 9.4). The implied equivalency between the pressure and volume in the ventricular chambers is often not correct and depends on the compliance or distendability of the ventricle. During acute or chronic myocardial ischemia, sepsis, valvular dysfunction states, and even in simple tachycardia, the ventricles may become less compliant and may not fully relax during diastole. Any changes in intrathoracic pressures (pneumothorax, hemothorax, positive pressure ventilation, distending airway pressures) will affect the ventricular compliance, as well as the pressure required to fill the ventricle and ultimately the ventricular volume. This pathologic diastolic dysfunction reduces the chamber size and decreases volume load at end-diastole, and a smaller EDV may continue to be expressed in terms of a high filling pressure, therefore misleading the provider into assuming adequate volume loading.

Afterload. Afterload is the resistance or pressure load that the ventricle must overcome in order to shorten the myofibrils, generate an opening pressure and eject the ventricular volumes into the outflow artery (right ventricle to pulmonary artery and left ventricle to aorta). This amount of tension that is required to eject volume into the arterial bed is not measurable and is referred to as afterload. Afterload is traditionally documented with basic or complex calculations for vascular resistance. The tension or power that the ventricle must develop directly opposes the valvular–arterial resistance. The higher the afterload, the more tension the ventricle must develop, therefore due to the increased workload, the less efficient the contraction may become. The integrity of the

Exhibit

9.4 Factors Affecting Ventricular Compliance

1. Heart Rate
2. Positive Pressure Ventilation
3. Outlet Valve Stenosis/Regurgitation
4. Alteration in Arterial Resistance
5. Tension Development of the Ventricle (Afterload)
6. Ischemia
7. Remodeling

ventricular wall, the compressing thoracic and pleural pressure, valvular (semilunar) function, and the outflow vascular tone affect the tension development required. The preload volume-stretch affects the afterload as the filling volumes must be moved via tension development.

Compensatory Mechanisms

Three major compensatory mechanisms designed to sustain tissues are: increasing the CO, vasoconstriction of the vessels supplying organs that do not require a high level of oxygen, and releasing more of the bound oxygen. This is critical in maintaining and preserving tissue oxygenation (demand or consumption known as VO_2) (Figure 9.8).

A profound neuroendocrine response stimulates both the beta and alpha receptors begins with α stimulation which in an intact endothelium will promote vasoconstriction and ultimately redirects blood flow from high flow, low oxygen requiring organs (i.e., skeletal muscles, peripheral nervous system) toward oxygen dependent organs (i.e., heart, brain, diaphragm). The beta-1 (β-1) stimulation effects will primarily affect heart rate and myocardial contractility. If the

9.8

Increasing Cardiac Output and Compensatory Oxygen Dissociation from HgB (Must be measured in venous or capillary circulation.)

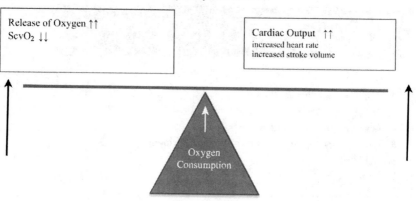

receptor sites are intact and not opposed by circulatory mediators, tachycardia, increased contractility and vaso-constriction will ensue. The correlating clinical measure of "cold hands and feet" is associated with this compensatory mechanism in shock, although those subjective indicators may lose value in the presence of complex disease and variable compensatory mechanisms. The significant increase in CO is limited solely by the intrinsic volume status, as well as the endogenous and exogenous cardiac dynamics. Other processes, such as the release of renin, vasopressin, and other hormonal communicators, lead to a decreased excretion of water, preserving the water load in an attempt to increase the circulating volume and hopefully the oxygen delivery (Figure 9.9).

The second compensatory component, increasing the rate of release of oxygen off-load from the Hgb at the capillary level (shift to the right) requires that indeed the blood flows into the capillary, the cell signals its need for oxygen (presence of acidosis), and there is adequate releasing product to separate the oxygen from the Hgb (2,3-diphosphoglycerate). The patient will not be able to acutely increase oxygen content (CaO_2: Hgb [1.34] saturation in the decimal) by increasing his own red cell count, although this is exactly what the chronic patient will do, as evidenced by patients with disease and polycythemia (Figure 9.10 on page 338).

9.9

Failure of Oxygen Dissociation and Compensatory Increase in Cardiac Output

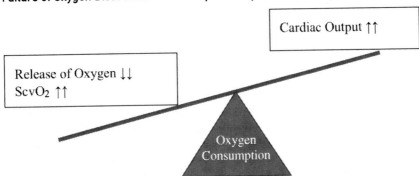

Cardiac Output ↑↑

Release of Oxygen ↓↓
$ScvO_2$ ↑↑

Oxygen Consumption

9.10

Failure of Cardiac Output and Compensatory Increase in Oxygen Dissociation

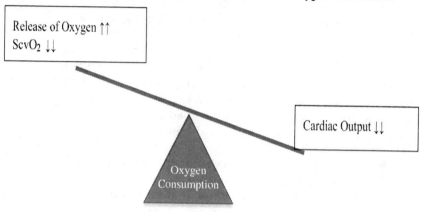

When supporting oxygen delivery, the ACNP should consider volume, inotropic enhancement, and administration of packed red blood cells. Consideration should be taken for the risk of any of these therapies. If the patient has refractory, unexplained acidosis, and/or continued compensatory mechanisms, all three may be necessary.

Monitoring of mixed, central venous or local oximetry as well as indicators of tissue hypoxia (metabolic acidosis) may provide insight toward alterations in oxygenation. The stimulation of central and peripheral chemoreceptors via the presence of metabolic acid drives a shift toward the easily manipulated CO_2. A rapid respiratory rate "blows off" the excess acid in an attempt to maintain the required electrically neutral blood pH.

Confirmation of adequacy of either or both of these compensatory mechanisms can be supported with combinations that include compensatory measures such as heart rate, respiratory rate, blood pressure, pulse pressure, stroke volume, stroke volume variation, as well as indicators of appropriate tissue oxygenation including SvO_2, StO_2 anion gap, base deficit, serum CO_2, bicarbonate, and serial lactic acid levels. The three major variables that ensure oxygen delivery are CO, Hgb (mg/dl), and arterial saturation (SpO_2 or SaO_2).

Methodology for Monitoring and Evaluation

In recent years, there has been significant reduction in the utilization of invasive monitoring catheters and a greater emphasis on minimally and noninvasive methods of evaluating the dynamics of oxygenation and blood flow. The utilization of pulmonary artery (PA) catheters was attributed to an increased mortality and morbidity in catheterized patient groups (Connors et al., 1996). Other studies have challenged these results. There continues to be controversy over whether or not the utilization of PA catheter-based information is beneficial in the management of specific disease states.

Measuring Cardiac Output

In most clinical circumstances, tachycardia should be considered a compensatory attempt to increase oxygen delivery to the cellular level. Optimal management calls for increasing the stroke volume and thereby decreasing the heart rate. The ability to evaluate the stroke volume or CO may significantly impact the treatment measures and patient outcome. Contractility is generally assumed by the CO. Contractility is highly dependent on preload and afterload and is difficult to measure as an independent variable. Evidence of low contractility may cause an imbalance in the oxygen delivery or demand response. Evidence of a higher CO usually indicates a compensatory mechanism for an increased demand or the functional inability to utilize oxygen at the cellular level. Following are some of the current methods utilized for CO measurement.

Bioimpedence. Noninvasive hemodynamic assessment in heart failure has been either unreliable or difficult to obtain. Bioimpedance relies on the proportional change in the conduction of alternating current applied across the thorax as a function of blood volume in the heart and great vessels. Stroke volume, CO, thoracic fluid volume and measures of diastolic function can be determined with bioimpedance, but the presence of extravascular lung fluids significantly impacts the validity of the readings. Although not generally utilized in critical care, the use of bioimpedence has been strongly supported in outpatient clinics and emergency departments.

Volumetric End-Tidal CO$_2$. Any gas that diffuses across the alveolar capillary membrane can be utilized in the Fick calculation. Continuous monitoring of end-tidal CO$_2$ (PETCO$_2$) reflects the arterial partial pressure of CO$_2$, and minute ventilation is used to calculate the actual estimated CO$_2$ production. The rate of CO$_2$ clearance is then used to estimate perfusion, and correction testing is done to eliminate alterations in ventilation as a CO$_2$ source. This methodology utilized in intubated patients, evaluates only the blood flow that is processed and does not include shunted blood; therefore, in shunt disease states, the accuracy of actual CO may underestimate cardiac function and volume indicators.

Esophageal Doppler Probes. Using a Doppler transducer on the tip of a probe, the esophageal Doppler measures aortic blood velocity that is then converted into systemic stroke volume. Recent studies advocate the use of Doppler technology to evaluate fluid resuscitation in high-risk patients and have been correlated to improved outcomes. Compared with ultrasound transit time measures, the esophageal Doppler has accurately evaluated the aortic blood flow and therefore the left ventricular (LV) stroke volume. The probe may be placed by a qualified ACNP; however, even with experienced clinicians, accurate placement and position may be difficult to achieve and maintain.

The Arterial Pressure Wave. Arterial waveform analysis uses the complete pressure waveform for analysis and and to predict stroke volume. The shape of the waveform, the systolic component, velocity, ejection time, arterial resistance (age, gender, and weight based) and the overall pulse pressure are all indicators that should be considered. These measurements rely on an intact arterial catheter, a transducer system, and a viable waveform. Different products offer a different palate of calculated measures in addition to CO, stroke volume (standard and indexed), and stroke volume variability (see Figure 9.11). Additional measures depend on either operator input of fixed values (Hgb, hematocrit [Hct], central venous pressure [CVP]) or direct measurements that are either required (central line) or independent (central line with oximetry or input data). Some of the available methods require external calibration using an indicator washout curve or thermodilution.

9.11

Arterial Waveform Analysis

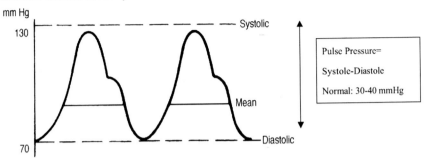

Pulse Pressure=
Systole-Diastole
Normal: 30-40 mmHg

Monitoring Pressures and Assuming Volumes. CVP, which estimates the right ventricular (RV) EDP, is considered less invasive than intrapulmonary artery monitoring and may also be utilized to provide direct oxygenation information that allows for Fick calculation of CO and other measures designed for goal direction in therapy. Normal CVP is traditionally 4–8 mmHg; however, when treating patients who are in a pre-shock or shock state, CVP goals may need to be driven higher (8–12 mmHg or higher when there is evidence of compliance loss of the ventricle) (Hofer et al., 2005; Kincaid, Meredith, & Chang, 2001; Kramer, Zygun, Hawes, Easton, & Ferland, 2004; Michard et al., 2003; Rivers et al., 2001) Normal or high CVP measurements must be evaluated cautiously, as pressure may not be an accurate predictor of actual preload volume.

An indwelling arterial catheter allows for beat-to-beat determination of blood pressure, pulse volume or pressure (which trends with cardiac stroke volume), mean arterial pressure, arterial blood gases, and arterial based CO monitoring. The catheter is never used for infusion of any medications or fluids and must be continuously monitored via a specialized pressure monitoring setup. The calculation of the mean is based on area under the curve and is most significantly effected by diastolic pressure and time (heart rate effect).

Recently, the effects on variation of systolic pressure and/or stroke volume related to pleural and thoracic pressure changes have received significant notice as indicators of both tension development and volume responsiveness in critical patients on positive pressure ventilatory support. There is increasing interest in the evaluation of the inspiratory effects on the arterial pulse pressure in order to predict the probable hemodynamic response to a fluid challenge. This variation reflects the ability of the ventricular system to maintain optimum ejection despite changes in pleural, thoracic, and myocardial pressure (Figure 9.12).

The cyclic variations in intrathoracic and pleural pressure during positive pressure breaths produce corresponding variations in the central venous and arterial waveforms (De Waal, Rex, Kruitwagen, Kalkman, & Buhre, 2008). The intrathoracic pressure is transmitted to the vascular space and affects the intravascular pressure by altering the compliance of the ventricles. The digital reading of the filling pressures during inspiration will vary accordingly and may profoundly misrepresent volume load. In general, low intravascular

9.12

Stroke Volume Variation with Positive Pressure Ventilation

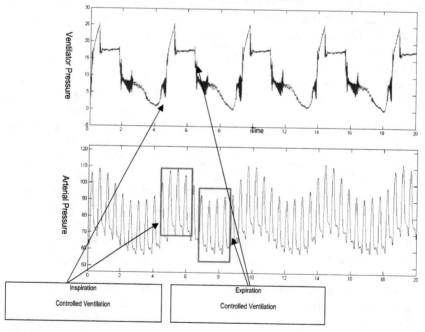

volume will be accompanied by a significant reproducible drop in pressure, stroke volume when positive inspiratory pressures are applied. The variable of inspiratory pressure must be controlled in order for the reduction of pulse volume following the positive pressure breath to be meaningful.

Monitoring Tissue Oxygenation

The more recent development of a centrally placed triple lumen catheter with an oximeter on the tip is significantly less invasive than the PA and allows clinicians to actually evaluate tissue oxygenation in both the ICU and non-ICU environment. This tool assists in directing goals toward tissue perfusion rather than blood pressure. Because tissue oxygenation is so profoundly affected in patients with shock, it becomes the most meaningful indicator, even in the presence of normal blood pressure (it is important to remember that central or mixed venous monitoring reflects global oxygenation, not regional or local). Some organs may still be hypoperfused in the face of a normal $ScvO_2$ or SvO_2.

The measurement of the (de)saturation of Hgb reflects the dissociation of oxygen, a function that uniquely occurs in an environment where the cells are using oxygen and perfusion is optimized. As the red cells deform and flow into the capillaries a constant dissociation occurs when the capillary partial pressure of oxygen decreases as the cells uptake oxygen. Measurement of the saturation of Hgb in the central vein at right atrial inflow provides a view of the leftover oxygen still bound to the hemoglobin. As the Hgb, via blood flow, moves into the right atria and mixes with the acutely desaturated Hgb from the coronary sinus (the myocardium) and the inferior vena cava (IVC), the blood mix mobilizes into the right ventricle, mixes again, and is ejected into the pulmonary artery. The monitoring and evaluation of central venous oximetry ($ScvO_2$, measured just before the inflow vessel of the right atrial via a triple lumen catheter with an oximeter on the distal tip) has been significantly popularized since the work of Rivers (2001) was published. Two of the unique components of this study were the instrumentation and measurement of central venous oximetry in the emergency department. The study also hypothesized the promotion of increased oxygen delivery with the end goal of tissue oxygenation prior to (if possible) a mitochondrial failure state, such as occurs in severe sepsis, as a method of prevention rather than intervention. Normal values range from 65%–85% and should always be evaluated and treated when persistently below 70%. Any sustained decrease in the $ScvO_2$ should be considered as a compensatory mechanism (shift to the righ of the oxyhemoglobin dissociation curve) and is evidence that the patient is in a critical state, sustained only by their oxygen reservoir. The goal is to maintain the reservoir at a normal level, therefore always having an adequate protective mechanism. However, ACNPs should be aware that normal values of $ScvO_2$ may be misleading in the presence of microcirculatory deficits.

Concerning Adequacy of Tissue Oxygenation

To objectively and proactively identify the patient at risk, the traditional parameters, heart rate, blood pressure, respiratory rate, urine output, the monitoring of the saturation of continuous central or mixed venous Hgb, and serum creatinine should be correlated to the most available and simple method of confirming appropriate tissue oxygenation is the serial evaluation of lactic acid and the anion gap.

Lactic Acidosis. Arterial lactate concentration is dependent on the balance between its production and clearance. In the critically ill septic population, increased glucose metabolism, increased energy expenditures and profound catabolism are the norm (Tappy & Chiolero, 2007; Revelly et al., 2005). The corresponding lactic acidosis signals physiologic stress, but may not necessarily be evidence of tissue hypoxia. The concomitant energy expenditures, along with metabolic dysfunction, will increase lactate production. These conditions, in addition to an exaggerated inflammatory response and increasing oxygenation dysfunction at the tissue level, combine to produce a profound tissue acidosis. The lactate production is further increased via other abnormal pathways specifically related to metabolic dysfunction, even in the absence of tissue hypoxia (Type B lactic acidosis). The main cause of the significantly increased lactate is unknown (Table 9.4), but one factor that contributes to lactic acidosis is the failure of adenosine triphosphate (ATP) production that clearly occurs in the presence of a profound oxygen supply–demand imbalance (Type A lactic acidosis). The mitochondrial ability to utilize pyruvate, is indicative

9.4 — Common Causes of Elevated Lactate in Acute and Critical Patients

Lactic Acid Checklist			
Nonhypoxic Lactic Acidosis	Problem Metabolic Dysfunction	Problem Regional/local Hypoperfusion	Hypoxic (Ischemic) Lactic Acidosis
Liver Dysfunction	υ	υ	Cardiogenic Shock
Renal Dysfunction	υ	υ	Hypovolemic Shock
Malignancies	υ	υ	Hemmorrhagic Shock
Accelerated Aerobic Glycosis DKA	υ	υ	Hyperglycemic Hyperosmolar Syndrome
Methanol, Ethanol	υ	υ	Severe Pulmonary Dysfunction
Antiretrovirals, INH	υ	υ	Carbon Monoxide Poisoning
Cyanide Poisoning	υ	υ	Cardiac Arrest
Valproic Acid	υ	υ	Any Condition Where Oxygen Delivery is Inadequate
Early Sepsis Pyruvate Dehydrogenase Deficiency	υ	υ	Severe Sepsis Profound Tissue Hypoxia and metabolic dysfunction

of a profound metabolic hyperlactatemia, an elevated lactate/pyruvate ratio, increased glucose, and low-energy production. Always be aware dynamic liver clearance of lactate may mask this disturbing trend.

Ultimately, as severe sepsis progresses and evolves, a mediator induced cardiac failure, or profound intra-arterial hypovolemia occurs. The presence of elevated lactate levels should be treated first with volume resuscitation (20 ml/kg of isotonic crystalloids, with continued volume resuscitation as necessary). It may be necessary to support the CO with low-dose inotropes to prevent the evolution of profound tissue hypoxia. Goal: Lactate < 2.0 mEq/L, $ScvO_2 \geq 70\%$.

Single lactate measurements are not significantly beneficial in the continued treatment and evaluation of severe sepsis (Nguyen et al., 2004). In patients with sepsis, persistent hyperlactatemia has been linked to mortality and morbidity (Levraut et al., 1993). Bakker et al., coined the phrase "lac time" as the time during which lactate remains >2 mmol/L and observed that this duration of lactic acidosis was predictive of organ failure and survival. Nguyen et al., proved a significant correlation between normalization of elevated lactate in the first 24 hours of therapy and survival (100%), regardless of whether or not metabolic deficits or profound hypoxia (or a combination thereof) were the primary causes.

Anion Gap. Metabolic acidosis is a condition that generally occurs from an addition of H^+, the primary expression of tissue respiration and metabolism (normal and abnormal). The increased H+ binds to bicarbonate causing a fall in the primary serum bicarbonate level, In this simple chemical and reversible equation, H^+ represents tissue acid, bicarbonate (H_2CO_3) represents the primary buffer, CO_2 represents the gaseous carbonic acid, H_2O: water, and HCO_3 (carbonic acid) represents the traditional combination of the acid and the neutralizing components. The level of carbonic acid inversely affects the pH. Initially, in most metabolic acidotic environments, hydrogen goes up, bicarbonate goes down, carbonic acid increases and shifts to the H_2O and CO_2 side. As long as the patient can hyperventilate, the increased CO_2 will be blown off and the pH should be compensated.

$$(H^+ + HCO_{3-}) \leftrightarrow H_2CO_3 \leftrightarrow (H_2O + CO_2)$$

For every 1 mEq/L drop of HCO_{3-} below 25, the p_aCO_2 should decrease by ~1 torr in order to compensate for the increase in metabolic acid. Therefore a compensatory p_aCO_2 in the face of HCO_{3-} of 10 would be around 25 mmHg. If the pH is not normalized because of failure of the opposing system to adequately regulate the offending product, that is known as a mixed disorder.

The combination of metabolic acidosis with a widening of the serum anion gap (AG) is one of the most important confirmation of metabolic acidosis. Extreme elevations of the AG is predicated on the concept of physiological electroneutrality: the assumption that the sum of all available cations (positively charged ions) is equal to the sum of all available anions (negative charged ions). This is quite simply evaluated as

$$(Na)^+ - (Cl^- + HCO_3) = AG = 12-14.$$

A wide gap can appear in various clinical settings and are usually associated with serious metabolic problems. The by-product of tissue respiration is hydrogen ion (+). Hydrogen binds to the bicarbonate (or serum CO_2) and chloride causing a decrease in the measured anions. This now will produce a "gap" in the measured cations and anions (Table 9.5). An AG of >20 mEq/L is suggestive of ketoacidosis and/or lactic acidosis. The anion gap is only performed when confirming or evaluating metabolic acidosis.

Serum albumin contributes ~one half of the total anion equivalency of the the unmeasured anion pool. Assuming normal electrolytes, a 1 gm/dl decline in serum albumin increases the AG measurement by 3 mEq/L and needs to be accounted for and manually corrected when suspicious of the patient's condition (Rocktaeschel et al., 2003; Kaplan & Kellum, 2004).

Therefore an AG of 12 mEq/L is corrected to 17–18 mEq/L when the serum albumin is half of normal; this is an important correction factor in settings of chronic illness, malnourished patients, or in the hypermetabolic stress response of severe sepsis.

9.5 Gap and Acidosis

Endogenous Acidosis	Wide Gap
Uremia (uncleared organic acids)	No
Ketoacidosis	Yes
Lactic acidosis (increased organic acid production)	Yes
renal failure	Not necessarily

The normal value of lactate identified by Shoemaker (1998) is <2.5 ml/dl. However, more recent literature tells us to be vigilant in any individual with a lactate level >1.5 ml/dl (Nguyen, 2004). In mediator shock, (as in anaphylaxis or severe sepsis) the presence of normal to elevated SvO_2 in the face of persistent lactic acidosis is an ominous sign and requires immediate resuscitation.

The value of lactate is obviously limited due to lactate concentrations that are affected by both production as well as elimination. Individuals who have hepatic dysfunction and hypoperfusion may have higher lactate levels than the person who does not have liver disease, and both may have a significant degree of stress. Therefore, lactate levels by themselves will not give as much beneficial information as those in the presence of wide anion gap and low or normal $ScvO_2$.

Recently, Nguyen et al., (2004) validated that the higher the clearance of lactate in the first 6 hours after resuscitation, the more significant the reduction in mortality. The statistical significance of improved survival for individuals who could clear their lactate levels >10% in the first 6 hours of resuscitation was sustained across all cause mortality at 60 days out. In those first hours following resuscitation, achieving a normal $ScvO_2$ along with increasing lactate clearance is a desired therapeutic end point and achieving these endpoints safely and rapidly may significantly reduce the potential for multiple organ dysfunction.

Shock and MODS

The two overarching categories of shock: Oxygen Delivery and Oxygen Use failures generally present with tachycardia, hypotension, and even lactic acidosis. The limitation of these presentations depends on the patient's history and medication regimen (for example, beta-blocker therapy). Extreme caution must be utilized when evaluating patients presenting with shock. As a compensatory mechanism, a surge in catecholamines and neural regulation maintains arterial pressure via a regional vasoconstrictive response and tachycardia may sustain or increase the cardiac indices, although the actual ventricular efficiency may be depressed. This response may mask how serious the situation is.

The more traditional divisions of cardiogenic, hypovolemic, and hemorrhagic shock can be classified as failure of the mechanics of oxygen delivery. This failure includes three basic oxygenation delivery parameters including CI, Hgb, and Hgb saturation as well as pure vascular tonal deficits (such as acute spinal cord injury, anaphylaxis, vasodilator overdose, severe sepsis). The therapies involved are relatively traditional and are aimed at restoring oxygen delivery to a normal level in respect to oxygen demand. Patients with mechanical shock will compensate via sympathetic discharge and a catecholamine surge, shifting blood away from nonessential organs to essential organs. The nonessential organ uses <50% of oxygen delivered to them and are generally not profoundly affected by a short period of ischemia. The redirected blood flow sustains the oxygen dependent organs, including the heart, the brain, and the lung parenchyma as well as the diaphragm.

Hypovolemic Shock

Hypovolemic shock occurs when either total body, intravascular or intra-arterial volumes are significantly decreased. This depletion may be a result of hemorrhage, which not only affects the volume load, but also the oxygen carrying capacity associated with the Hgb. Loss of effective arterial volume can occur with third-space losses, salt-wasting disorders, diabetic shock syndromes (diabetic ketoacidosis [DKA] and hyperosmolar hyperglycemic state [HHS]) vomiting, diarrhea, and/or dehydration. The hemodynamic findings in hypovolemic shock are typically tachycardia, decreased CO, decreased stroke volume, narrow pulse pressures, increased calculated SVR, normal to low ventricular filling pressures, and a very low SvO_2. When hemorrhage is the culprit, the Hgb and Hct may underpredict the severity of bleeding as those two measures might be affected by the concurrent dehydration. Index of suspicion and serial Hct, as well as BUN and creatinine measures, may differentiate bleeding from pure hypovolemia, particularly after volume resuscitation, as hemorrhagic shock may initially be misconstrued. Postural vital signs should be measured in the upright or semi-Fowler's position, with narrowing pulse pressure and tachycardia noted as one of the primary signs of decreased CO and compensatory vasoconstriction.

The primary compensatory mechanism is to conserve oxygen for the essential organs and allow the nonessential organs to generate some metabolic failure, lactic acidosis, and hydrogen ion accumulation. In the inadequate delivery state, the essential organs, to escape ischemia and infarction, will maintain the level of oxygen consumption necessary for preservation via dissociation of oxygen. The evaluation of venous Hgb saturation via continuous monitoring SvO_2 or $ScvO_2$ determines the reservoir level and facilitates the therapeutic goal of reducing tissue demands and improving oxygen delivery.

When the oxygen saturated Hgb in the continuous central or mixed venous compartment is less than normal, the issues are clear: demand is higher than supply can keep up with. There are three common issues with oxygen delivery and tissue demand: decreased content, decreased CO/CI, and increased demand. The inability of oxygen delivery to match oxygen demand (consumption) will result in a desaturation of Hgb (Rivers, 2001). As tissue demand exceeds the arterial supply (supply–demand imbalance), Hgb will more aggressively desaturate to maintain tissue consumption, causing a drop in the measured venous saturation of Hgb (SvO_2/$ScvO_2$). Along with more traditional parameters (MAP, heart rate, respiratory rate, CVP, pulse pressure, or stroke volume and the corresponding variation), this shift to the right provides a therapeutic end point and a window of opportunity for therapy.

Relative Hypovolemic Shock

Distributive. Relative hypovolemic shock occurs primarily when sympathetic tone is lost (as in acute spinal cord injury), when there is a profound mediator vasodilation syndrome (Anaphylaxis an late Sepsis or septic shock) or as an incidental symptom in acute acidostic environments (pH < 7.25), hypokalemia, and hypocalcemia states. As loss of vascular tone ensues, there is a substantial inability to maintain capillary perfusion pressures, and the compensatory mechanism will be assisted by a neuroendocrine mediated cardio renal response designed to preserve volume and increase CO. If sympathetic tone is lost or opposed, as in acute spinal cord injury, the failure of the cardiac compensatory response (relative bradycardia in an acute hypotensive state) must alert the clinican to the potential for cell death. When there is opposition at the vascular surface, as in histamine-related anaphylaxis or mediator (such as nitric oxide) induced vasodilation, the cardiac compensation is generally inadequate to maintain blood pressure, as the volume input from LV ejection cannot supplant the vascular tonal requirement for blood pressure management. This is frequently known as distributive shock, an uncontrolled vascular dilation with inability to shunt bloods adequately towards the oxygen dependent organs (heart, brain, lung parenchyma, and kidney, in that order).

Microcirculatory and Mitochondrial

Unlike all the other forms of shock, this unique process presents with increasing evidence of lactic acidosis and organ dysfunction in the face of an initial increase in oxygen delivery. With adequate volume and an initially normal cardiac function, primary compensation is to increase the CO. As time progress, the inverse relationship between measured CO and the increasing SvO_2 (indicating available, unutilized oxygen) coupled with the evidence of tissue dysfunction (organ indicators, increasing lactic acidosis) complicates the treatment and resolution of severe sepsis.

Early stages were previously known as compensated or warm shock and the later stage, which is similar to cardiogenic shock (and in fact may be heart failure), as late, cold, or decompensated shock. The critical point is early recognition and intervention during the compensatory stage, to limit endothelial and mitochondrial, and therefore organ, dysfunction. The development of critical hypotension, unresponsive to fluid resuscitation in the face of SIRS and index of suspicion, may actually portend vascular tonal loss. Tonal loss most frequently occurs with acidotic environments, hypocalcemia and endothelial production of nitric oxide. In these situations, the patient may be refractory to α stimulation type vasopressors. After volume resuscitation, vasopressor management, and evaluation and treatment of the first two conditions, consideration of continuous intravenous vasopressin or IV bolus dose cortisol, which may potentiate vascular tone, should be considered.

Summary

In the severely septic state, circulating mediators, and communicators change the capillary integrity and cause capillary leak, promoting microcoagulopathies in multiple small vessels, therefore, limiting the ability of the Hgb to move into the capillary and release the oxygen. Proinflammation, procoagulation, endothelial dysfunction, and neutrophil sequestration are the hallmarks of septic shock. Despite an adequate Hgb level and often times an increased CI, the microcirculatory blood flow is limited by nondeformable red blood cells, fibrin clots, and platelet plugs. This condition sets up a systemic shunt, or a shift to the left of the oxyHgb dissociation curve, in the face of significant tissue level hypoxia. That ongoing tissue hypoxia perpetuates and sustains more inflammatory stimulation. Vasopressors and uncontrolled hyperglycemia may also impact the capillary dynamics, therefore, the early compensatory mechanism is to increase the CO.

The tissues signal for sympathoadrenal response as tissue hypoxia and lactic acidosis mounts. Despite available oxygen reservoirs (reflected by normal to elevated SvO_2 or $ScvO_2$), there is an ongoing state of microcirculatory deficits, evidenced by increasingly elevated lactate levels, wide anion gap, base deficit, and evolving organ dysfunction. As the oxygen delivery increases (via increasing CO) to meet tissue demands, the proportional oxygen extraction ($S_aO_2 - ScvO_2/ S_aO_2$) ratio will decrease. In the most basic sense, the patient needs and has oxygen, but is not using it proportionately.

At this point, the effect on the oxyHgb curve may be very misleading. Despite persistent lactic acidosis, these patients may present with a normal to high normal or even high SvO_2. Along with more traditional measurable parameters, this shift to the left in the presence of lactic acidosis provides a window for therapy. In severe sepsis and septic shock, the primary compensatory mechanism is to increase the delivery of oxygen primarily via an increase in CO. The cardiac response relates to the systemic microcirculatory shunt and the compounding tissue hypoxia. However, the more oxygen delivery increases, the more profoundly one may see a failure of oxygen utilization. Our earliest identification of patients at risk may well be related to these global indicators of tissue perfusion. A mixed venous or central monitoring technique will communicate the availability of reserve oxygen, whether or not it has been appropriately utilized, and lactic acid levels will differentiate the adequacy of the oxygen dissociation.

The identification of the early subtle and less subjective indicators of hypoperfusion is critical. When delivery of oxygen is poor or inadequate to meet the cellular needs, there will be a significant drop in the $ScvO_2$ or SvO_2. This is generally accompanied by rapid heart rate and/or rapid respiratory rate. Coupled with an increasing lactic acidosis and wide anion gap, these parameters warn of impending danger and possible severe organ dysfunction. This patient requires very focused early goal direction aimed at tissue perfusion.

The patient in mediator shock is even more difficult to diagnose in the early stages, presenting initially with delivery dependent consumption and then spiraling toward an extraction deficit. The elevated $ScvO_2$ with persistent lactic acidosis forewarns the possibility of a microcirculatory deficit.

In summary, individuals with primary delivery deficit will traditionally have a low SvO_2 or $ScvO_2$ and may or may not have elevated lactate. Without early aggressive resuscitation, a severe lactic acidosis will develop. The mediator shock syndrome, in the earliest stage presents with a low $ScvO_2$, but later presents with normal to elevated SvO_2 or $ScvO_2$. Hgb desaturates to maintain cellular oxygenation when demand is high and delivery poor. In the inverse, the Hgb does NOT desaturate when demand is low, delivery is high, or there are microcirculatory deficits. The astute provider evaluates the venous saturations in the presence of serial lactic acid levels, determining whether or not the patient has an adequate reservoir of oxygen.

Supporting tissue demand and providing stability, prior to endothelial damage may prevent end organ death. The ability to closely monitor the oxygen delivery, the release of oxygen from the Hgb and the adequacy of both forms of compensation via serial lactic acid levels and anion gap facilitates earlier, more appropriate therapies for the acute patient at risk for MODS.

References

Aird, W. C. (2002). Endothelial cell dynamics and complexity theory. *Critical Care Medicine, 30*(Suppl. 5), S180–S185.

American College of Chest Physicians/Society of Critical Care Medicine Consensus Conference (1992). Definitions for sepsis and multiple organ failure and guidelines for the use of innovative therapies in sepsis. *Critical Care Medicine, 20*, 864–874.

Bakker, J., Gris, P., Coffernils, M., Kahn, R. J., & Vincent, J. L. (1996). Serial blood lactate levels can predict the development of multiple organ failure following septic shock. *American Journal of Surgery, 171*, 221–226.

Bone, R. C., Balk, R. A., Cerra, F. B., Dellinger, R. P., Fein, A. M., Knaus, W. A., et al. (1992). Definitions for sepsis and organ failure and guidelines for the use of innovative therapies in sepsis. The ACCP/SCCM Consensus Conference Committee. American College of Chest Physicians/Society of Critical Care Medicine. *Chest, 101*, 1644–1655.

Connors, A. F., Jr., Speroff, T., Dawson, N. V., Thomas, C., Harrell, F. E., Jr., Wagner, D., et al. (1996). The effectiveness of right heart catheterization in the initial care of critically ill patients. *JAMA, 276*, 889–897.

Cunneen, J., & Cartwright, M. (2004). The puzzle of sepsis: Fitting the pieces of the inflammatory response with treatment. *AACN Clinical Issues, 15*(1), 18–44.

De Waal, E. E., Rex, S., Kruitwagen, C. L., Kalkman, C. J., & Buhre, W. F. (2008). Stroke volume variation obtained with FloTrac/Vigileo fails to predict fluid responsiveness in coronary artery bypass graft patients. *British Journal of Anaesthesia, 100*(5), 725–726.

Hofer, C. K., Muller, S. M., Furrer, L., Klaghofer, R., Genoni, M., & Zollinger, A. (2005). Stroke volume and pulse pressure variation for prediction of fluid responsiveness in patients undergoing off-pump coronary artery bypass grafting. *Chest, 128*(2), 848–854.

Kaplan, L. J., & Kellum, J. A. (2004). Initial pH, base deficit, lactate, anion gap, strong ion difference, and strong ion gap predict outcome from major vascular injury. *Critical Care Medicine, 32*(5), 1120–1124.

Kincaid, E. H., Meredith, J. W., & Chang, M. C. (2001). Determining optimal cardiac preload during resuscitation using measurements of ventricular compliance. *Journal of Trauma–Injury, Infection, and Critical Care, 50*(4), 665–669.

Kramer, A., Zygun, D., Hawes, H., Easton, P., & Ferland, A. (2004). Pulse pressure variation predicts fluid responsiveness following coronary artery bypass surgery. *Chest, 126*(5), 1563–1568.

Kreymann, G., Grosser, S., Buggisch, P., Gottschall, C., Matthaei, S. & Greten, H. (1993). Oxygen consumption and resting metabolic rate in sepsis, sepsis syndrome, and septic shock. *Critical Care Medicine, 21*, 1012–1019.

Kumar, A., Roberts, D., Wood, K. E., Light, B., Parrillo, J. E., Sharma, S., et al. (2006). Duration of hypotension before initiation of effective antimicrobial therapy is the critical determinant of survival in human septic shock. *Critical Care Medicine, 34*, 1589–1596.

Levraut, J., Ciebiera, J. P., Chave, S., Robary, O., Jamboy, P., Charles, M., et al. (1998). Mild hyperlactatemia in stable septic patients is due to impaired lactate clearance rather than overproduction. *American Journal of Respiratory Critical Care Medicine, 157*, 1021–1026.

Levy, M. M., Fink, M. P., Marshall, J. C., Abraham, E., Angus, D., Cook, D., et al. (2003). 2001 SCCM/ESICM/ACCP/ATS/SIS International Sepsis Definitions Conference. *Critical Care Medicine, 31*(4), 1250–1256.

Marshall, J. C., Cook, D. J., Christou, N. V., Bernard, G. R., Sprung, C. L., & Sibbald, W. J. (1995). Multiple organ dysfunction score: A reliable descriptor of a complex clinical outcome. *Critical Care Medicine, 23*, 1638–1652.

Michard, F., Alaya, S., Zarka, V., Bahloul, M., Richard, C., & Teboul, J. L. (2003). Global end-diastolic volume as an indicator of cardiac preload in patients with septic shock. *Chest, 124*(5), 1900–1908.

Nguyen, H. B. Rivers, E. P., Knoblich, B. P., Jacobsen, G., Muzzin, A., Ressler, J. A., et al. (2004). Early lactate clearance is associated with improved outcome in severe sepsis and septic shock. *Critical Care Medicine, 32*(8), 1637–1642.

Revelly, J. P., Tappy, L., Martinez, A., Bollmann, M., Cayeux, M. C., Berger, M. M., et al. (2005). Lactate and glucose metabolism in severe sepsis and cardiogenic shock. *Critical Care Medicine, 33*, 2235–2240.

Rivers, E., Nguyen, B., Havstad, S., Ressler, J., Muzzin, A., Knoblich, B., et al., (2001). Early goal-directed therapy in the treatment of severe sepsis and septic shock. *New England Journal of Medicine, 345*, 1368–1377.

Reinhart K. Kuhn, H. J., Hartog, C., & Bredle, D. L. (2004). Continuous central venous and pulmonary artery oxygen saturation monitoring in the critically ill. *Intensive Care Medicine*, 30:1572–1578

Reinhart K. Meisner M. Brunkhorst F. M. (2006) Markers for sepsis diagnosis: what is useful? *Critical Care Clinics. 22(3): 503–19, ix–x*

Rocktaeschel, J., Morimatsu, H., Uchino, S., & Bellomo, R. (2003). Unmeasured anions in critically ill patients: Can they predict mortality? *Critical Care Medicine, 31*, 2131–2136.

Shoemaker, W. C., Appel, P. L., Kram, H. B., Waxman, K., & Lee, T. S. (1998). Prospective trial of supranormal values of survivors as therapeutic goals in high-risk surgical patients. *Chest, 94*, 1176–1186.

Tappy, L., & Chioléro, R. (2007) Substrate utilization in sepsis and multiple organ failure. *Critical Care Medicine, 35*(Suppl. 9), S531–S534.

Suggested Readings

De Castro, V., Goarin, J. P., Lhotel, L., Mabrouk, N., Perel, A., & Coriat, P. (2006). Comparison of stroke volume (SV) and stroke volume respiratory variation (SVV) measured by the axillary artery pulse-contour method and by aortic Doppler echocardiography in patients undergoing aortic surgery. *British Journal of Anaesthesia, 97*(5), 605–610.

Dellinger, R. P., Levy, M. M., Carlet, J. M., Bion, J., Parker, M. M., Jaescke, R., et al. (2008). Surviving sepsis campaign: International guidelines for management of severe sepsis and septic shock. *Critical Care Medicine, 36*(1), 296–327.

Feldman, M., Soni, N., & Dickson, B. (2005). Influence of hypoalbuminemia or hyperalbuminemia on the serum anion gap. *Journal of Laboratory and Clinical Medicine, 146*(6), 317–320.

Headley, J. M. (2006). Arterial pressure-based technologies: A new trend in CO monitoring. *Critical Care Nursing Clinics of North America, 18*(2), 179–187.

Jonas, M. M., & Tanser, S. J. (2002). Lithium dilution measurement of cardiac output and arterial pulse waveform analysis: an indicator dilution calibrated beat-by-beat system for continuous estimation of cardiac output. *Current Opinion in Critical Care, 8*(3), 257–261.

Magder, S. (2004). Clinical usefulness of respiratory variations in arterial pressure. *American Journal of Respiratory and Critical Care Medicine, 169*(2), 151–155.

Marx, G., Cope, T., McCrossan, L., Swaraj, S., Cowan, C., Mostafa, S. M., et al. (2004). Assessing fluid responsiveness by stroke volume variation in mechanically ventilated patients with severe sepsis. *European Journal of Anaesthesiology, 21*(2), 132–138.

Pinsky, M. R. (2003). Hemodynamic monitoring in the intensive care unit. *Clinics in Chest Medicine, 24*(4), 549–560.

Reuter, D. A., Kirchner, A., Felbinger, T. W., Weis, F. C., Kilger, E., Lamm, P., et al. (2003). Usefulness of left ventricular stroke volume variation to assess fluid responsiveness in patients with reduced cardiac function. *Critical Care Medicine, 31*(5), 1399–1404.

Vincent, J. L., Dufaye, P., Berre, J., Leeman, M., Deqaute, J. P., & Kahn, R. J. (1983). Serial lactate determinations during circulatory shock. *Critical Care Medicine, 11*, 449–451.

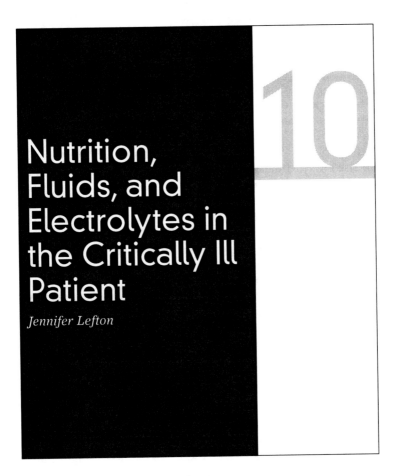

Nutrition, Fluids, and Electrolytes in the Critically Ill Patient

Jennifer Lefton

Introduction

Critically ill patients experience metabolic changes that include hypermetabolism, and net protein catabolism that can lead to depletion of lean body mass. (American Society for Parenteral and Enteral Nutrition [A.S.P.E.N.], 2002). The goal of nutrition support in the critical care setting is to minimize nitrogen losses. Critically ill patients requiring nutritional support must be monitored closely because both underfeeding as well as overfeeding can result in adverse outcomes. This chapter reviews metabolism, fluid, electrolyte, and nutrient needs, and nutrition support therapies for critically ill patients.

Metabolism

The metabolic response to conditions leading to critical illness is divided into three phases: shock/resuscitation, acute catabolic, and anabolic. During the shock/resuscitation phase, patients are hypometabolic. The reaction to the initial insult or injury leads to low cardiac output, hypotension, reduced oxygen consumption, poor tissue perfusion, and eventual shock. Lower energy expenditure and low insulin levels also occur. After 24–48 hours, the acute catabolic phase ensues with a sharp rise in counter-regulatory hormones (glucagon, cortisol, epinephrine, and norepinephrine).

During the acute catabolic phase, the rise in glucagon stimulates glycogenolysis and gluconeogenesis, (Chiolero, Revelly, & Tappy, 1997). An increase in production of proinflammatory cytokines such as tumor necrosis factor (TNF), and interleukins (IL) 1, 2, and 6 also leads to many of the changes that occur during this phase (Hill, 2000). Protein becomes a preferred energy source resulting in increased proteolysis and ureagenesis and protein losses cannot be corrected with nutrition support (Cerra, Siegel, & Coleman, 1980). Oxygen consumption and energy expenditure rise, and significant catabolism occurs.

The metabolic response is a key part of the systemic inflammatory response syndrome (SIRS) and about 50% of critically ill patients have SIRS (Brun-Buisson, 2000). SIRS is defined as having two of the following (Muckart & Bhagwanjee, 1997):

- Temperature > 38°C or <36°C
- Heart rate > 90 beats/min
- Respiratory rate > 20 breaths/min or $PaCO_2$ < 32 torr
- WBC > 12,000 cells/mm^3 or <4,000 cells/mm^3, or >10% immature band cells

During the anabolic phase, counter regulatory hormones and energy expenditure return to normal levels. Additional energy may be needed to replenish losses or support the increases in activity. Patients often still require nutritional support therapy while they begin their transition back to a regular diet.

Nutrient Requirements

Energy. Assessment of energy needs in the critically ill patients continue to be challenging to clinicians, especially in patients with extremes of age or body size. Failure to meet caloric needs can impair wound healing, organ function, and immune function (Cresci & Martindale, 2000), whereas excess calories can result in azotemia (Gault, Dixon, Doyle, & Cohen, 1968), electrolyte abnormalities, hepatic steatosis (Kaminski, Adams, & Jellinek, 1980), hyperglycemia (Rosmarin, Wardlaw, & Mirtallo, 1996), pulmonary compromise (Askanazi, Elwyn, Silverberg, Rosenbaum, & Kinney, 1980; Covelli, Black, Olsen, & Beekman, 1982), and failure to wean from the mechanical ventilator (Dark, Pingleton, & Kerby, 1985).

The use of indirect calorimetric methods to measure energy expenditure are the gold standard for determining energy needs. However, conducting these tests requires time, expensive equipment, and well-trained personnel to conduct the study and interpret the results. Because not all health care facilities are equipped to conduct indirect calorimetry studies, several equations have been developed to predict the energy needs of critically ill patients. Over 100 different predictive equations are available for use, but clinicians must find the equation that best meets the patient's needs.

Based on the current research, the American Dietetic Association's Critical Illness Guidelines recommend equations that have the highest predictive accuracy in the critically ill patients. Recommended predictive equations are shown in Table 10.1. Those no longer recommended for use include the Harris–Benedict equation (with or without stress factors), the 1997 version of the Ireton–Jones equation, and the Fick method. In addition, the Mifflin–St. Jeor equation, which is recommended to determine energy needs in the healthy population, has not been validated for use in the critically ill population (Frankenfield, Hise, Malone, Russell, Gradwell, & Compher, 2007). Predictive equations recommended for use to predict energy needs of the critically ill obese patient are shown in Table 10.1.

10.1 Predictive Equations Used to Predict Calories Needs

Critically Ill Patients

Penn State Equation (2003a)	$EE = HBEE\ (0.85) + V_E\ (33) + T_{max}\ (175) - 6433$
Swinamer	$EE = 945\ (BSA) - 6.4\ (A) + 108\ (Temp) + 24.2\ (f) + 817\ (VT) - 4349$
Ireton–Jones Equation (1992)	$EE\ (v) = 1925 - 10(A) + 5\ (W) + 281(S) + 292(T) + 851(B)$ $EE\ (s) = 629 - 11(A) + 25(W) - 609(O)$

Critically Ill Obese Patients

Ireton–Jones (1992)	$EE\ (v) = 1925 - 10(A) + 5\ (W) + 281(S) + 292(T) + 851(B)$ $EE\ (s) = 629 - 11(A) + 25(W) - 609(O)$
Penn State (1998)	$EE = HBEE(1.1) + V_E(32) + T_{max}(140) - 5340$

EE = energy expenditure; HBEE = Harris–Benedict energy expenditure; V_E = minute ventilation (liters per minute); T_{max} = maximum temperature (degrees Celsius); BSA = body surface area (m²); Temp = current temperature (degrees Celsius); f = respiratory rate (breath per minute); VT = tidal volume (liters per minute); s = spontaneously breathing; A = age (years); W = weight (kg); O = obesity (present = 1; not present = 0); v = ventilated; S = sex (male = 1; female = 0); T = trauma (present = 1; not present = 0); B = burn (present = 1; not present = 0).

Source: Frankenfield, D., Hise, M., Malone, A., Russell, M., Gradwell, E., & Compher, C. (2007). Prediction of resting metabolic rate in critically ill adult patients: results of a systematic review of the evidence. *Journal of the American Diatetic Association.* p. 1552.

Hypocaloric feeding regimens have gained attention in recent years, particularly in the obese population. Studies of hypocaloric regimens in obese patients have found that patients achieve positive nitrogen balance (Dickerson, Rosato, & Mullen, 1986), heal wounds (Dickerson, Rosato, & Mullen, 1986), and have better glucose control (Choban, Burge, Scales, & Flancbaum, 1997), shorter length of stay (LOS) in ICU, and shorter duration of antibiotic days (Dickerson, Boschert, Kudsk, & Brown, 2002). There is no agreed-upon definition of hypocaloric feeding regimens, but the studies have used anywhere from 50% of the patients' measured energy expenditure (MEE) to 14 cal/kg actual weight or <20 cal/kg adjusted ideal body weight. All of the studies provided approximately 2.0 grams protein/kg ideal body weight. Initial studies are promising, and A.S.P.E.N. suggests the use of hypocaloric feeding regimens with supplemental protein in mild to moderately stressed obese patients (A.S.P.E.N., 2002); however, it is not yet known whether this can be applied to other patient populations including the nonobese. One study in the nonobese population did not find benefit to hypocaloric total parenteral nutrition (TPN) regimens (McCowen et al., 2000). An additional observational study linked more infectious complications to critically ill patients with the greatest cumulative energy deficit (Villet et al., 2005).

Carbohydate. Carbohydrates are the main source of calories in most diets and provides energy to all cells in the body, providing 4 cal/g. Cells in the central nervous system (e.g., brain) and those that rely on anaerobic glycolysis (e.g., red blood cells) have an absolute carbohydrate requirement (Otten, Hellwig, Meyers, 2006a).

Underfeeding carbohydrates in critically ill patients further exacerbates protein breakdown. Without adequate carbohydrates, adipose and muscle tissue are broken down and are used as fuel source, entering gluconeogenic pathways to provide glucose to the body. Protein catabolism leads to loss of skeletal muscle mass and loss of body proteins, which may lead to impaired immune response and poor wound healing.

Excessive carbohydrates in critically ill patients affects glycemic response, respiratory function, and long term liver function. Hyperglycemia causes a rise in insulin levels that can shift electrolytes intracellularly (e.g., potassium and phosphorus), and this is reflected by a drop in serum levels. Excess carbohydrate intake has also been reported to contribute to respiratory distress (Askanazi et al., 1980), hypercapnia during weaning from mechanical ventilation (Dark et al., 1985), and respiratory failure (Covelli et al., 1982). Death has been reported as a complication of overfeeding (75 kcals/kg per day as carbohydrate) in malnourished patients (Weinsier & Krumdieck, 1981). Potential signs of overfeeding include increased carbon dioxide (CO_2) production, increased minute ventilation, difficulty weaning from the ventilator, acute respiratory acidosis or metabolic alkalosis, and a respiratory quotient (RQ) >1.0 (Klein, Stanek, & Wiles, 1998). When overfeeding is suspected, a reduction in carbohydrate and total calories may prevent respiratory compromise (Talpers, Romberger, Bunce, & Pingleton, 1992). Patients at risk of being overfed are the elderly, those with unusual body sizes (malnourished or extremely obese), and those on dialysis using a dialysate containing dextrose (Klein et al., 1998).

The adequate intake established for carbohydrates is 130 g/day (Otten et al., 2006a). Additional suggestions for carbohydrate intake in critically ill patients range from 30% to 70% of total calories (Cerra et al., 1997). Critically ill patients should receive no more than 4 $mg \cdot kg^{-1} \cdot min^{-1}$ of carbohydrates. For burn patients, no more than 5 $mg \cdot kg^{-1} \cdot min^{-1}$ is acceptable (Jacobs et al., 2004). It has been suggested to limit this to 2.5–4.0 $mg \cdot kg^{-1} \cdot min^{-1}$ in patients with hyperglycemia or those receiving steroid therapy (Klein, Stanek, & Wiles, 1998). Additional suggestions are to limit dextrose to 100–150 g/day in malnourished patients who are at risk of developing refeeding syndrome (Chan, McCown, & Blackburn, 1999). The ideal dose of carbohydrates is the amount that can allow for maximal protein sparing while minimizing hyperglycemia.

Fat. Fat is a concentrated source of energy providing 9 cal/g. It functions in cell signaling and helps with absorption of fat soluble vitamins (Otten, Hellwig, & Meyers, 2006b). The only essential fatty acids are linoleic acid and alpha-linolenic acid.

Limiting fat can impair growth in children. When combined with inadequate intake of carbohydrate and protein, a negative energy balance develops leading to malnutrition. Insufficient fat intake can lead to essential fatty acid deficiency. Three weeks of TPN without added fat was reported to result in essential fatty deficiency (EFAD) (Richardson & Sgoutas, 1975). Signs and symptoms of EFAD include scaly dermatitis, alopecia, thrombocytopenia, anemia, and impaired wound healing; the deficiency can be confirmed by checking a triene-to-tetraene ratio.

Excess fat intake may lead to hypertriglyceridemia. Overfeeding parenteral sources of fat may also contribute to immunosuppression, because the omega-6 fatty acids desaturate and elongate to form arachidonic acid, a precursor to proinflammatory eicosanoids (Alexander, 1998). The use of sedatives such as propofol are provided in a lipid emulsion providing 1.1 cal/ml, which contributes to fat and total calorie intake of critically ill patients. Any long-term use of this sedative requires adjustments be made to the nutrition regimen to avoid overfeeding fat and total calories.

The acceptable macronutrient distribution range for total fat is 20% to 35% of total calories (Otten et al., 2006b). At least 2% to 4% of total calories should be provided as essential fatty acids (1%–2% linoleic acid and 0.5% from alpha-linolenic acid) to prevent development of EFAD (A.S.P.E.N., 2002). Fat intake should not exceed 1 g/kg body weight per day (A.S.P.E.N., 2002). Overfeeding fat calories can easily be prevented by aiming for 15%–30% total calories coming from fat. Contraindications in providing a parenteral source of fat include egg allergy and hypertriglyceridemia. Parenteral sources of fat are generally considered safe to provide as long as triglyceride levels are <400 mg/dl (A.S.P.E.N., 2002). When triglycerides are >400 mg/dl, the minimum amount of fat needed to avoid EFAD should be given (250 ml 20% IV lipid emulsion 1–2 times/week).

Protein. Protein is a main structural and functional component of every cell in the body. Enzymes, membrane carriers, blood transport molecules, intracellular matrices, hair, fingernails, keratin, collagen, many hormones, and a large portion of membranes are actually proteins. All body proteins are continuously degraded and resynthesized in a process referred to as protein turnover (Otten, Hellwig, & Meyers, 2006d). Protein can provide 4 cal/g when used for energy.

Underfeeding protein can result in greater protein losses and impaired wound healing. Protein deficiency can affect all organs and many systems in the body. Although the risk of excessive intake of protein from foods is very low, there have been reports of adverse events from overfeeding protein in patients requiring enteral and parenteral nutrition (Otten et al., 2006d). Any excess protein is deaminated, and the ammonia is excreted as urea (Frankenfield, 2001). Because water is required for the excretion of urea, dehydration can result when excess protein is provided (Gault et al., 1968). Protein intake in excess of 1.5 g/kg body weight per day is more likely to result in azotemia for older adults rather than younger adults (Frankenfield, Cooney, Mith, & Rowe, 2000; Clevenger et al., 1992). A rising blood urea nitrogen (BUN) that is not proportional to changes in creatinine levels and/or a rising ammonia level with worsening encephalopathy indicate a need to reduce protein intake (Cerra et al., 1997).

Although the recommended dietary allowance (RDA) for protein in healthy adults is 0.8 g/kg body weight per day (Otten et al., 2006d), protein needs can be almost twice this amount in critically ill patients. Studies have found that providing 1–1.2 g/kg of body weight per day was optimal in the first 2 weeks of critical illness (Ishibashi, Plank, Sando, & Hill, 1998) and that 1.25 g protein/kg body weight/d was ideal in the 1st week post trauma (Larsson, Lennmarken, Martensson, Sandsedt, & Vinnars, 1990). The goal of providing nutrition support therapy, including an exogenous source of protein, during critical illness is to minimize nitrogen losses. Provision of more than 1.5 g/kg body weight per day does not further lead toward attaining this goal (Ishibashi et al., 1998; Hoffer, 2003; Larsson, Lennmarken, Martensson, Sandsedt, & Vinnars, 1990; Shaw, Wildbore, & Wolfe, 1987). Patients with open wounds (e.g., open abdomens or burn patients) and with significant gastrointestinal losses (e.g., enterocutaneous fistulas) may be an exception. High-protein regimens (over 1.5 g/kg body weight per day) are recommended for patients with burn wounds until significant healing is achieved (A.S.P.E.N., 2002). Studies in patients with burns have shown that high protein regimens help attain nitrogen balance (Kagan, Matsuda, Hanumadass, Castillo, & Jonasson, 1982; Matsuda, Kagan, Hanumadass, & Jonasson, 1983), increase the rate of restored body weight and muscle function (Demling & DeSanti, 1998), and improve immune function and survival in burned children (Alexander et al., 1980).

Fluid. Daily fluid needs vary greatly in the critical care setting. In general, fluid administration is adjusted to maintain normal urine output, blood pressure, and organ perfusion. An easy estimate for stable ICU patients is 30–40 ml fluid/kg body weight or 1–1.5 ml/cal consumed, but this may require adjustments based on age, size, and organ function (Lucarelli, Pell, Shirk, & Mirtallo,

2005). Familiarity with electrolyte composition of body fluids and intravenous fluids is essential when ordering intravenous fluids for critically ill patients (Tables 10.2 and 10.3).

Vitamins and Minerals. It is unknown whether the vitamin and mineral needs of critically ill patients differs from the needs of the healthy population. Patients should receive a minimum of the RDA for vitamins and mineralsand most enteral formulations provide this amount once patients have reached their prescribed goal volumes. However, in some cases when these needs are not met, a multivitamin with minerals should be prescribed (Lefton, Esper, & Kochevar, 2007). On the other hand, some enteral formulations provide supplemental amounts of vitamins and minerals beyond RDA amounts. For ICU patients requiring PN, standard amounts of vitamins and trace elements are added to the PN daily (Mirtallo et al., 2004).

The potential benefit of antioxidant supplementation in critically ill patients has been of recent interest. Studies have shown that antioxidant supplementation can decrease the incidence of organ failure (Nathens et al., 2002; Porter, Ivatury, Azimuddin, & Swami, 1999), result in fewer infectious complications (Porter et al., 1999), and reduce 28-day mortality (Crimi et al., 2004). However, these studies have varied in terms of the ICU population studied, the antioxidant regimens studied (including route of administration and dosage). Therefore, arriving at conclusions regarding widespread use would be premature at this time.

Selenium has also been studied in the critically ill population. Patients with low selenium levels at the time of admission had a threefold increase in ventilator association pneumonia (VAP), organ dysfunction, and mortality (Forceville et al., 1998). In another study, patients randomized to receive selenium supplementation had a reduced incidence of renal failure (Angstwurm, Schottdorf, Schopohl, & Gaertner, 1999). Further research is needed to determine the clinical significance of low selenium levels and whether replacement improves outcomes.

Electrolytes. Electrolyte needs must be individualized and vary tremendously among critically ill patients. Table 10.4 shows general recommendations for electrolyte needs, but this may need to be adjusted depending on body size, organ function, and electrolyte losses.

10.2 Composition of Gastrointestinal Secretions

	Volume (ml/24 hours)	Sodium (mmol/L)	Potassium (mmol/L)	Chloride (mmol/L)	Bicarbonate (mmol/L)
Saliva	1500 (500–2000)	10	20	10	20
Stomach	1500 (100–4000)	60	10	130	0
Duodenum	100–2000	140	5	104	0
Ileum	3000 (100–9000)	140 (80–150)	5 (2–8)	104 (43–137)	30
Colon		60	30	40	
Pancreas	(100–800)	140 (113–185)	5 (3–7)	75 (54–95)	115
Bile	(50–800)	145 (131–164)	5 (3–12)	100 (89–180)	35

Reprinted with permission from Shires III, G. T., Barber, A., & Shires, G. T. (1999). Fluid and electrolyte management of the surgical patient. In S. I. Schwartz (Ed.). *Principles of surgery* (7th ed., pp. 55–56). New York: McGraw–Hill.

10.3 Composition of Intravenous Fluids

	Glucose (g/dl)	Sodium (mEq/L)	Potassium (mEq/L)	Calcium (mEq/L)	Chloride (mEq/L)	Lactate (mEq/L)	Osmolarity (mOsm/L)
Lactated Ringers	—	130	4	3	109	28	273
0.9% NaCl (normal saline)	—	154	—	—	154	—	308
0.45% NaCl (half normal saline)	—	77	—	—	77	—	154
5% dextrose in water	5	—	—	—	—	—	253
5% dextrose in 0.45% NaCl	5	77	—	—	77	—	407
5% dextrose in 0.9% NaCl	5	154	—	—	154	—	560
3% sodium chloride	—	513	—	—	513	—	1026

Reprinted with permission from Shires III, G. T., Barber, A.., & Shires, G. T. (1999) Fluid and electrolyte management of the surgical patient. In S. I. Schwartz (Ed.). *Principles of surgery* (7th ed., pp. 55–56). New York: McGraw–Hill.

10.4 Daily Electrolyte Requirements

Electrolyte	Enteral	Parenteral
Sodium	500 mg (22 mEq)	1–2 mEq/kg body weight
Potassium	2 g (51 mEq)	1–2 mEq/kg body weight
Chloride	750 mg (21 mEq)	As needed to maintain acid–base balance
Acetate	—	As needed to maintain acid–base balance
Calcium	1200 mg (60 mEq)	10–15 mEq
Magnesium	420 mg (35 mEq)	8–20 mEq
Phosphorus	700 mg (23 mmol)	20–40 mmol

Note: This table gives general ranges for safe administration of nutrients in generally healthy people. Nutrient prescriptions must be individualized for each patient and clinical situation.

Reprinted with permission from A.S.P.E.N. Board of Directors and Clinical Guidelines Task Force. (2002). Guidelines for the use of parenteral and enteral nutrition in adult and pediatric patients. *Journal of Parenteral and Enteral Nutrition, 26,* pp. 1SA–138SA.

Nutrition Support

Enteral nutrition (EN) continues to be the preferred route of nutritional support over parenteral nutrition (PN). The popular phrase "if the gut works, use it" is well known among clinicians. Historically, PN had been the preferred route of nutrition support in the 1970s and early 1980s. During the late 1980s, studies in trauma patients began reporting reduced infectious complications with EN when compared with PN (Moore & Jones, 1986; Moore, Moore, & Jones, 1989; Kudsk et al., 1992; Moore, et al., 1992). More recent meta-analysis of the use of PN compared with EN have found no effect on mortality (Heyland, MacDonald, Keefe, & Drover, 1998) (Peter, Moran, & Phillips–Hughes, 2005). However, PN results in greater infectious complications, catheter related blood stream infections (CRBSI), and hospital length of stay (Peter,

Moran, & Phillips–Hughes, 2005). When EN is not possible, PN may be beneficial in patients with preexisting malnutrition, but care must be taken to avoid overfeeding and prevent complications associated with refeeding syndrome (Heyland et al., 1998; Jeejeebhoy, 2001). EN is also cheaper compared with PN (American Dietetic Association [ADA], 2007).

Enteral Nutrition

Enteral Access. Several options are available for enteral feeding access in critically ill patients. Nasoenteric devices are used initially to meet the patients' short-term needs. There is considerable debate over whether the tip of the feeding tube should be in the stomach or the small bowel. Several studies have found that patients fed via postpyloric feeding access receive more nutrition earlier (Kearns et al., 2000; Kortbeek, Haigh, & Doig, 1999; Minard, Kudsk, Melton, Patton, & Tolley, 2000; Montecalvo et al., 1992; Taylor, Fettes, Jewkes, & Nelson, 1999). This improved nutrient delivery is likely a result of less frequent interruptions of the feedings, because gastric feedings are frequently withheld for high gastric residual volumes (GRV), nursing care, and tests or procedures in which the patient must lay flat. Feeding into the jejunum is associated with lower GRV (ADA, 2007; Davies et al., 2002; Montejo et al., 2002). Feedings into the small bowel have not been shown to result in less aspiration (Kearns et al., 2000; Neumann & DeLegge, 2002) or a lower incidence of pneumonia (Kearns et al., 2000; Kortbeek et al., 1999; Montecalvo et al., 1992; Montejo et al., 2002), but these studies evaluated duodenal feedings. To prevent aspiration, the tip of the feeding tube should be placed in the jejunum beyond the ligament of Treitz. The ability to place small bowel feeding tubes into the jejunum varies among institutions and depends on the skill level of the personnel who will insert feeding tubes or the availability of portable fluoroscopy or endoscopy. Patients who require multiple abdominal surgeries should have a small-bowel feeding access placed during surgery. Small-bowel feeding access has been recommended when two or more risk factors for aspiration are present. These risk factors include, but are not limited to, endotracheal intubation, decreased level of consciousness/sedation, persistently high GRV/vomiting, need for supine position, and presence of nasoenteric tubes, all of which are common in critically ill patients (McClave et al., 2002).

Prior to initiation of enteral feedings, radiographic confirmation of feeding tube placement is recommended for any
blindly placed feeding tubes (gastric or small bowel). It is
also useful to mark the exit site of the feeding tube when the
initial radiograph is done because any increase in the external length would be a clue that the feeding tube is dislodged
(Bankhead et al., 2008).

Patients requiring long-term enteral feedings should
have a more permanent feeding access placed such as a percutaneous endoscopic gastrostomy (PEG) or a percutaneous
endoscopic jejunostomy (PEJ).

Enteral Formulations. Adult enteral formulations are considered "medical foods" by the U.S. government and are therefore not subject to the same regulatory standards as drugs
or PN. Most critically ill patients can tolerate a standard
intact formula. Very few patients with altered digestion and
absorption may require a formula that is partially hydrolyzed
or elemental. However, there is insufficient evidence to suggest that elemental formulas result in better outcomes when
compared with standard polymeric formulas in patients with
maldigestion or malabsorption (Makola, 2005).

Some products contain fiber. The recommended fiber
intake for healthy individuals is 14 g/1,000 cal (Otten, Hellwig, & Meyers, 2006c); however, there is no recommendation
for fiber intake in the critically ill population. Some studies
have found that feeding formulas with added soluble fiber
may help alleviate or prevent diarrhea, because it increases
sodium and water absorption (Spapen et al., 2001; Rushdi,
Pichard, & Khater, 2004). Insoluble fiber may reduce transit
time (Malone, 2005). Patients who are receiving fiber-supplemented formulas should be monitored closely for bowel
function, because cases of small bowel obstruction have been
reported in patients who were given fiber-supplemented
feeding formulas (McIvor, Meguid, Curtas, & Kaplan, 1990;
Scaife, Saffle, & Morris, 1999).

Several disease-specific formulas (e.g., diabetic, renal,
and hepatic formulas) are available, but the efficacy of their
use should be evaluated in conjunction with their increased
cost. There is very little evidence to support the routine use of
many of these products in the critically ill population (Russell
& Charney, 2002).

The category of "immune-enhancing" formulas that contain supplemental amounts of arginine, nucleic acids, omega-3 fatty acids, or vitamins and minerals has received the most attention. Potential benefits include reduced infection rates (Beale, Bryg, & Bihari, 1999; Heyland et al., 2001; Heys, Walker, Smith, & Eremin, 1999), fewer ventilator days (Beale et al., 1999), and shorter length of hospital stay (Beale et al., 1999; Heys et al., 1999). Evidence-based guidelines have not recommended the routine use of these products in all critically ill patients (ADA, 2007), but others have suggested their use in severely injured trauma patients (Jacobs et al., 2004; Kudsk et al., 2001) or in patients requiring GI surgery (Kudsk et al., 2001) There is difficulty arriving at a conclusion based on available research, because the studies enrolled different patient populations, used different feeding formulations, compared study products with control products that were not isonitrogenous, used different feeding protocols, and studied different outcome variables.

Initiation and Advancement of EN. Critically ill patients should be started on EN once they have been adequately resuscitated and are hemodynamically stable. Patients should be able to sustain a mean arterial pressure (MAP) of 70 mmHg or more before starting feedings (ADA, 2007). Patients with a cardiac index <2 L·min–1·m², MAP <70 mmHg, and oxygen saturation <95% when requiring FiO_2 >60% and PEEP >5 cm are not likely to tolerate EN (Skipper, Peloquin, Gregoire, & Tangney, 2001).

The goal is to start enteral feedings within 24–48 hours of injury or ICU admission (ADA, 2007; Heyland et al., 2003). Additional research suggests that enteral feedings should be started within 24 hours of injury or admission (Marik & Zaloga, 2001). Starting "early" enteral feedings compared with "late" feedings has been associated with reduced infectious complications and may reduce LOS (ADA, 2007). The benefit of early enteral feedings is mostly seen in surgical, trauma, and burn population. One study found increased infectious complications and longer LOS in medical ICU patients started on early EN versus late EN (Ibrahim et al., 2002). In surgical patients, the presence of flatus or a bowel movement is not needed prior to initiating EN (Bankhead et al., 2008).

Enteral feedings should be initiated at full strength but often are initiated at a lower infusion rate that is advanced to a "goal rate" once tolerance to the enteral feeding has been established. Whether patients are started at 20 ml/hr or at 50 ml/hr and how tolerance is defined, varies among institutions. To keep the initial amount of tube feeding delivered in perspective, one must consider that 15 ml of formula is the equivalent of one tablespoon of formula.

Enteral feedings are most often delivered at a continuous rate in the ICU setting as opposed to bolus or intermittent feeding regimens. The increasingly common use of insulin drips in the critical care setting combined with intermittent enteral feedings would make achievement of optimal glucose control challenging.

Enteral Feeding Protocols. With an increasing emphasis on patient safety, many facilities have been developing protocols to improve the overall quality of care. These include protocols for initiating and advancing enteral feedings in ICU patients, which tend to focus on when feedings should be initiated and how much EN should be delivered. Studies of enteral feeding protocols have shown that more patients reach their "goal" volume within 72 hours of admission (Spain et al., 1999), required fewer ventilator days and had a lower risk of death (Barr, Hecht, Flavin, Khorana, & Gould, 2004), and received more EN and had shorter LOS (Martin, Doig, Heyland, Morrison, & Sibbald, 2004). An average intake of 60% to 70% of goal enteral feedings during the 1st week of critical illness has been associated with a decreased LOS, fewer days on the ventilator, and reduced infectious complications (ADA, 2007).

Enteral feeding protocols can be developed into standard order forms that can help guide the clinician prescribe enteral nutrition to best meet each patients' needs. Orders for EN should include but is not limited to the following: patient identifiers, enteral formulation, enteral access delivery site, and the administration method and rate (Bankhead et al., 2008)

Complications Associated with EN. The most common complications associated with EN in critically ill patients include diarrhea (Cataldi-Betcher, Seltzer, Slocum, & Jones, 1983; Smith, et al.,1990) and high GRV (Cataldi-Betcher et al., 1983). These and other complications associated with EN are shown in Exhibit 10.1.

Exhibit

10.1 Troubleshooting Complications Associated with EN

Complication	Etiology	Prevention	Treatment
Aspiration	▓ Feeding access dislodged or migrated back into esophagus ▓ Emesis ▓ Gastroesopheal reflux or elevated GRV	▓ Monitor or confirm proper feeding tube placement. ▓ Refer to reflux, elevated GRV below	▓ Replace feeding access as needed. ▓ Refer to reflux, elevated GRV below
Clogged feeding tube	▓ Insufficient water flushes ▓ Administering medications via feeding tube	▓ 30 ml water flush any time that the feedings are interrupted ▓ 30 ml water flush before and after residual check ▓ 30 ml water flush before and after each medication administered ▓ Use liquid form of medications when feasible.	▓ Flush with 30 ml warm water. ▓ Avoid use of juices and sodas for flushing feeding tubes. ▓ If not cleared with water, flush 5 ml water mixed with viokase and sodium bicarbonate, or use commercially available declogging solution. ▓ Replace feeding access if unable to clear.

(continued)

Exhibit

| 10.1 | Troubleshooting Complications Associated with EN *(continued)* |

Complication	Etiology	Prevention	Treatment
Constipation	▪ Inadequate fiber intake	▪ Use fiber-containing formula if appropriate and tolerated. ▪ Provide adequate fluid.	▪ Change to a fiber-containing formula if appropriate and tolerated. ▪ Provide adequate fluid.
	▪ Dehydration	▪ Add appropriate water flushes to meet fluid need.	▪ Rehydrate
	▪ Lack of activity	▪ Encourage ambulation if possible.	▪ Encourage ambulation if possible.
Diarrhea	▪ Concurrent drug therapy (antibiotics, sorbitol-containing elixir medications, magnesium-containing antacids, phosphorus supplements)	▪ Avoid enteral route of administration for meds with high sorbitol content. ▪ Dilute medications with high osmolarity in water when given via enteral route. ▪ Avoid enteral magnesium and phosphorus supplementation; opt for parenteral route.	▪ Discontinue causative agent if possible. ▪ Replace electrolyte losses by IV route.

Complication	Etiology	Prevention	Treatment
	▓ Disease or condition associated with malabsorption	▓ Pancreatic enzymes if indicated	▓ Treat underlying condition. ▓ Pancreatic enzymes if indicated ▓ Semi-elemental formula if indicated
	▓ Inadequate fiber intake		▓ Change to fiber-containing enteral products.
	▓ Infectious source (e.g., *C. difficile*)		▓ Check for *C. difficile* toxin and provide antiobiotics if positive.
Elevated GRV	▓ Decreased bowel motility, ileus, narcotics, electrolyte disorder	▓ Minimize use of narcotics ▓ Monitor electrolytes; keep magnesium >2.0 and potassium >4.0.	▓ Stool softeners as needed ▓ Treat underlying issue causing ileus. ▓ Reduce use of narcotics. ▓ Replace potassium and magnesium levels if needed.
	▓ Delayed gastric emptying		▓ Promotility agents if problem is persistent
	▓ Feeding tube dislodged or migrated back into esophagus	▓ Confirm feeding access by x-ray.	▓ Replace feeding access if needed.

Source: Lefton, J. (2002). Management of common gastrointestinal complications in tube-fed patients. *Support Line*, 19–25.

The etiology of diarrhea in critically ill tube-fed patients is typically multifactorial and most often is not related to the feeding formulation itself. The use of antibiotics and delivery of medications that may contain sorbitol or those that have a high osmolarity via the enteral route can lead to diarrhea. Laxatives, stool softeners, promotility agents, phosphorus supplements, and magnesium-containing antacids have been implicated as causing diarrhea. Careful review of the medication administration record in conjunction with tolerance to enteral feedings during daily rounds may help avoid diarrhea. The presence of enteric pathogens such as *Clostridium difficile* should be ruled out prior to administering antidiarrheal agents (Lefton, 2002).

High GRV or delayed gastric emptying is thought to increase the risk of reflux and aspiration of gastric contents. Possible causes of high GRV include ileus, sepsis, use of narcotics, and obstruction. One single episode of a high GRV does not equate to feeding intolerance, and persistently low GRV does not mean that the patient is always tolerating the enteral feeding regimen (Lefton, 2002). One issue of much debate is the GRV threshold at which feedings should be temporarily discontinued. Recent guidelines have suggested that feedings should be held after GRV are 250 ml in two consecutive measurements (ADA, 2007). Others have suggested that feedings should not be held unless GRV are >500 ml (McClave, et al., 2002). For patients with persistently high GRV, promotility agents should be added and consideration should be given to small-bowel feeding access (ADA, 2007). However, if increasing gastric output is accompanied by worsening abdominal pain and distension, feedings should be held, and a workup to determine the etiology of feeding intolerance is warranted.

Additional complications may include hyperglycemia, refeeding syndrome, and electrolyte abnormalities although these tend to be more dramatic with PN. Changing to an enteral formulation marketed for use in hyperglycemic patients has not been adequately studied in the critically ill population (Lampert & Lefton, 2008); therefore, standard enteral formulations, avoiding overfeeding, and exogenous insulin when needed is the preferred management for hyperglycemic critically ill patients who are receiving EN. Refeeding syndrome can be avoided by initiating EN at a lower rate and advancing the feedings slowly while monitoring electrolyte levels. These complications and electrolyte abnormalities are shown in Exhibit 10.2.

Exhibit

10.2 Troubleshooting Metabolic Complications Associated with EN and PN

Complication	Etiology	Prevention	Treatment
Azotemia	▨ Catabolism ▨ GI bleed ▨ Excess protein administration	▨ Keep protein administration to <2 g·kg·day and <1.5 g·kg·day for older adults.	▨ Reduce protein in EN or PN if indicated. ▨ Increase fluid intake.
Elevated liver enzymes	▨ Overfeeding (dextrose >4–5 mg·kg^{-1}·min^{-1} or lipids >1 gm·kg·day)	▨ Avoid overfeeding.	▨ Reduce total calories delivered to provide no more than 25 cals·kg·day. ▨ Reduce dextrose and/or lipid content of PN.
	▨ Long-term PN use		▨ Cycle PN if patient is stable on PN (glucose well controlled without use of insulin).
	▨ Lack of GI stimulation in patients unable to eat orally		▨ Provide some nutrition via the enteral route if possible.
Hyperglycemia	▨ Stress response or infection ▨ Steroid therapy		▨ Provide exogenous insulin if needed.
	▨ Preexisting history of diabetes mellitus	▨ Initiate PN with 2.5 mg·kg^{-1}·min^{-1} dextrose and follow glucose levels.	▨ Provide exogenous insulin if needed.

(continued)

Exhibit 10.2 Troubleshooting Metabolic Complications Associated with EN and PN *(continued)*

Complication	Etiology	Prevention	Treatment
	■ Excessive glucose administration	■ Avoid overfeeding. ■ Keep dextrose administration in PN to 1 <4 $mg \cdot kg^{-1} \cdot min^{-1}$. ■ Assess dextrose administration from other sources (e.g., IVFs and meds)	■ Reduce EN feeding rate if indicated (keep to <25–30 kcals·kg·day) ■ Reduce dextrose in PN if indicated. ■ Remove dextrose from other sources (e.g., IVF) if indicated. ■ Provide exogenous insulin if needed.
	■ Results falsely elevated because of blood drawn from PN line		■ Recheck laboratories
Hypoglycemia	■ EN interrupted, but insulin infusion continues.	■ Close monitoring of glucose levels	■ Adjust insulin dose.
	■ Excess insulin in TPN	■ Cautiously add insulin to TPN if indicated—add 2/3 of previous day's insulin requirements.	■ Discontinue PN until new bag is available with less insulin; provide source of dextrose (usually $D_{10}W$ at same rate as PN or per hospital policy). per hospital policy).

Complication	Etiology	Prevention	Treatment
Hypernatremia	▓ Fluid imbalance —excess water loss ▓ Inadequate free water	▓ Add H_2O flushes for patients on EN; enteral formulation is not intended to meet fluid needs.	▓ Assess fluid needs ▓ Calculate H_2O deficit** (L) = ([serum Na^+/140] − 1) × wt (kg) × 0.6 ▓ Adjust IVF composition and/or rate
	▓ Excess sodium intake		▓ Reduce sodium in PN and/or IVF if indicated
Hyponatremia	▓ Fluid overload ▓ Adrenal insufficiency ▓ CHF ▓ SIADH ▓ Cirrhosis/Ascites ▓ Renal failure ▓ Pseudohypo-natremia (for every 100 mg/dl glucose above normal, serum Na+ will drop by 1.6–2.0 mEq/L)	▓ Usual dose of Na^+ in PN is 100–150 m Eq/day	▓ Restrict fluid as needed
	▓ GI losses ▓ Inadequate Na+ in PN	▓ Anticipate increased sodium losses with ileostomies/ jejunostomies	▓ Increase sodium in PN if indicated (hypovolemic, hyponatremic with low osmolality) ▓ Sodium deficit **(mEq) = (140 − serum Na^+) × wt (kg) × 0.6
Hyperkalemia	▓ Renal failure	▓ Anticipate reduced K+ need for renal failure patients	▓ Use K+ binders if needed

(continued)

Exhibit

10.2	Troubleshooting Metabolic Complications Associated with EN and PN *(continued)*

Complication	Etiology	Prevention	Treatment
	▥ Metabolic acidosis ▥ Excess K+ in EN/PN		▥ Correct acidosis ▥ Change to a lower K+ content enteral formulation if high K+ levels persist ▥ Reduce or eliminate K+ in PN
	▥ Hemolyzed blood sample ▥ Catabolism		▥ Recheck K+ result
Hypokalemia	▥ Refeeding syndrome ▥ Increased GI losses ▥ Increased K+ excretion from certain meds (e.g., Amphotericin B, Furosemide) ▥ Inadequate K+ in PN	▥ Usual dose of K+ in PN is 60–120 mEq/d (for patients with normal K+ levels and good renal function) ▥ Anticipate higher K+ needs when initiating PN in malnourished patients or patients with higher than normal K+ losses	▥ Correct acute hypokalemia with IV K+ source separate from PN (generally 20 mEq K+ will increase serum K+ level by 0.2 mEq/L) ▥ Increase K+ in PN for chronic hypokalemia or for those with increased requirements
	▥ Hyperglycemia ▥ Metabolic alkalosis	▥ Control glucose levels	▥ Provide insulin if needed ▥ Correct alkalosis

Complication	Etiology	Prevention	Treatment
Hyperchloremia	▪ Excessive administration of Cl− or Cl− containing IVF (e.g., normal saline)	▪ For TPN, give Na+ and Cl− in a 1:1 ratio and other anions in acetate form	▪ Change IVF to give less Cl− ▪ Reduce Cl− in TPN
	▪ Increased loss of HCO_3-	▪ Anticipate higher bicarbonate needs with high GI losses	▪ Calculate HCO_3- deficit** = 0.5 × wt (kg) (desired HCO_3- minus measured HCO_3-)
Hypochloremia	▪ High gastric losses (NG suctioning, vomiting) ▪ Chronic diarrhea ▪ Inadequate Cl− in PN	▪ Usual dose of Cl− in PN is 100–150 mEq/day	▪ Provide more chloride w/ IVF if additional fluid is needed. ▪ Increase Cl− in TPN. ▪ Calculate Cl− deficit**(mEq) = 0.5 × wt (kg) × (103 − measured Cl−)
	▪ Metabolic alkalosis		▪ Volume and K+ repletion
Hyperphosphatemia	▪ Renal failure	▪ Anticipate reduced PO_4 needs for renal failure patients.	▪ Reduce or eliminate PO_4 administration.
	▪ Excess PO_4 administration		▪ Change to a lower PO_4 content enteral formulation if high PO4 levels persist. ▪ Reduce or eliminate PO_4 administration in PN. ▪ PO_4 binders if indicated (for enterally fed patients)

(continued)

Exhibit

10.2 Troubleshooting Metabolic Complications Associated with EN and PN *(continued)*

Complication	Etiology	Prevention	Treatment
Hypophos-phatemia	▨ Refeeding syndrome ▨ Inadequate PO_4 in TPN	▨ Usual dose of PO_4 in PN is 15–30 mmol/day ▨ Anticipate higher PO_4 needs when initiating PN in malnourished patients.	▨ Correct acute hypophosphate-mia with IV PO_4 source separate from TPN (0.16–0.64 mmol PO_4/kg wt depen-ding on severity of hypophospha-temia)* ▨ Increase PO_4 in PN for chronic hypophosphate-mia or those with increased requirements
	▨ Hyperglycemia ▨ Patients requiring CRRT ▨ Alcoholism ▨ Hyperpara-thyroidism ▨ Hyperglycemia	▨ Control glucose levels	▨ Provide exogenous insulin as needed
Hypermagna-semia	▨ Renal failure ▨ Excess Mg in TPN ▨ Adrenal insufficiency ▨ Hypothyroidism	▨ Anticipate reduced Mg needs in renal failure patients (exception is patients on CRRT).	▨ Reduce Mg in PN if indicated.
	▨ Severe acidosis		▨ Correct acidosis.

Complication	Etiology	Prevention	Treatment
Hypomagnasemia	▓ Inadequate Mg in PN ▓ Refeeding syndrome ▓ High GI losses ▓ Increased losses from meds (Amphotericin B)	▓ Usual dose of Mg in PN is 8–24 mEq/day ▓ Anticipate higher needs when initiating PN in malnourished patients or those with higher than normal Mg losses.	▓ Correct acute hyopmagnesemia with IV Mg source separate from PN ▓ Increase Mg in PN for chronic hypomagnesemia, patients at risk of refeeding syndrome, and those with high losses
Hypercalcemia	▓ Alcoholism ▓ Excess Ca+ in PN		▓ Supplement Mg. ▓ Reduce Ca+ in PN if indicated.
	▓ Prolonged immobilization ▓ Cancer with bone metastisis ▓ Renal failure ▓ Hyperparathyroidism ▓ Excessive Vitamin D	▓ Encourage activity if feasible.	
Hypocalcemia	▓ Inadequate Ca+ in PN ▓ Ca+ wasting drugs ▓ Hypoalbuminemia	▓ Usual dose of Ca+ in PN is 9–22 mEq/day	▓ Correct acute hypocalcemia separate from PN ▓ Increase Ca+ in PN if indicated ▓ Correct Ca+ level for low albumin = (4.0 g/dl − albumin level) × 0.8 + measured calcium ▓ Check ionized calcium to confirm low Ca+ level

(continued)

Exhibit

10.2 Troubleshooting Metabolic Complications Associated with EN and PN (continued)

Complication	Etiology	Prevention	Treatment
	▪ Reduced vitamin D intake		▪ Supplement vitamin D (although not in PN)

* 1 mEq potassium phosphate = 0.68 mmol phosphate; 1 mEq sodium phosphate = 0.75 mmol phosphate

Abbreviations: EN = enteral nutrition; PN = parenteral nutrition; IVF = intravenous fluid; GI = gastrointestinal; wt = weight; kg = kilograms; Na+ = sodium; K+ = potassium; CHF = congestive heart failure; SIADH = syndrome of inappropriate ADH secretion; Cl− = chloride; HCO₃− = bicarbonate; IV = intravenous; NG = nasogastric; PO₄ = phosphorus; mEq = milliequivalent; mmol = millimoles; Mg = magnesium; Ca+ = calcium; CRRT = continuous renal replacement therapy.

Sources: Klein, Stanek, & Wiles, (1998), Kraft, Btaiche, Sacks, & Kudsk, (2005), Clark, Sacks, Dickerson, Kudsk, & Brown, (1995), Piazza–Barnett & Matarese, (1999), Schmidt, (2000), Klein, et al., (2002), Hamilton & Austin, (2006).

Parenteral Nutrition

Parenteral nutrition (PN) is a complex admixture that may contain more than 40 different components. It ranks second behind anti-infective agents as a class of medications with errors in preparation or administration. Serious harm and even death has been reported from improperly prepared or administered PN solutions. A.S.P.E.N. has published "Safe Practices for Parenteral Nutrition" to help avoid some of the potential complications that can occur with PN (Mirtallo et al., 2004).

Parenteral nutrition in critically ill patients is reserved for those who are unable to be fed enterally. This may include patients with malabsorption, short bowel syndrome, complete bowel obstruction, severe necrotizing pancreatitis, high-output gastrointestinal fistulas, hemodynamic instability, and intolerance to enteral feedings. When considering PN, it should be anticipated that patients will require the therapy for at least 5 days. (Mirtallo, 2007).

Parenteral Access. Parenteral nutrition can be administered through a peripheral or a central line. The ability to meet patients' nutrient needs with peripheral PN (PPN) is limited because of restraints in osmolarity of the solution. Patients must have good peripheral venous access and be able to tolerate large volumes of fluid (Mirtallo, 2007). PPN is not an appropriate choice for patients requiring fluid restrictions (e.g., renal, cardiac, or liver failure) and patients with metabolic stress or malnutrition. The use of PPN is also considered to be a short-term therapy, and patients should be given total PN (TPN) if they continue to require PN for more than 2 weeks. Typically, no >10% dextrose solution (100 g dextrose/liter) can be given via a peripheral IV site, but amino acids, vitamins, minerals, and electrolytes in the PPN will also contribute to the osmolarity of the solution.

More concentrated PN solutions with higher osmolarities can be administered through a central line with the tip of the catheter placed in the superior vena cava. Most critically ill patients have central lines in place for administration of other medications and/or fluids. One major complication associated with central lines and TPN is the development of catheter-related blood stream infections (CRBSI). Prevention and treatment of CRBSI are discussed in Chapter 11.

Parenteral Formulations. Parenteral formulations contain dextrose, lipids, and amino acids to make up the macronutrient content of the formula. Dextrose and fat are energy sources providing 3.4 and 9 cal/g, respectively. Amino acids provide 4 cal/g if used for energy. Patients with critical illness, requiring large amounts of propofol (delivered in a fat emulsion that provides 1.1 cal/ml) for sedation, may not need additional fat with their PN formula. Formulas may be provided as a 2-in-1 solution in which the lipids are provided separately or as a 3-in-1 solution where the lipids are mixed in with the dextrose and amino acids.

Institutions may require prescription of PN macronutrients as percent stock solution, percent final concentration, grams per day, grams per kilogram of body weight per day, or calories per day. This can lead to a great deal of confusion when patients transfer from one facility to another, and significant errors can occur. Therefore, A.S.P.E.N. has suggested PN macronutrients be prescribed in grams per day or grams per kilogram of body weight per day. The use of percent concentration to prescribe PN should be avoided (Mirtallo, et al., 2004). Sample TPN macronutrient calculations are shown in Exhibit 10.3.

Exhibit

10.3 Sample Calculations to Determine Macronutrient Content of PN Formulation

There is no single measure of nutritional status or adequacy of nutrient intake.

Patient JD is critically ill and has been assessed to need approximately 2,000 ml fluid, 1,800 cal, and 80 g of protein daily. The following steps will help determine the macronutrient content of the PN solution that would provide the estimated calorie and protein needs.

1. Determine calories to be provided as protein.
   80 g protein × 4 cal/g = 320 cal
2. Determine calories remaining to be provided as fat and dextrose.
   1,800 total calories − 320 protein calories = 1,480 calories
3. Determine the amount of calories to be provided as fat
   (an easy estimate is 30% calories as fat and 70% calories as dextrose).
   1,480 × 0.30 = 444 calories as fat
   Determine grams of fat to be added to PN solution.
   444 cal as fat ÷ 9 cal/g = 49.3 g or ~50 g fat/day
4. Determine calories left to be provided as dextrose.
   1,800 − (320 protein cal + 444 fat cal) = 1,036 dextrose cal
5. Determine grams of dextrose to be added to the PN solution.
   1,036 cal as dextrose ÷ 3.4 cal/g = 304 grams or ~300 g dextrose/day

The PN prescription would then be for 2,000 ml (or 2 L) containing 80 g amino acids/day, 50 g fat/day, and 300 g of dextrose/day. The amount of dextrose should be initiated as 150 g/day and eventually increased to 300 g/day if glucose levels are well controlled and electrolytes stable.

The following electrolytes may be added to PN solutions: sodium, potassium, calcium, phosphorus, and magnesium. Sodium and potassium may be added as chloride, acetate, or phosphate salt. Bicarbonate is not stable in PN solutions, and acetate is used for base needs. The amount of chloride and acetate added to the PN formulation depends on the acid–base balance of the patient. For example, patients with high gastric losses will most likely need chloride, whereas renal failure patients may benefit from some acetate in the solution. Electrolytes should be prescribed as a total amount per day rather than per liter (Mirtallo, et al., 2004).

There are limitations in regard to the total amount of phosphorus and calcium that can safely be added to the PN formulation. Excess calcium and phosphorus could result in patients' harm or death, because calcium phosphate precipitates leading to diffuse microvascular pulmonary emboli (Mirtallo et al., 2004). Institution policy regarding PN compounding and compatibility issues should be followed.

A multiple vitamin infusion (MVI) and a multiple trace element (MTE) solution should be added daily to the PN prescription (Mirtallo et al., 2004). Tables 10.5 and 10.6 show daily vitamin and mineral requirements for adults requiring PN. Patients with significant GI losses through ostomies or fistulas or other malabsorptive states requiring long-term PN may need additional zinc, copper and chromium supplementation. Long-term PN patients with cholestasis or bile duct obstruction should have copper and manganese monitored, and supplementation may need to be adjusted or eliminated from the PN solution (Misra & Kirby, 2000).

10.5 Daily Requirements for Adult Parenteral Vitamins

Vitamin	Requirement
Thiamin (B$_1$)	6 mg
Riboflavin (B$_2$)	3.6 mg
Niacin (B$_3$)	40 mg
Folic acid	600 mcg
Pantothenic acid	15 mg
Pyridoxine (B6)	6 mg
Cyanocobalamin (B$_{12}$)	5 mcg
Biotin	60 mcg
Ascorbic Acid (C)	200 mg
Vitamin A	3300 IU
Vitamin D	200 IU
Vitamin E	10 IU
Vitamin K	150 mcg

Source: Food and Drug Administration.

10.6 Daily Trace Element Supplementation to Adult PN Formulations

Trace Element	Standard Intake
Chromium	10–15 mcg
Copper	0.3–0.5 mg
Iron	Not routinely added
Manganese	60–100 mcg
Selenium	20–60 mcg
Zinc	2.5–5 mg

Source: Mirtallo, J., Canada, T., Johnson, D., Kumpf, V., Peterson, C., Sacks, G., et al. (2004). Safe practices for parenteral nutrition. *Journal of Parenteral and Enteral Nutrition,* S39–S70.

Little is known about the compatibility of drugs in PN solutions. H2 blockers and insulin are the only medications that are added to PN solutions. When insulin is added to the PN regimen, regular insulin should be used. There are several suggested methods for calculating insulin needs to be added to the PN. One easy method is to add two thirds of what the patient required from the previous day's sliding scale insulin regimen. However, some ICUs may prefer not to add insulin to the PN solution and continue with unit specific insulin drip protocols.

Initiation and Advancement of PN. Baseline laboratory values including electrolytes, BUN, creatinine, glucose, hepatic function, and triglyceride levels should be obtained prior to initiating PN. Any acute electrolyte abnormalities (e.g., low K+, PO4, and magnesium levels) or hyperglycemia should be corrected prior to initiation of PN. When glucose levels are >300 mg/dl, BUN is >100 mg/dl, sodium level is >150 mEq/L, chloride level is >115 mEq/L, or phosphorus levels are <2.0 mg/dl, it would be prudent to delay initiation of PN until these levels are corrected (Mirtallo J. et al., 2007).

Amino acids and IV fat emulsions can be initiated at "goal" amounts, whereas dextrose is typically initiated at half the goal amount. Large amounts of dextrose provided too quickly to patients who may be at risk of refeeding syndrome or those with hyperglycemia will exacerbate these complications. By providing half the dextrose in the initial PN formula, clinicians can monitor tolerance and incrementally increase the amount of dextrose over a few days if glucose levels are maintained <150 mg/dl and phosphorus levels >2.0 mg/dl.

Complications Associated with PN. There are several complications associated with PN including mechanical complications because of central line insertion and CRBSI. However, this section will focus on the metabolic complications that may occur and are largely avoidable when PN prescriptions are developed by clinicians who are knowledgeable in PN support therapy.

Hyperglycemia is probably the most common complication associated with PN use. Providing a mixed fuel substrate solution and keeping the dextrose to <4 mg·kg^{-1}·min^{-1} will help avoid hyperglycemia associated with overfeeding (Khaodhiar & Bistrian, 1999; Jacobs et al., 2004). However, many critically ill patients experience hyperglycemia as part of their metabolic response and will require exogenous sources of insulin regardless of the amount of dextrose prescribed in the PN. Additional sources of dextrose such as those in additional IVFs should be limited.

Patients who have exhibited poor nutritional intake prior to initiation of PN or that have been assessed to have a poor nutritional status are at risk for developing refeeding syndrome with initiation of PN. When refeeding syndrome develops, potassium, phosphorus, and magnesium will shift intracellularly, and serum levels will drop requiring replacement. Even a starvation period as short as 48 hours has been reported to predispose critically ill patients to refeeding hypophosphatemia (Marik & Bedigian, 1996). Sodium retention and fluid overload can also occur as a result of refeeding syndrome. An additional 50–100 mg IV or 100 mg oral thiamine over 5–7 days has also been suggested for patients at risk of refeeding syndrome (Kraft, Btaiche, & Sacks, 2005).

Electrolyte abnormalities can also occur in patients requiring PN (see Exhibit 10.2, pages 377 through 384). Careful monitoring of daily electrolyte levels and adjustments in the PN prescription can help to avoid these complications. Further details about electrolyte disorders have been addressed in great detail elsewhere (Kraft et al., 2005).

Most metabolic complications associated with use of PN are related to overfeeding the patient or providing too much nutrition too soon. When starting patients on PN, consultation with the nutrition support clinician will offer a thorough evaluation of nutrition status, nutrient needs, and suggestions for initiation and advancement of the regimen to help avoid these complications.

Monitoring Nutrition Support Therapy

There is no single measure that is indicative of patients' nutritional status nor the adequacy of nutrients provided. Albumin is a transport protein with a long half life (about 21 days) that has often been used in nutrition assessment. However, its application in the assessment of critically ill patients is inappropriate because serum levels will fall with fluid resuscitation, capillary leakage, blood loss, and the acute phase response (APR). During the APR, such as that which occurs with SIRS, sepsis, trauma, burn, and other sources of inflammation, protein synthesis is altered. The liver will synthesize more positive acute phase reactants (e.g., C-reactive protein) and less negative acute phase reactants (e.g., albumin) (Gabay & Kushner, 1999).

Transthyretin (or prealbumin) has a much shorter half-life (about 3 days), but similar to albumin is a negative acute phase reactant (Gabay & Kushner, 1999). Prealbumin levels will be low during periods of inflammation, regardless of adequate nutrition support provision. Studies of albumin and prealbumin levels in critically ill patients have found that they are better indicators of the severity of injury and prognosis rather than nutritional status (Boosalis et al., 1989).

Another monitoring tool used in nutrition assessment is nitrogen balance. Nitrogen balance is simply the difference between nitrogen input and output. The equation is as follows:

$$N_2 \text{ balance} = (\text{grams protein intake}/6.25) - (\text{urine urea nitrogen} + 4)$$

An additional 4 g of nitrogen losses is added to account for nonurine urea losses (feces and sweat). A nitrogen balance result that is +2–4 is theoretically indicative of anabolic metabolism; however, nitrogen balance really reflects the difference between protein intake and renal excretion of nitrogen-containing compounds. Additional protein to achieve a positive nitrogen balance may not always mean that patients will become anabolic (Russell & Mueller, 2007). Extremely catabolic patients may not reach a point of anabolism until they have recovered from their initial insult or injury. The test also requires an accurate record of protein intake, accurate urine collection, and good renal function (Russell & Mueller, 2007).

Because there is no single indicator of a patients' nutritional status or the adequacy of nutrient intake, clinicians must consider the whole picture of how patients are progressing. Outcomes suggesting adequate nutritional intake in the critical care setting include:

- Tolerance of enteral feedings without complications or frequent interruptions
- Healing of wounds
- Resolution of infections
- Weaning from mechanical ventilation
- Trend toward improvement in acute phase proteins (prealbumin)

Conclusion

Critically ill patients experience a myriad of metabolic changes and require nutrition support therapy to avoid excessive losses of protein and lean tissue. Both enteral and parenteral nutrition support therapies are employed in the critical care setting although EN remains the preferred route. Both therapies require skilled and knowledgeable clinicians to prescribe, administer, and monitor therapy to avoid possible complications. Nutritional needs, current nutritional support, and tolerance should be reviewed by the ICU team (including the nutrition support clinician) daily during team rounds.

Evidence-Based Practice Guidelines

Initiate nutritional support within 24–48 hours of ICU admission. Enteral route is preferable to parenteral.

Start enteral feeds only when patient is hemodynamically stable (MAP ≥ 70).

Administer enteral nutrition via a postpyloric nasoenteric tube when feasible.

Initiate nutritional support at half (or less) of goal rate to minimize complications.

Do not administer nutritional support greater than calculated needs in response to low nutritional laboratory values.

Online Resources

American Society for Parenteral and Enteral Nutrition (A.S.P.E.N.) (http://www.nutritioncare.org) Enteral Nutrition Practice Recommendations Guidelines for the Use of Parenteral and Enteral Nutrition in Adult and Pediatric Patients Safe Practices for Parenteral Nutrition

American Dietetic Association (ADA) (http://www.adaevidence library.com) Critical Illness Guidelines

Canadian Clinical Practice Guidelines (http://www.criticalcare nutrition.com)

References

American Society for Parenteral and Enteral Nutrition (A.S.P.E.N.) Board of Directors and the Clinical Guidelines Task Force. (2002). Guidelines for the use of parenteral and enteral nutrition in adult and pediatric patients. *Journal of Parenteral and Enteral Nutrition*, 1SA–138SA.

American Dietetic Association. (2007). *Critical Illness Guidelines*. Retrieved February 20, 2008, from ADA Evidence Analysis Library at http://www.adaevidenceanalysis.org

Alexander, J. (1998). Immunonutrition: The role of omega-3 fatty acids. *Nutrition*, 627–633.

Alexander, J., MacMillan, B., Stinnett, J., Ogle, C., Bozian, R., Fischer, J., et al. (1980). Beneficial effects of aggressive protein feeding in severely burned children. *Annals of Surgery*, 505–517.

Angstwurm, M., Schottdorf, J., Schopohl, J., & Gaertner, R. (1999). Selenium replacement in patients with severe systemic inflammatory response syndrome improves clinical outcome. *Critical Care Medicine*, 1807–1813.

Askanazi, J., Elwyn, D., Silverberg, P., Rosenbaum, S., & Kinney, J. (1980). Respiratory distress secondary to high carbohydrate load: A case report. *Surgery*, 596–598.

Bankhead, R., Boullata, J., Brantley, S., Corkins, M., Guenter, P., Krenitsky, J., et al. (2008). Enteral nutrition practice recommendations. *Journal of Parenteral and Enteral Nutrition*, 122–167.

Barr, J., Hecht, M., Flavin, K., Khorana, A., & Gould, M. (2004). Outcomes in critically ill patients before and after the implementation of an evidence-based nutritional management protocol. *Chest*, 1446–1457.

Beale, R., Bryg, D., & Bihari, D. (1999). Immunonutrition in the critically ill: A systematic review of clinical outcome. *Critical Care Medicine*, 2799–2805.

Boosalis, M., Ott, L., Levine, A., Slag, M., Morley, J., Young, B., et al. (1989). Relationship of visceral proteins to nutritional status in chronic and acute stress. *Critical Care Medicine*, 741–747.

Brun-Buisson, C. (2000). The epidemiology of the systemic inflammatory response. *Intensive Care Medicine*, S64–S74.

Cataldi-Betcher, E., Seltzer, M., Slocum, B., & Jones, K. (1983). Complications occurring during enteral nutrition support: A prospective study. *Jounal of Parenteral and Enteral Nutrition*, 546–552.

Cerra, F., Benitez, M., Blackburn, G., Irwin, R., Jeejeebhoy, K., Katz, D., et al. (1997). Applied nutrition in ICU patients: A consensus statement of the American College of Chest Physicians. *Chest*, 769–778.

Cerra, F., Siegel, J., & Coleman, B. (1980). Septic autocannabolism: A failure of exogenous nutritional support. *Annals of Surgery*, 570–580.

Chan, S., McCown, K., & Blackburn, G. (1999). Nutrition management in the ICU. *Chest*, 145S–148S.

Chiolero, R., Revelly, J., & Tappy, L. (1997). Energy metabolism in sepsis and injury. *Nutrition*, 45S–51S.

Choban, P., Burge, J., Scales, D., & Flancbaum, L. (1997). Hypoenergetic nutrition support in hospitalized obese patients: a simplified method for clinical application. *The American Journal of Clinical Nutrition*, 546–550.

Clark, C., Sacks, G., Dickerson, R., Kudsk, K., & Brown, R. (1995). Treatment of hypophosphatemia in patients receiving specialized nutrition support using a graduated dosing scheme: results from a prospective clinical trial. *Critical Care Medicine*, 1504–1511.

Clevenger, F., Rodriguez, D., Demarest, G., Osler, T., Olson, S., & Fry, D. (1992). Protein and energy tolerance by stressed geriatric patients. *The Journal of Surgical Research*, 135–139.

Covelli, H., Black, J., Olsen, M., & Beekman, J. (1982). Respiratory failure precipitated by high carbohydrate loads. *Annals of Internal Medicine*, 579–581.

Cresci, G., & Martindale, R. (2000). Nutrition Support in Trauma. In M. M. Gottschlich (Ed.), *The science and practice of nutrition support: A case-based core curriculum* (pp. 445–460). Dubuque, IA: Kendall/Hunt Publishing.

Crimi, E., Liguori, A., Condorelli, M., Cioffi, M., Astuto, M., Bontempo, P., et al. (2004). The beneficial effects of antioxidant supplementation in enteral feeding in critically ill patients: A prospective, randomized, double-blind, placebo-controlled trial. *Anesthesia and Analgesia*, 857–863.

Dark, D., Pingleton, S., & Kerby, G. (1985). Hypercapnia during weaning: a complication of nutritional support. *Chest*, 141–143.

Davies, A., Froomes, P., French, C., Bellomo, R., Gutteridge, G., Nyulasi, I., et al. (2002). Randomized comparison on nasojejunal and nasogastric feeding in critically ill patients. *Critical Care Medicine*, 586–590.

Demling, R., & DeSanti, L. (1998). Increased protein intake during the recovery phase after severe burns increases body weight and muscle function. *The Journal of Burn Care and Rehabilitation*, 161–168.

Dickerson, R., Boschert, K., Kudsk, K., & Brown, R. (2002). Hypocaloric enteral tube feeding in critically ill obese patients. *Nutrition*, 241–246.

Dickerson, R., Rosato, E., & Mullen, J. (1986). Net protein anabolism with hypocaloric parenteral nutrition in obese stressed patients. *The American Journal of Clinical Nutrition*, 747–755.

Forceville, X., Vitoux, D., Remy, G., Combes, A., Lahilaire, P., & Chappuis, P. (1998). Selenium, systemic immune response syndrome, sepsis, and outcome in critically ill patients. *Critical Care Medicine*, 1536–1544.

Frankenfield, D. (2001). Energy and macrosubstrate requirements. In M. M. Gottschlich (Ed.), *The science and practice of nutrition support: A case-based core curriculum* (pp. 31–52). Dubuque, IA: Kendall/Hunt.

Frankenfield, D., Cooney, R., Mith, J., & Rowe, W. (2000). Age-related differences in the metabolic response to injury. *The Journal of Trauma*, 49–57.

Frankenfield, D., Hise, M., Malone, A., Russell, M., Gradwell, E., & Compher, C. (2007). Prediction of resting metabolic rate in critically ill adult patients: Results of a systematic review of the evidence. *Journal of the American Diatetic Association*, 1552–1561.

Gabay, C., & Kushner, I. (1999). Acute-phase proteins and other systemic responses to inflammation. *The New England Journal of Medicine*, 448–454.

Gault, M., Dixon, M., Doyle, M., & Cohen, W. (1968). Hypernatremia, azotemia, and dehydration due to high-protein tube feeding. *Annals of Internal Medicine*, 778–791.

Hamilton, C., & Austin, T. (2006). Liver disease in long-term parenteral nutrition. *Support Line*, 10–18.

Heyland, D., Dhaliwhal, R., Drover, J., Gramlich, L., Dodek, P., & Committee, a. t. (2003). Canadian clinical practice guidelines for nutrition support in mechanically ventilated, critically ill adult patients. *Journal of Parenteral and Enteral Nutrition*, 355–373.

Heyland, D., MacDonald, S., Keefe, L., & Drover, J. (1998). Total parenteral nutrition in the critically ill patient—a meta-analysis. *The Journal of American Medical Association*, 2013–2019.

Heyland, D., Novak, F., Drover, J., Jain, M., Su, X., & Suchner, U. (2001). Should immunonutrition become routine in critically ill patients? A systematic review of the evidence. *The Journal of American Medical Association*, 944–953.

Heys, S., Walker, L., Smith, I., & Eremin, O. (1999). Enteral nutrition supplementation with key nutrients in patients with critical illness and cancer: A meta-analysis of randomized controlled clinical trials. *Annals of Surgery*, 467–477.

Hill, A. (2000). Initiators and propagators of the metabolic response to injury. *World Journal of Surgery*, 624–629.

Hoffer, L. (2003). Protein and energy provision in critical illness. *The American Journal of Clinical Nutrition*, 906–911.

Ibrahim, E., Mehringer, L., Prentice, D., Sherman, G., Schaiff, R., Fraser, V., et al. (2002). Early versus late enteral feeding of mechanically ventilated patients: results of a clinical trial. *Journal of Parenteral and Enteral Nutrition*, 174–181.

Ishibashi, N., Plank, L., Sando, K., & Hill, G. (1998). Optimal protein requirements during the first 2 weeks after the onset of critical illness. *Critical Care Medicine*, 1529–1535.

Jacobs, D., Jacobs, D., Kudsk, K., Moore, F., Oswanski, M., Poole, G., et al. (2004). Practice management guidelines for nutritional support of the trauma patient. *The Journal of Trauma*, 660–679.

Jeejeebhoy, K. (2001). Enteral and parenteral nutrition: Evidence-based approach. *Proceedings of the Nutrition Society*, 399–402.

Kagan, R., Matsuda, T., Hanumadass, M., Castillo, B., & Jonasson, O. (1982). The effect of burn wound size on ureagenesis and nitrogen balance. *Annals of Surgery*, 70–74.

Kaminski, D., Adams, A., & Jellinek, M. (1980). The effect of hyperalimentation on hepatic lipid content and lipogenic enzyme activity in rats and man. *Surgery*, 93–100.

Kearns, P., Chin, D., Mueller, L., Wallace, K., Jensen, W., & Kirsch, C. (2000). The incidence of ventilator-associated pneumonia and success in nutrient delivery with gastric versus small intestinal feeding: a randomized clinical trial. *Critical Care Medicine*, 1742–1746.

Khaodhiar, L., & Bistrian, B. (1999). Avoidance and Management of Complications of Total Parenteral Nutrition. *Nutrition in Clinical Care*, 239–249.

Klein, C., Moser–Veillon, P., Schweitzer, A., Douglass, L., Reynolds, N., Patterson, K., et al. (2002). Magnesium, Calcium, Zinc, and Nitrogen Losses in Trauma Patients During Continuous Renal Replacement Therapy. *Journal of Parenteral and Enteral Nutrition*, 77–93.

Klein, C., Stanek, G., & Wiles, C. (1998). Overfeeding macronutrients to critically ill adults: metabolic complications. *Journal of the American Dietetic Association*, 795–806.

Kortbeek, J., Haigh, P., & Doig, C. (1999). Duodenal versus gastric feeding in ventilated blunt trauma patients: a randomized controlled trial. *The Journal of Trauma*, 992–998.

Kraft, M., Btaiche, I., & Sacks, G. (2005). Review of refeeding syndrome. *Nutrition in Clinical Practice*, 625–633.

Kraft, M., Btaiche, I., Sacks, G., & Kudsk, K. (2005). Treatment of electrolyte disorders in adult patients in the intensive care unit. *American Journal of Health-System Pharmacy*, 1663–1682.

Kudsk, K., Croce, M., Fabian, T., Minard, G., Tolley, E., Poret, H., et al. (1992). Enteral versus parenteral feeding. Effects of septic morbidity after blunt and penetrating trauma. *Annals of Surgery*, 503–513.

Kudsk, K. A., Schloerb, P. R., DeLegge, M. H. et al. (2001). Concensus recommendations from the U.S. summit on immune-enhancing enteral therapy. *Journal of Parenteral and Enteral Nutrition*, 561–562.

Lampert, T., & Lefton, J. (2008). Inquire Here: What is the evidence to support the use of diabetic formulas in acutely ill patients? *Support Line*, 23–24.

Larsson, J., Lennmarken, C., Martensson, J., Sandsedt, S., & Vinnars, E. (1990). Nitrogen requirements in severely injured patients. *The British Journal of Surgery*, 413–416.

Lefton, J. (2002). Management of common gastrointestinal complications in tube-fed patients. *Support Line*, 19–25.

Lefton, J., Esper, D., & Kochevar, M. (2007). Enteral formulations. In M. Gottschlich, *The A.S.P.E.N. nutrition support core curriculum: A case-based approach— the adult patient* (pp. 209–232). Silver Spring, MD: A.S.P.E.N.

Lucarelli, M., Pell, L., Shirk, M., & Mirtallo, J. (2005). Fluid, electrolyte, and acid–base requirements. In G. Cresci, *Nutrition support for the critically ill patient—a guide to practice* (pp. 125–149). Boca Raton, FL: CRC Press.

Makola, D. (2005). Elemental and semi-elemental formulas: Are they superior to polymeric formulas? *Practical Gastroenerology*, 59–72.

Malone, A. (2005). Enteral formula selection: a review of selected product categories. *Practical Gastroenerology*, 44–74.

Marik, P., & Bedigian, M. (1996). Refeeding hypophosphatemia in critically ill patients in an intensive care unit. *Archives of Surgery*, 1043–1047.

Marik, P., & Zaloga, G. (2001). Early enteral nutrition in acutely ill patients: A systematic review. *Critical Care Medicine*, 2264–2270.

Martin, C., Doig, G., Heyland, D., Morrison, T., & Sibbald, W. (2004). Multicentre, cluster–randomized clinical trial of algorithms for critical-care enteral and parenteral therapy (ACCEPT). *Canadian Medical Association Journal*, 197–204.

Matsuda, T., Kagan, R., Hanumadass, M., & Jonasson, O. (1983). The importance of burn wound size in determining the optimal calorie–nitrogen ratio. *Surgery*, 562–568.

McClave, S., DeMeo, M., DeLegge, M., DiSario, J., Heyland, D., Maloney, J., et al. (2002). North American Summit on Aspiration in the Critically Ill Patient: consensus statement. *Journal of Parenteral and Enteral Nutrition*, S80–S85.

McCowen, K., Friel, C., Sternberg, J., Chan, S., Forse, R., Burke, P., et al. (2000). Hypocaloric total parenteral nutrition: Effectiveness in prevention of hyperglycemia and infectious complications—a randomized clinical trial. *Critical Care Medicine*, 3606–3611.

McIvor, A., Meguid, M., Curtas, S., & Kaplan, D. (1990). Intestinal obstruction from cecal bezoar: A complication of fiber-containing tube feedings. *Nutrition*, 115–117.

Minard, G., Kudsk, K., Melton, S., Patton, J., & Tolley, E. (2000). Early verus delayed feeding with an immune-enhancing diet in patients with severe head injuries. *Journal of Parenteral and Enteral Nutrition*, 145–149.

Mirtallo, J. (2007). Overview of parenteral nutrition. In Gottschlich, MM (Ed.), *The A.S.P.E.N. nutrition support core curriculum: A case-based approah—The adult patient* (pp. 264–276). Silver Spring, MD: A.S.P.E.N.

Mirtallo, J., Canada, T., Johnson, D., Kumpf, V., Peterson, C., Sacks, G., et al. (2004). Safe practices for parenteral nutrition. *Journal of Parenteral and Enteral Nutition*, S39–S70.

Misra, S., & Kirby, D. (2000). Micronutrient and Trace Element Monitoring in Adult Nutrition Support. *Nutr Clin Pract*, 120–126.

Montecalvo, M., Steger, K., Farber, H., Smith, B., Dennis, R., Fitzpatrick, G., et al. (1992). Nutritional outcome and pneumonia in critical care patients randomized to gastric versus jejunal tube feedings. *Critical Care Medicine*, 1377–1387.

Montejo, J., Grau, T., Acosta, J., Ruiz-Santana, S., Planas, M., Garcia–de-Lorenzo, A., et al. (2002). Multicenter, prospective, randomized, single-blind study comparing the efficacy and gastrointestinal complications of early jejunal feeding with early gastric feeding in critically ill patients. *Critical Care Medicine*, 796–800.

Moore, E., & Jones, T. (1986). Benefits of immediate jejunal feeding after major abdominal trauma: A prospective randomized study. *Journal of Trauma*, 874–881.

Moore, F., Feliciano, D., Andrassy, R., McArdle, A., Booth, F., Morgenstein–Wagner, T., et al. (1992). Early enteral feeding, compared with parenteral, reduces postoperative septic complications. The results of a meta-analysis. *Annals of Surgery*, 172–183.

Moore, F., Moore, E., & Jones, T. (1989). TEN versus TPN following major abdominal trauma reduced septic morbidity. *Journal of Trauma*, 916–922.

Muckart, D., & Bhagwanjee, S. (1997). American College of Chest Physicians/Society of Critical Care Medicine Consensus Conference definitions of the systemic inflammatory response syndrome and allied disorders in relation to critically injured patients. *Critical Care Medicine*, 1789–1795.

Nathens, A., Neff, M., Jurkovich, G., Klotz, P., Farver, K., Ruzinski, J., et al. (2002). Randomized, prospective trial of antioxidant supplementation in critically ill surgical patients. *Annals of Surgery*, 814–822.

Neumann, D., & DeLegge, M. (2002). Gastric versus small-bowel feeding in the intensive care unit: A prospective comparison of efficacy. *Critical Care Medicine*, 1436–1438.

Otten, J., Hellwig, J., & Meyers, L. (Eds.). (2006a). Dietary carbohydrates: sugars and starches. In J. Otten, J. Hellwig, & L. Meyers (Eds.), *Dietary reference intakes: The essential guide to nutrient requirements* (pp. 102–109). Washington, DC: The National Academies Press.

Otten, J., Hellwig, J., & Meyers, L. (Eds.). (2006b). Dietary fat: Total fat and fatty acids. In J. Otten, J. Hellwig, & L. Meyers (Eds.), *Dietary reference intakes—The essential guide to nutrient requirements* (pp. 122–139). Washington, DC: The National Academies Press.

Otten, J., Hellwig, J., & Meyers, L. (Eds.). (2006c). Fiber. In J. Otten, J. Hellwig, & L. Meyers (Eds.), *Dietary reference intakes: The essential guide to nutrient requirements* (pp. 110–121). Washington, DC: The National Academies Press.

Otten, J., Hellwig, J., & Meyers, L. (Eds.). (2006d). Protein and amino acids. In J. Otten, J. Hellwig, & L. Meyers (Eds.), *Dietary reference intakes: The essential guide to nutrient requirements* (pp. 145–155). Washington, DC: The National Academies Press.

Peter, J., Moran, J., & Phillips–Hughes, J. (2005). A meta-analysis of treatment outcomes of early enteral versus early parenteral nutrition in hospitalized patients. *Critical Care Medicine*, 213–220.

Piazza-Barnett, R., & Matarese, L. (1999). Electrolyte management in total parenteral nutrition. *Support Line*, 8–15.

Porter, J., Ivatury, R., Azimuddin, K., & Swami, R. (1999). Antioxidant therapy in the prevention of organ dysfunction syndrome and infectious complications after trauma: Early results of a prospective randomized study. *The American Surgeon*, 478–483.

Richardson, T., & Sgoutas, D. (1975). Essential fatty acid deficiency in four adult patients during total parenteral nutrition. *The American Journal of Clinical Nutrition*, 258–263.

Rosmarin, D., Wardlaw, G., & Mirtallo, J. (1996). Hyperglycemia associated with high, continuous infusion rates of total parenteral nutrition dextrose. *Nutrition in Clinical Practice*, 151–156.

Rushdi, T., Pichard, C., & Khater, Y. (2004). Control of diarrhea by fiber-enriched diet in ICU patient on enteral nutrition: A prospective randomized controlled trial. *Clinical Nutrition*, 1344–1352.

Russell, M., & Charney, P. (2002). Is there a role for specialized enteral nutrition in the intensive care unit? *Nutrition in Clinical Practice*, 156–168.

Russell, M., & Mueller, C. (2007). Nutrition Screening and Assessment. In M. Gottschlich (Ed.), *The A.S.P.E.N. nutrition support core curriculum: A case-based approach—the adult patient* (pp. 163–186). Silver Spring, MD: A.S.P.E.N.

Scaife, C., Saffle, J., & Morris, S. (1999). Intestinal obstruction secondary to enteral feedings in burn trauma patients. *The Journal of Trauma*, 859–863.

Schmidt, G. (2000). Guidelines for managing electrolytes in total parenteral nutrition solutions. *Nutrition in Clinical Practice*, 94–109.

Shaw, J., Wildbore, M., & Wolfe, R. (1987). Whole body protein kinetics in severely septic patients. *Annals of Surgery*, 288–294.

Skipper, A., Peloquin, T., Gregoire, M., & Tangney, C. (2001). Validation of objective criteria for predicting tolerance to enteral feeding in medical intensive care unit patients. *Nutrition in Clinical Practice*, 139–143.

Smith, C., Marien, L. B., Faust–Wilson, P., Lohr, G., Gerald, K., & Pingleton, S. (1990). Diarrhea associated with tube feeding in mechanically ventilated critically ill patients. *Nursing Research*, 148–152.

Spain, D., McClave, S., Sexton, L., Adams, J., Blanford, B., Sullins, M., et al. (1999). Infusion protocol improves delivery of enteral tube feeding in the critical care unit. *Journal of Parenteral and Enteral Nutrition*, 288–292.

Spapen, H., Diltoer, M., Van Malderen, C., Opdenacker, G., Suys, E., & Huyghens, L. (2001). Soluble fiber reduces the incidence of diarrhea in septic patients receiving total enteral nutrition: A prospective, double-blind, randomized, and controlled trial. *Clinical Nutrition*, 301–305.

Talpers, S., Romberger, D., Bunce, S., & Pingleton, S. (1992). Nutritionally associated increased carbon dioxide production: excess total calories vs high proportion of carbohydrate calories. *Chest*, 551–555.

Taylor, S., Fettes, S., Jewkes, C., & Nelson, R. (1999). Prospective, randomized, controlled trial to determine the effect of early enhanced enteral nutrition on clinical outcome in mechanically ventilated patients suffering head injury. *Critical Care Medicine*, 2525–2531.

Villet, S., Chiolero, R., Bollman, M., Revelly, J., Cayeux, M., Dalarue, J., et al. (2005). Negative impact of hypocaloric feeding and energy balance on clinical outcome in ICU patients. *Clinical Nutrition*, 502–509.

Weinsier, R., & Krumdieck, C. (1981). Death resulting from overzealous total parenteral nutrition: The refeeding syndrome revisited. *The American Journal of Clinical Nutrition*, 393–399.10.2

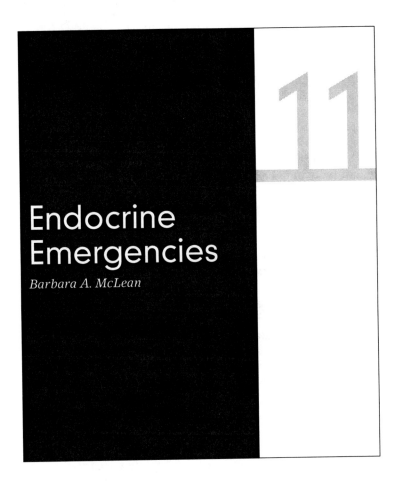

Endocrine Emergencies

Barbara A. McLean

Introduction

Electrolyte and metabolic disturbances are common in critically ill and injured patients. These disturbances alter physiologic function and contribute to morbidity and mortality. Although these disturbances are commonly encountered, the insidious failure of the hormonal balancing act in critical illness may precipitate a life-threatening crisis. The metabolic effects related to acute endocrine dysfunction have gained a considerable amount of interest in the last decade. The most common life threatening hormonal and electrolyte disturbances in critically ill patients present as glucose/insulin deregulation, cortisol deficiencies, and vasopressin deregulation. The ensuing metabolic disturbances that accompany many systemic disease processes or result from altered endocrine function are complex and threatening, but the most concerning of these is the presence of lactic acidosis and refractory hypotension. With early recognition and treatment of these abnormalities, life-threatening complications, such as multiple organ dysfunction related to hypoperfusion might be avoided and outcomes may improve. These abnormalities will be discussed in this chapter.

Pathophysiology

The physiologic stress response is controlled largely by the hypothalamic–pituitary–adrenal (HPA) axis and the sympatho-adrenal system (SAS), which includes the sympathetic nervous system and the adrenal medulla (Marik, 2006). The HPA axis and the SAS are functionally related. Activation of the HPA and SAS systems provides a survival foundation for the host. The ability to compensate in hypermetabolic states depends on the balancing act and integrated response of the two systems.

These two systems are activated by cellular triggers, which communicate primarily to the hypothalamus initiating a range of releasing, limiting, or stimulating responses. This response controls the internal milieu, that is, increased sympathetic activity, increased circulating catecholamines, increased glucagon and cortisol, which all contribute to increased gluconeogenesis, metabolic alterations, and exhaustion of the HPA. The mechanisms leading to dysfunction of the HPA axis during critical illness are complex and poorly understood and likely include increased or decreased production of releasing, regulating, stimulating hormones (hypothalamic and pituitary), as well as an altered response of the target organs and distal receptor sites. The appropriate responses ultimately answer the triggering cellular call, which, in return, creates a negative feedback loop (Figure 11.1). Understanding these essential stimulation-inhibition mechanisms provides the basis for bedside and laboratory evaluation. With early recognition and treatment of these abnormalities, life-threatening complications such as multiple organ dysfunction might be avoided and patient outcomes may improve.

The primary hormonal disturbances in critically ill patients to be discussed here include altered glucose regulation and insulin reactivity; relative (situational) adrenal

11.1

The Organ Connection

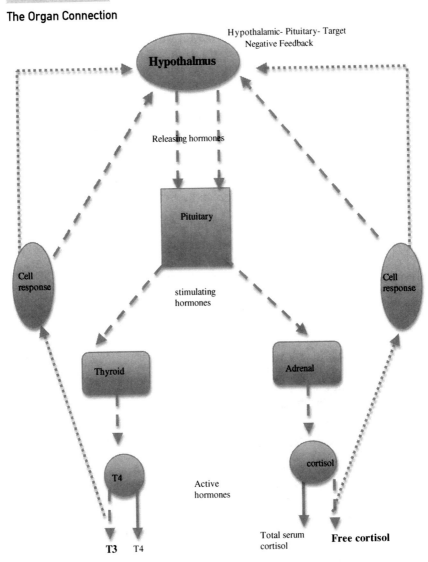

Hypothalamic- Pituitary- Target
Negative Feedback

insufficiency; relative pituitary or receptor dysfunction (vasopressin) and alterations in thyroid response.

Critical Illness Hyperglycemia

Hyperglycemia with or without diabetes is associated with increased mortality and morbidity. It is rare for patients to be admitted to the hospital for primary management of diabetes, but relatively common for elevated blood sugar to complicate the initial diagnosis. A recent study by Umpierrez and Kitabchi (2004) showed 1,886 patients admitted to a community hospital met criteria for the diagnosis of hyperglycemia (defined as an admission or in-hospital fasting glucose levels exceeding 126 mg/dl [7 mmol/L]). According to Umpierrez and Kitabchi, 38% of patients presented with hyperglycemia, 26% of the total with known diabetes, and the remaining 12% with no prior history of diabetes. Stress or new hyperglycemia was associated with a higher in-hospital mortality rate (16%) as compared with those patients with a prior history of diabetes and therefore managed (3%) and the remaining 1,177 patients with normoglycemia (1.7%). Even after risk adjustment for confounding variables and factors, patients with new hyperglycemia had an 18.3-fold increase in mortality rate compared with a 2.7-fold increase in the known diabetes group. Providers often perceive hyperglycemia as a compensatory consequence of stress and acute illness and therefore do not recognize the significance. This misunderstanding will often delay treatment until blood glucose (BG) exceeds 200–250 mg/dl.

Glucose Regulation

Glucose transport into cells occurs as facilitated diffusion using one of the five different glucose transporter (GLUT) channel proteins. GLUT-1–mediated insulin-independent transport occurs in most tissues and accounts for basal glucose uptake, whereas the membrane presence of GLUT-4 is specifically and reversibly up regulated by insulin. The role of insulin at this level is essential to the maintenance of cellular levels of glucose. Insulin is produced by the beta cells of the islets of Langerhans of the pancreas under the influence of the BG level. At the cellular level, insulin interacts with a protein on the cell surface. The ultimate reaction is the production of the glucose transporter (GLUT-4) in muscle cells, which passes or migrates to the surface and facilitates the entrance of larger molecular nutrients such as glucose. At this level, insulin binds to the insulin receptor sites, requiring them to be responsive. Insulin bound to the sites create a second messenger response molecules which then mobilizes other responses. (1 and 2 insulin receptor substrate (IRS). IRS-1 activates other systems required to mobilize stored GLUT-4 transporter molecules to the cell membrane). During moderate hyperglycemia, cells usually shift and hold GLUT transport molecules (intracellularly) decreasing the cellular uptake of glucose and therefore protecting themselves from glucose overload.

Glucose uptake related to the glucose transporters GLUT-1, GLUT-2, or GLUT-3 is profoundly effected in stress and illness. Cytokines, angiotensin II, endothelin-1, vascular endothelial growth factor, transforming growth factor, and hypoxia, have all been proven to significantly affect and upregulate the expression and availability of GLUT-1 and GLUT-3 in different cell types, which often over rides the normal hyperglycemic protection mechanisms. GLUT-2 and GLUT-3 allow glucose to enter cells directly proportional to the extracellular glucose level which may be significantly higher in critical illness states (Clerici & Mathay, 2000; Sánchez–Alvarez, Tabernero, & Medina, 2004).

Hyperglycemia in septic patients is partially related to the presence of proinflammatory cytokines, counterregulatory hormones, and excessive glucose availability (hyperglycemia). Hepatic insulin resistance and increased gluconeogenesis are major contributors to hyperglycemia. Total body glucose uptake is typically increased in critical illness due to alterations in the cellular protection process which normally limit uptake in the non-insulin dependent cells such as the central nervous system or blood cells (see Table 11.1 on page 404).

The physiologic response to injury, trauma, sepsis, or with major operations is heralded by hypermetabolism and catabolism, both leading to peripheral protein waste, compromise of the immune system and the skin, and eventually, multiorgan dysfunction. The liver plays a crucial role in this process. During normal physiologic conditions, the liver synthesizes mainly constitutive-hepatic proteins, such as

11.1 Some Proposed Causes of Critical Illness Induced Hyperglycemia

Cause	Response	Effect
pro-HPA and sympathetic activation: catecholamines and glucagon↑↑	↑ hepatic glucose production	↑ glycogenolysis and gluconeogenesis
↓ Glut-4 (cell protection)	Impaired peripheral glucose uptake	hyperglycemia and insulin resistance
↑glucose uptake in non–insulin-dependent tissues	Brain and blood cells most prominently affected	↓ immunocompetence ↑ red cell lysis ↓ neurologic function

albumin, prealbumin, or transferrin. After profound stress (surgery, trauma, sepsis), the liver shifts to a hepatic acute-phase response, now synthesizing many different proteins, such as C-reactive protein (CRP). The goal of this response is to restore homeostasis; however, a prolonged, exaggerated output promotes increased and continuous hypermetabolism and catabolism. Mediators of the acute-phase response are proinflammatory cytokines, such as interleukin-1 (IL-1 beta), interleukin-6 (IL-6), interleukin-8 (IL-8), tumor-necrosis factor (TNF), and/or the anti-inflammatory cytokine interleukin-10 (IL-10) (Moshage, 1997; Livingston, Mosenthal, & Deitch, 1995; Selzman et al., 1998; De Maio, Mooney, Matesic, Paidas, & Reeves, 1998; Pruitt, Copeland, & Moldawer, 1995; & Williams & Giroir, 1995). The presence of these communicators ensures that the patient's normal protein stores will be low when measured.

The presence of hyperglycemia in a patient with *any* critical illness should always be considered to indicate inflammation and compensation that may rapidly become maladaptive. Serious metabolic complications of uncontrolled hyperglycemia resulting from the inflammatory mediated loss of cellular protection mechanisms (GLUT-4) coupled with increased production of counter regulatory hormones such as glucagon, catecholamines (epinephrine), cortisol, and others, affects multiple systems and sends out a signal that must not be ignored. Van den Berghe (2001), and the Leuven 1 group, hypothesized that even moderate sustained hyperglycemia, was directly or indirectly harmful to vital organs and systems and contributed to adverse outcomes (Table 11.2).

The Leuven 1 group actively studied the benefit of tighter glycemic controls (TGC) in critically ill patients with hyperglycemia and those without diabetes. The Leuven protocol demonstrated that a BG target of 80–110 mg/dl in the intensive insulin group yielded benefits in morbidity, including decreased blood transfusion requirements, decreased need for dialysis, increased immunocompetence, and decreased length of stay, as well as a 30% reduction in mortality when compared with a more traditional approach to hyperglycemia (see Table 11.3 on page 406). Although the trial was introduced in a mixed medical–surgical unit, 71% of patients were predominantly cardiothoracic patients and all required mechanical ventilation. The Leuven I study reported an increase in the number of patients with severe hypoglycemia from 0.8% to 5.1%; however, there were no associated adverse consequences reported.

11.2 The Proposed Effects of Insulin on the Endothelium

Endothelial Protection	Response
↓ nitric oxide production	↑ vascular tone
	↑ response to fluids/vasopressors
↓ oxyradicals	endothelial protection

Other effects	Response
↓ C-reactive protein	↑ anti-inflammation
↓ mannose-binding lectin	↓ proinflammation
↓ TNF-α	
↓ superoxide radicals	
↓ cellular energy metabolism	↑ Glut-4 uptake

11.3   Safe Effective Glucose Control

Protocol target	Appropriate to skills, experience, and tools available to the ICU
	Concern for nurse work burden
80–150 mgm/dl	Successful implementation drives a decreasing level of glycemic control
Data monitoring tools	Essential for collection of efficiency and time required to achieve goals
	Record hypoglycemia
	Collection of clinical outcomes

Hyperglycemia in the critically ill patient, whether in a known diabetic or stress-induced, has long been known to increase morbidity and mortality (Sung, Bochicchio, Joshi, et al., 2005). Negative effects include longer lengths of stay, increased incidence of infection, and in-hospital death (Whitcomb, Pradhan, Pittas, et al., 2005). Observational studies and early randomized trials have suggested that lowering glucose levels can improve outcomes, especially in critical care patients treated with intravenous insulin to a range of 80–110 mg/dl (Capes, Hunt, & Malmberg, et al., 2001; Kingsley et al., 1999; McCowen, Malhotra, Bistrian, et al., 2001). In 2001, a large scale trial of ICU patients reported that reducing blood glucose concentrations to 4.4–6.1 mmol/L lessened in-patient mortality (Van der Berghe, Wouters, Weekers, 2001). More recent studies in the critical care population were unable to replicate earlier studies, and identified severe hypoglycemia as a significant risk of intensive glucose control (van der Berghe, Wilmer, Hermans, et al., 2006; Arabi, Dabbagh, Tanmin, et al., 2008; Brunkhorst, Engel, Donado, Restrepo, et al., 2008; Devos, Preiser, Melot, 2007). Wiener, Wiener, & Larson (2008) concluded in a meta-analysis that such therapy was not a factor in reduction of mortality among critically ill hospitalized patients. Severe hypoglycemia was evident and resulted in the termination of large scale study in Germany (Brunkhorst, F., Engel, C.,

Bloos, F., et al., 2008) and Europe (Devos, P., Preiser, J., Melot, C., 2007). The American Diabetes Association (2008) and the American Association of Clinical Endocrinologists (2007) have recommended intensive insulin therapy even in the presence of conflicting data. The Normoglycemia in Intensive Care Evaluation-Survival Using Glucose Algorithim Regulation (NICE-SUGAR) study was a large scale international study including 6104 hospitalized critically ill patients (Finfer et al., 2009). They reported 1580 deaths.

Following the NICE-SUGAR findings, Griesdale et al. (2009) conducted a meta-analysis of existing randomized trials of intensive insulin regimes in critically ill patients. They explored the effects of this therapy in relation to hypoglycemia and death. The researchers reviewed 26 international studies involving more than 13,500 patients. Their findings supported that there is no mortality benefit related to intensive insulin regimes except in surgical ICU patients.

While both hyperglycemia and hypoglycemia are correlated to poor outcomes in critically ill patients, intensive insulin therapy is not ideal for every patient. Griesdale et al. (2009) emphasized that trials of intensive insulin therapy were distinctly different and the demographics of patients, units, and treatment protocols varied. The method of blood glucose measurement included central lines, arterial lines, and capillary measurement. Administration of insulin varied dramatically from subcutaneous to peripheral and central line IV dosing. Finally the researchers cited extremes in achieving target goals based on health care teams and thus the term "intensive insulin therapy" were not consistent. The authors emphasize that differences in outcomes may be secondary to existing hyperglycemia prior to therapy and accuracy in glucose measurement and intervention. Suggestions for future research include identification of optimal targets for blood sugar in distinct patient populations.

The ADA and the AACE issued a statement regarding the findings of the NICE-SUGAR study and urge that practitioners should not abandon the concept of good glucose management in the hospital setting. (ADA/AACE, 2009). The two organizations maintain that strategies must be identified to help hospitals establish structured protocols for safe and effective management of blood glucose in both intensive care units and other hospital settings. A task force representing the ADA/AACE is

11.4 Proposed Differences in Pathophysiology of Diabetic Mellitus

Pathology	Type 1	Type 2
↓Insulin Production from Islet β-type cells	Auto-immune destruction	Not generally present in the early disease, occurs as disease progresses
Insulin deficiency	Yes	Not generally in early disease
Glucose intolerance	Yes	Yes
Insulin resistance*	5%–30% of adult patients, not the common cause	Yes
Central obesity*	Not generally/causative	Yes
Dyslipedemia*	Not generally/causative	Yes
Hypertension*	Not generally/causative	Yes

currently attempting to identify "reasonable, achievable, and safe glucose targets, and to describe the protocols, procedures, and system improvements to achieve optimal glucose control efficiently and safely." (Korytkowski, 2009). Current recommendations suggest reasonable attempts to treat critical care patients in a less intensive yet "good" range similar to the conventional arm of the NICE-SUGAR trial." (ADA/AACE, 2009). This equates to a blood sugar of 8-10mmol/L. Krinsley (2006) and Devos et al., (2008) recommend a method of glucose control that promotes a stepwise approach system appropriately coined : Safe, Effective, Glucose Control (SEGC). This methodology targets an *intermediate* BG level to protect the patient from the negative effects of both hyper and hypoglycemia and meets the current post NICE-SUGAR guidelines. Application of tight control methodologies is not recommended (Table 11.4).

Whatever lower range is chosen, the risk of hypoglycemia is increased if the insulin dosing scheme is not properly constructed and vigilant, accurate evaluation is not performed

(Krinsley, 2006). Sliding scale subcutaneous and regular insulin regimens are not useful in the critical care setting in achieving goal control, because the insulin dose is determined *after* the blood sugar has already increased, not in a predictive, prophylactic method.

Targets can be achieved with frequent analysis of blood from an arterial catheter or finger-stick BG determinations and an when the insulin infusion rate is dictated by a dosing algorithm. There is complexity involved in controlling the BG to any target ranges and teamwork is absolutely essential. Patient safety concerns dictate that bedside providers should follow a single protocol based on frequent BG determinations and properly adjust the therapy accordingly. One of the most important methods for evaluation may include using arterial blood (both point of care [POC] as well as in patient laboratory analysis) whenever possible (Kanji et al., 2005).

Managing Diabetics in Acute States

Insulin Basics

Insulin is necessary for the transport of glucose into the cells for use as fuel and also to provide mechanisms for excessive fuel storage I. The ability to utilize and breakdown these stored units (glycogenolysis) is an insulin dependent process. This breakdown of storage substances is normal and vital to the metabolic process. The liver also promotes the catabolism of protein and to a lesser extent, the glycerol produced in fat breakdown to support gluconeogenesis. Glucose production by the liver is one of the most important contributors to the hyperglycemia of diabetes and is profoundly affected by the presence or absence of insulin.

Type 1 Diabetes Mellitus. Type 1 insulin-dependent diabetes (T1DM) occurs when there is a primary damage/death of the beta cells resulting in an *absolute insulin deficiency*. Absolute insulin deficiency results in a primary failure of the glucose to be utilized or even stored by the cell. Fat breakdown results in the release of free fatty acids (FFAs). FFAs travel to the liver and are converted into acetone, acetoacetic acid, and betahydroxybuteric acid or ketone bodies. The presence of excess acids will affect the homeostatic, neutral blood environment (blood pH). Historically, T1DM was diagnosed at an early age and was referred to as juvenile or thin diabetes. When the condition is a birth defect or genetic deficit triggered by an autoimmune response, this may still be the case; however, over the last 50 years, the evolution of the sedentary, supersize mentality in western cultures has promoted a greater increase in causative factors for the T1DM.

Type 2 Diabetes Mellitus. Type 2 insulin-dependent diabetes (T2DM) is more difficult to understand and describe. T2DM combines both insulin resistance and insulin deficiency and is frequently diagnosed on a continuum. This evolutional process is both genetic and environmental and continues to be the subject of significant discussion and ongoing research.

Genetic Issues in T2DM

Genes control several chemical steps in beta cell action, including the secretion, action, and transportation of insulin. Genetic defects can prevent enzyme production and block the action of insulin. The insulin block then affects glucose uptake, gluconeogensis, and increases the breakdown of the triglycerides.

Insulin Resistance

Insulin resistance (the first defect) occurs in the peripheral cells (primarily muscle and fat) of the muscles and the liver. Genetic factors affect this resistance; but the roles of environmental factors are what unveil and elevate the condition. Environmental factors include aging, sedentary lifestyle, obesity, and particularly central obesity. As insulin resistance develops, decreasing the transport of glucose to the cell, the beta cells respond to the cellular "starvation" by increasing insulin production. Insulin resistance that persists or increases over time causes the beta cells to fail secondary to genetic defects, glucose and/or fat toxicity, and/or exhaustion. Frequently a complete or absolute deficiency that was not diagnosed at an early age is related to a combination of all these factors. When insulin resistance persists over time, the insulin secretion may begin to decrease and BG levels begin to rise, clinical signs and symptoms will begin to proliferate.

People who suffer from obesity already have a degree of insulin resistance and compensatory hyperinsulinemia. The presence of central obesity places patients at risk because of their abdominal adipose tissue that becomes increasingly resistant to insulin as it accumulates. However, only those individuals with central obesity plus genetic deficits go on to develop diabetes. This condition is commonly referred to as *metabolic syndrome*.

Insulin Deficiency

The insulin deficiency in T2DM is frequently due to beta cell exhaustion from the constant hypersecretion of insulin, and glucose/lipid toxicity. The toxicity of high levels of glucose is profoundly expressed in nervous system, vascular and beta cells. Bardsley, and Want (2004) showed that 50% of beta-cell insulin production is lost by the time that the diagnosis of T2DM is made. For most T2DMs, insulin therapy will be needed within 3–5 years after diagnosis (Bardsley & Want). Diabetic ketoacidosis (DKA) and hyperglycemic hyperosmolar syndrome (HHS) are the most serious acute complications of diabetes mellitus. Although these disorders are not absolutely related to the type of diabetes, most commonly, diabetic ketoacidosis (DKA) occurs in the T1DM and HHS in the T2DM. Both are characterized by insulinopenia and are differentiated primarily, although not always, via the severity of hyperglycemia, acidosis, and dehydration. In critical illness states, the high concentrations of catecholamines, cortisol, and growth hormone may cause a relative insulin deficiency ($\uparrow$hormones/$\uparrow\uparrow$glucose/insulin) and thus further worsen hyperglycemia. When administering any or all of these agents exogenously, the provider must be aware of these effects and adjust insulin therapy accordingly.

As the glucose concentration and osmolality of extracellular fluid increases (5.6 mOsm/kg for every 100 mg/dl increase in plasma glucose), an osmolar gradient is created that draws water out of the cells. The diuresis of the hyperosmolar glucose molecule initially increases glomerular filtration and limits the profound accumulation of serum glucose. Through the renal filtration process, glucose, water, and most electrolytes will be wasted in the urine. Careful analysis of the patient's laboratory results is required to prevent errors. The fluid flux and acidosis will significantly impact the serum concentration of sodium as well as the intracellular presence of potassium. When evaluating dehydration, the common formula for calculating the serum osmolality must be performed and corrected. The measure of sodium content (135–145 mEq/dl) may return from the laboratory as normal, low, or elevated. However, the sodium concentration is profoundly affected by the renal glomerular filtration rate (GFR). When the patient persists in an osmotic diuresis the serum sodium is being lost at an alarming rate and the measured content without regard to corrected concentrations may under predict how dehydrated the patient actually is.

A measured and calculated sodium concentration (2[Na⁺] + [serum glucose/18] + BUN/2.8 = serum osmolality. Normal 275–295 mOsm/L) is frequently performed to evaluate dehydration and the concentration gradient for electrophysiological conduction. Blood urea nitrogen (BUN) is not always included in the formula because it is freely permeable through the intracellular wall and therefore does not exert pressure in the osmolar gradient.

To determine the *true* concentration and, therefore, not underestimate the volume loss that has occurred, a correction of the serum sodium and the concentration gradient is absolutely necessary in hyperglycemic patients. For every 100 mg/dl BG measured above the normal of 100 mg/dl, add 1.6 mEq back to the measured sodium. This correction is used to determine dehydration, not true sodium.

Example:

1. Patient A has a blood glucose of 500 mgm/dl.
2. Patient A has a serum sodium of 138 mEq/dl.

In order to determine true dehydration:

3. Glucose of 500 = 500 − 100 = 400 (four 100s above the normal glucose)
4. 4(1.6 mEq) = 6.4 mEq to be added to correct the sodium
5. Corrected sodium= 2(138 + 6.4) = 144.4

The corrected sodium is then utilized in the osmolar calculation

2(144) + (500/18) is 288 + 27.7 = 315 corrected osmolality reflecting dehydration.

In addition, serum potassium concentration is generally elevated in relationship to cellular potassium due to the extracellular shift of potassium caused by insulin deficiency, acidemia, and hypertonicity. When the patient has metabolic acidosis (from ketosis as well as lactic acidosis), the H+ (metabolic acid) moves across the cellular wall and shifts the intracellular ion K+ out of the cell into the serum. The measured serum K+ may then over predict the patient's true ionic state.

While the patient is in a hyperglycemic osmotic diuresis state, K+ moves from cell to serum to urine in a profound K+ dumping mode. Volume and insulin are given to manage both ketosis and hypovolemia. The H+ will exchange (to serum) with the K+ (to cell) and if the provider has not been cautious, profound serum hypokalemia may occur. Potassium is required for electrical and mechanical response of cells, muscles, heart, and nervous system cells. Great care must be applied in managing a hyperglycemic crisis in a low–normal or low serum potassium state.

The serum phosphate level in patients with DKA, like serum potassium, does not truly reflect the actual body deficit.

Diabetic Ketoacidosis. Diabetic ketoacidosis (DKA) is an acute complication of diabetes mellitus that can be life threatening. The basic underlying mechanism for diabetic ketoacidosis is an *absolute* insulin deficiency coupled with elevated levels of counter regulatory hormones, such as glucagon, cortisol, catecholamines, growth hormone, proinflammatory cytokines. These hormones are frequently over stimulated by an infectious processes. Elevated cortisol levels stimulate protein catabolism increasing circulating levels of amino acids that become the fuel for gluconeogenesis in the liver. The hypersecretion and concentration of catecholamines, cortisol, and growth hormone, both endogenous and exogenous, combined with the resulting ketosis and acidosis impair cellular glucose uptake as well as insulin action and secretion, thus the vicious cycle of hyperglycemia persists and worsens (Umpierrez & Kitabchi, 2004). The serum glucose continues to elevate as cellular inability to process and transport glucose continues and glycogenolysis and gluconeogenesis begins.

DKA is expressed by marked hyperglycemia, ketosis, acidosis, and dehydration. The renal transport rate of the hyperosmolar glucose molecule is significant, causing the profound initial diuresis and loses of a significant amounts of fluids and electrolytes. These are both effected by the rate of glucose wasting in the urine (see Table 11.5 on page 414). DKA can cause significant abdominal pain that resolves with appropriate measures of treatment; however, caution should be taken, as the pain could be a result or indication of the precipitating

11.5 Signs and Symptoms of DKA

Signs	Symptoms	Analysis
Dehydration	Polyuria/polydypsia/ polyphagia	History most important
Dry mucus membranes	Weight loss	Serum glucose >250 mg/dl (in the absence of insulin administration)
Decreased skin turgor	Vomiting	Serum and urine ketones >3 mmol
Tachycardia	Abdominal pain	Blood pH <7.30 (beware of the compensation of rapid respiratory rate)
Kussmauls respirations	Weakness	Anion gap >20 (in the presence of normal chloride and albumin)
Hypotension	Drowsiness	Uncomplicated acidosis: for every 1 mmol ↑ in gap, there should be 1 mmol ↓ in bicarbonate
Alteration in mental status	Sleepy to comatose	Δ anion - Δ bicarbonate Normal with acidosis −6 to + 6

Note: Typically DKA is more commonly seen in T1DM, however, this is not a requirement for diagnosis.

cause of DKA. Further evaluation is needed if abdominal pain does not resolve with resolution of dehydration and metabolic acidosis (Umpierrez, Khajavi, & Kitabchi, 1996).

Hyperglycemic Hyperosmolar Syndrome (HHS). Although the hallmark of HHS is life-threatening dehydration and severe hyperglycemia, the pathophysiology is poorly understood. Currently, science points to the higher levels of endogenous insulin reserve in HHS than one might see in T1DM. Often there is adequate insulin concentration to prevent lipolysis (and therefore ketosis), but not enough insulin to inhibit hepatic glucose production and/or stimulate glucose use (Umpierrez & Kitabchi, 2004; Bardsley & Want, 2004).

There appears to be no limit on the level of BG that can be achieved during crisis. The rising level of blood glucose reflects that, glucose is produced but not used, and there appears to be enough insulin to store some glucose as glycogen which is then rapidly lysed (hence the very high levels) and also enough to *at least initially* limit the breakdown of nonglucose products (lipolysis). However, there is not enough to respond to the starving cell (transport) or limit liver production (Table 11.6).

11.6 Signs and Symptoms of HHS

Signs	Symptoms	Analysis
Dehydration	Profound	Serum osmolality >320 mOsm/L Serum sodium may be normal, low or high If measured (not corrected) sodium is elevated above normal, patient is in danger of terminal dehydration
Dry mucus membranes	Profound	Serum glucose >600 mg/dl (in the absence of insulin administration)
Decreased skin turgor	Profound	Serum and urine ketones usually negative, may have mild ketonemia
Tachycardia	Abdominal pain	Blood pH >7.30 (except if in hypovolemic shock)
Kussmaul's respirations	Not present	Anion gap <20 (except in hypovolemic shock)
Hypotension	Present	
Shock/coma	Present	Evaluate serum osmolality If <320 consider other causes for coma

Typically when glucose production is profoundly high, the GFR (osmotic diuresis) is abnormally active initially producing polyuria, and the patient may quite literally urinate themselves into a coma and subsequent death. The concomitant dehydration may significantly impact the presence of acids (H+ as well as Ketones), which explains the decreased diagnostic emphasis on presence or absence of metabolic acidosis.

The comparative analysis aside, both forms of hyperglycemic crisis are life threatening and appropriate treatment is emergent and critical. The treatment is focused on fluids, electrolytes, source control, and insulin replacement. Current

11.7 Comparing the Two Conditions

	DKA	HHS
Serum glucose	Usually <800	May be >1000
Serum and urine ketones	++++	May not be present
Serum K+	Serum levels over predict cellular, may be low (profound cellular hypokalemia)	Normal in the absence of acidosis
Serum Na+	Normal	Variable
Serum Osmolarity	elevated	Profoundly elevated
pH	Metabolic acidosis (presence of ketones [lipolysis] and lactic acid [glycogenolysis] and tissue hypoxia with dehydration)	Normal Metabolic acidosis primarily as an effect from lactic acidosis in severe dehydration and hypovolemic shock syndromes
Anion gap	wide	Normal or wide in the presence of lactic acidosis

recommendations for the treatment of patients with moderate or severe diabetic ketoacidosis and those with HHS are listed in Table 11.7.

Insulin therapy may need to be delayed in a few primary conditions, arterial hypotension and severe hyperglycemia, as well as significant hypokalemia states associated with dehydration and hyperglycemia (Umpierrez & Kitabchi, 2004). In hypotensive patients with severe hyperglycemia, if insulin is administered, this may generate vascular collapse and a significant fluid shift causing life-threatening hypotension. In addition, patients with low serum potassium (<2.5–3.0 mEq/L) are typically profoundly depleted at the intracellular level and must receive potassium replacement before insulin therapy commences (Exhibit 11.1).

Thyroid Dysfunction. Thyrotropin-releasing hormone (TRH), secreted by the hypothalamus, stimulates the pituitary to produce Thyrotropin, which then regulates the synthesis and secretion of thyroid hormones in the thyroid gland.

Exhibit

11.1 Recommended Treatment for Elevated Blood Glucose in Crisis

- initial intravenous bolus of regular insulin at a dose of 0.1 units/kg body weight, followed by
- continuous infusion of regular insulin at a dose of 0.1 units/kg until blood glucose levels reach 250 mg/dl
- once glucose is <250 add dextrose to the intravenous fluids and reduce insulin infusion to 0.05 units $\cdot$ kg^{-1} $\cdot$ hour^{-1}
- In HHS, convert to a standard glucose regulation strategy
- In DKA, continuous intravenous therapy until ketoacidosis is controlled. Two of the following normalized acid base requirements must be met:
  - serum bicarbonate ≥ 18 mEq/L
  - venous pH ≥ 7.3
  - anion gap ≤ 14 mEq/L
- capillary blood glucose is determined every 1–2 hours at the bedside using a glucose oxidase reagent strip.
- blood is drawn every 4 hours to determine serum electrolytes, glucose, blood urea nitrogen, creatinine, magnesium, phosphate, and venous pH

The thyroid hormones thyroxin (T4) and triiodothyronine (T3) are the active hormones produced by the thyroid gland (Table 11.8). The active circulating hormones control basal metabolism, glucose uptake and lipolysis, oxygen consumption and heat production. The normal levels of these hormones also increase protein synthesis in muscle, bone and brain and therefore affect growth. The thyroid hormones act in a synergistic manner with the circulating catecholamines, together creating a rise in heart rate and vascular tone, therefore the blood pressure. The ratio is 20% T3 to 80% T4, and T3, while more metabolically active, has a shorter effective response time. T3 and T4 must be transported by proteins (Thyroglobulin binding protein: TGBs) and the compound must be presented to the liver or skeletal muscle for cleavage to occur. The hormone secretion is controlled by Thyrotropin or the thyroid-stimulating hormone (TSH) released from the adeno-hypophysis of the pituitary. The pituitary response is controlled by hypothalamic Thyrotropin-releasing hormone (TRH) that in turn responds to cellular signals (Figure 11.2).

Thyroid disorders affect about 2% of the population and, along with diabetes, are the most common type of endocrine disorder. Signs and symptoms can be very generalized and may be confused with other medical disorders, not limited to the endocrine system. The signs and symptoms occur in concert with an increased hormone (tachycardia, atrial fibrillation, rapid metabolic and digestive rates) whereas hypothyroidism causes a marked reduction in the same clinical

11.8 Thyroid Measures

Measure	Normal	Target with Therapy
TSH	standard: 0.4 and 4.5 mIU/L consider: 0.4 and 2.5 mIU/L.	TSH to 0.4 to 2.5 mIU/L in T4-treated hypothyroid patients
free T4	60–170 nmol/l	standard with levothyroxine
T3	0.8–2.7 nmol/l	controversial

11.2

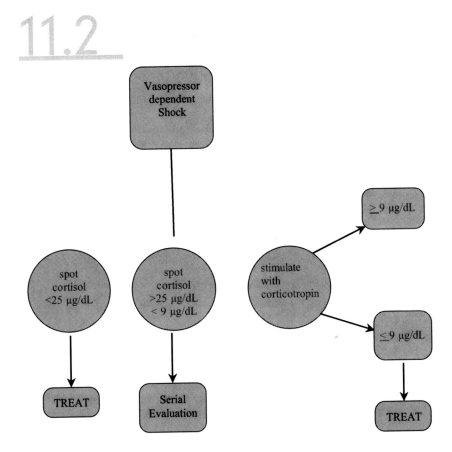

measures. In severe illness of any cause, down-regulation of the thyroid hormone system may occur.

The endocrine adaptations to critical illness are variable and much less than predictable. Illness in patients with pre-existing hypothyroidism or hyperthyroidism may precipitate extremes of the primary disorder such as Myxedema coma or thyroid storm. These conditions, although presenting with exaggerated nonspecific signs and symptoms, are in the end much more obvious than the simple diagnosis of hypothy-roidism or pre-hypothyroidism, which often is based on the relative suspicion that should be considered when patients present with refractory, exaggerated clinical states.

Abnormal laboratory analysis of thyroid function provides a relatively definitive diagnosis. Initial serum measurements should include a free T4 and TSH, but concerns regarding thyroidal dysfunction should be referred to a endocrinology specialist for a more thorough diagnostic panel.

Hypothyroidism. *Primary hypothyroidism,* the most common presenting form of thyroidal disorders, t is caused by thyroid suppressionfor any direct reason (i.e., cancer, radiation, autoimmune dysfunction). *Secondary hypothyroidism* is generated from deficiencies outside of the thyroid, and is related to the pitutitary gland. *Tertiary hypothyroidism* is related to hypothalamic deficiency related to the release of thyrotropin-releasing hormone (TRH). L less obvious may be the hypothyroidism which is diagnosed by the elevated of thyroid autoantibodies or caused by iodine containing agents.

In the setting of primary hypothyroidism, a decline in serum free T4 and a raised concentration of serum TSH support the definitive diagnosis. This negative feedback relationship between cells, hypothalamus, pituitary and thyroid is so responsive, that even slight shifts downward in free T4 associate dynamically with TSH (Figure 11.2 on page 419). This hyper vigilant, super sensitive response has led to the long and rich history of evaluating TSH levels in conjunction with free T4 to support diagnosis of both hypo and hyperthyroid states.

NOTE: The pituitary hormone should always reflect the presence or absence of free T4, i.e., when free T4 is elevated, TSH should be almost absent. Conversely, when free T4 is low, TSH should be elevated.

When the TSH of individuals in the U.S older than 12 were measured and evaluated, 86% had a serum TSH between 0.4 and 2.5 mIU/L (Hollowell, Staehling, & Flanders, et al., 2002). Therefore, the recommended methodology for appropriate treatment is to adjust T4 dosage to bring the TSH to optimal levels. Hollowell, et al., found that in tertiary care centers only 50% of patients received appropriate treatment, and nationwide, patients continue to be over or under treated.

In 2003, the American Association of Clinical Endocrinologists stated that treating patients with levothyroxine should be considered when the TSH >3.0 mIU/L (Wartofsky & Dickey, 2005). Other experts maintain that testing capability is not as precise as it must be to lower the limits from 4.5 mIU/L (Surks, Goswami & Daniels, 2005).

There are many reasons for a transient increase in serum TSH that requires serial testing to be measured at initial evaluation, at 1 month and again at 3 months. Those patients who have clinical symptomatology as well as a persistent TSH between 2.5 mIU/L and 4.5 mIU/L should be considered at risk, and an in depth family history, a specialist consult, and a more intensive and expensive measurement profile which includes anti-TPO antibodies. This profile allows for identification of patients at risk or those who are progressing slowly to a more overt form of hypothyroidism.

Hypothyroidism is eight times more common in women than men and often presents in the later decades of life. The patient often complains of non-specific clinical signs such as depression, lethargy, weight gain, swelling, constipation and some mental acuity delays, among others (see Table 11.9 on page 422). Because hypothyroidism presents with a depression of clinical signs (respiratory rate, heart rate, blood pressure, temperature, metabolic rate among others) the symptoms are frequently misdiagnosed. As metabolic effects decrease, blood glucose goes down along with most other important byproducts of metabolism. In fact, all measures of cardiovascular and metabolism decrease. The only frequently elevated metabolic measures that do not perform in this manner are cholesterol and triglycerides, which are often elevated.

Occasionally, elderly patients might present after a bout of pneumonia, severe sepsis, after a stroke or in relationship to aspiration. In acutely ill patients care must be taken to a.) evaluate situational hypothyroidism and b.) rule out euthyroid sick syndrome.

Individuals who are acutely or critically ill may suffer an extreme disruption of the normal thyroid axis, particularly related to the nocturnal surge that is normally seen with Thyrotropin. However, these patients will suffer a low T3 level even after the TSH is restored to normal (Langouche & Van den Berghe, 2006), and are commonly referred to as presenting with low T3 syndrome. Patients with poor heart function or more intense inflammatory reaction showed more pronounced down-regulation of the thyroid system. During sepsis, the pituitary gland is activated via blood-borne pro-inflammatory cytokines and through a complex interaction between the autonomic nervous system and the immune cells. Sepsis elicits a very reproducible pattern of pituitary hormone function causing a rapid inhibition of secretion of thyroid-stimulatory hormone.

The euthyroid sick syndrome (ESS) may manifest as a low T3, low T4, low TSH, or all three. ESS results from inactivation of 5'-Deiodinase, resulting in conversion of FT_4 to

11.9   Clinical Signs of Hypothyroidism

Sings and Symptoms of Hypothyroidism	Physical Examination
Less active than usual with loss of interest in things previously enjoyed.	Delayed relaxation time of deep tendon reflex
Lethargy, Fatigue and decreased mobility	Sluggish appearing slow responses
Dry skin	
Apathy and psychomotor retardation	Mental status change
Weakness, arthralgia, myalgia	Carotenemia: An orange or yellow tint without scleral icterus
Coarsening of the voice	Brittle nails and hair
Constipation	
Cold intolerance	Low body temperature
Edema, weight gain	Facial features that are puffy and coarse
Cardiovascular	Sinus bradycardia and a prolonged PR and QT intervals, flat T waves Low voltage Systolic hypotension with diastolic hypertension Pleural. Pericardial and peritoneal effusions
Respiratory and metabolic	CO_2 retention, hypoglycemia, hyponatremia Elevated cholesterol and triglycerides

rT_3 (a reverse form of T3 which is not metabolically active). ESS may occur in critically ill patients, but is also coexistent with DM, malnutrition, iodine loads, or medications (including Amiodarone, PTU, and glucocorticoids).

ESS should be considered when TSH and or T4 are normal, T3 is low and the patient presents with symptoms that suggest hypothyroidism (Docter, Krenning, de Jong & Henneman

(1993). Although there is some disagreement on management, currently practitioners are advised to terminate the causative agent and to allow resumption of normal thyroid function.

Myxedema Coma This exaggeration of the hypothyroid response may occur in undiagnosed hypothyroid patients or when an individual has not been optimally treated, or not treated appropriately during stressful situations (Exhibit 11. 2).

Clinically, hypoxemia, hypotension, hypoglycemia, hyponatremia, and confusion confound and delay the diagnosis of extreme hypothyroidism. The general signs and symptoms of profound hypothyroidsim are exacerbated, to the point of myxedema megacolon as well as myxedema madness.

Because myxedema coma is a life threatening event, rapid therapy must be considered. Outcome predictors that should facilitate prompt and aggressive treatment include advanced age, body temperature <93°F, hypothermic condition persisting more than three days, bradycardia <44 beats/minute profound hypotension and /or myocardial infarction.

Exhibit

11.2 Factors that Influence Myxedema Coma

Common Factors that Precipitate or Exacerbate Myxedema

Hypothermia (exposed to cold)	
Cerebrovascular accidents	
Congestive heart failure	
Infections	
Medications	Amiodarone (oral and over time) Lithium carbonate Sedatives, narcotics, anesthesia
Metabolism	Hypoglycemia Hyponatremia Acidosis Hypocalcemia
Respiratory	Hypercapnea, hypoxemia

The goal of immediate therapy is to support the thyroid hormone levels as well as intervene in the organ systems involved. Initial therapy must include immediate intravenous thyroid replacement (L-thyroxine (T4), 300 to 500 µg IV initially, then 1.7 mcg/kg/day intravenously until bowel function is normal, consider administration of T3 as 20 mcg IV bolus (loading dose 10–25 mcg), then 10 mcg Q8-12H until the patient can take oral therapy). Other primary interventions include, securing the airway and assuring ventilation, vigilant cardiac and respiratory monitoring, steroidst, passive rewarming, appropriate hydration and diuresis (with hyponatremia at the center of focus). Hydrocortisone 100 mg intravenously every 8 hours, is an adjunctive therapy that may also be essential. As soon as possible, oral therapy should be initiated. Care must be taken to assure that patients take medication on an empty stomach and at the same time each day.

Hyperthyroidism
Thyrotoxic Crisis (Thyroid Storm). The effects of hyperthyroidism are related to the continuous tissue exposure to excessive circulating thyroid hormone, which then produces a very hypermetabolic state. The most common cause of this syndrome is Graves' disease, followed by toxic multinodular goiter, and solitary hyperfunctioning nodules. Autoimmune postpartum and subacute thyroiditis, tumurs that secrete thyrotropin, and drug-induced thyroid dysfunction are also important causes. Hyperthyroid symptoms such as those expressed in Exhibit 11.3 are often positioned with opthalmic signs, at the more acute diagnostic point. Other indicators of hyperthyroidism may include osteoporosis, hypercalcemia, congestive heart failure, premature atrial contractions or atrial fibrillation, shortness of breath, muscle weakness, anxiety, or amenorrhea (Cooper, 2003). About 15% of elderly individuals with new onset atrial fibrillation have thyrotoxicosis. And Shimzu, et.al, (2002) found AF resistant to pharmacologic or electrical therapies until the thyroid condition was treated. 40% of the patients will present with ophthalmopathy, in particular exophthalmus. When thyrotoxicosis, goiter and ocular signs present in a triad, the diagnosis of Graves' disease is self evident. 50% of patients with Graves' disease may not have clinically detectable ophthalmopathy at presentation, which creates some concern for diagnosticians. The presence of profound hypothyroid states may create adrenal insufficiency and hypoglycemia as well.

Exhibit

11.3 Signs and Symptoms of Hyperthyroidism

Heat intolerance, sweating	Warm smooth moist skin
Purpura, pruritis	Palmar erythema
Dyspnea on exertion	Thin hair
Weight loss with hyperphagia	Lid retraction and lag
Abdominal pain or secretary diarrhea, hyper defecation	Myxedema of the pretibial areas
Tremulousness, tremor, weakness	Wide pulse pressure
Urinary frequency, nocturia, thirst	Increased systolic blood pressure
Cardiac	Angina pectoris Short PR Tachycardia and atrial fibrillation ST segment changes
Anxiety, emotional liability	Dementia, severe psychomotor dysfunction

Thyroid storm is a rare but potentially life-threatening complication of Graves disease. An acute decrease in thyroxine-binding globulin facilitates high levels of free and metabolically active hormone. The active thyroid hormone increases the density of beta-adrenergic receptors and alters the system responsiveness to catecholamines. The symptoms of hyperthyroidism are exaggerated and may include significant tachycardia, hyperpyrexia, congestive heart failure, neurological compromise, and gastroenterological or hepatic dysfunction. This profoundly exacerbated thyroid state presents as a *medical emergency*.

Although primarily a clinical assessment, laboratory diagnostic testing may reveal suppressed TSH levels and increased serum free T4, a significant increase in RAIU (radioactive iodide uptake), a markedly elevated erythrocyte sedimentation rate as well as other less obvious indicators. If the TSH is low and the free T4 is normal, evaluation of free T3 should be undertaken. The emergent therapeutic goal will be to immediately suppress the thyroid hormones and their Beta enhancing effects, as well as providing overall system support. Of vital concern is the administration of beta antagonists, generally Propranolol 1.0 to 10 mg VERY SLOWLY titrated intravenously over 30 minutes, or 40 to 120 mg orally every 6 hours. One may also consider intravenous Esmolol (0.25–0.5 mcg/kg loading, infusion of 0.05–0.1 mcg/kg/min. All therapies can be reviewed in Table 11.10. Once crises is over, the definitive treatment of Graves disease requires the historical triad that previous generations of clinicians have used; surgery, radioiodine, and antithyroid medications.

11.10	Interventions for Thyrotoxicosis (Thyroid Storm)	
Therapies	**Name of Medication**	**Dosing frequency and Route IV or (PO/NG)**
β-blockers: Antagonizes effects of increased adrenergic	Propranolol	1mg/min IV up to 10 mg (as required and titrated over time) and 60–80 mg
Tone, blocks T4-to-T3 conversion	Esmolol	every 4 h po or by NG tube
	Propylthiouracil	800 to 1200 mg orally initially, then begin 200–250 mg q4h for total daily dose of 1200–1500 mg
	Methimazole	30 mg po immediately, then 30 mg every 6 h
Iodinated contrast agents:	Iopanoic acid or ipodate	0.5–1.0 g/d po or by NG tube
Blocks T4-to-T3 conversion, blocks thyroid	Lugol's solution	10 drops tid po or by NG tube
Hormone release (via iodine release)	Potassium Iodide SSKI	5 drops every 6 h po or by NG tube
	Sodium iodine Hydrocortisone Dexmethasone	0.5–1.0 g intravenously every 12 hours
Cool patient	Cooling blankets	Acetaminephine only Salicylate converts T4 to T3
Hydrate as needed	Isotonic solutions	

Acute Adrenal Insufficiency

The ability to mount a compensatory, life-saving stress response is based on the complex interactions between the sympathetic nervous system and the pituitary expression of critical stress hormones, which stimulate the target organs. As stress increases, so does the expression of the hormonal cascade. Central to the stress response is the release of cortisol (see Figure 11.1 on page 401).

Cortisol has several important physiologic actions on metabolism, cardiovascular function and the immune system. The metabolic effects of cortisol include an increase in BG concentrations through the activation of key enzymes involved in hepatic gluconeogenesis and inhibition of glucose uptake in peripheral tissue. In addition, cortisol activates lipolysis in adipose tissue, which affects the release of free fatty acids into the circulation. Cortisol also has a permissive effect on other hormones including catecholamines and glucagon and may result in the development of a relative insulin resistance and hyperglycemia, at the expense of protein and lipid catabolism. The synergistic effects of cortisol on local catecholamine uptake essentially maintains vascular tone. Another possible cortisol effect is an inhibition of the nuclear factor-κB (NF-kappa B), which profoundly affects systemic inflammation through various mechanisms (Riad M et al., 2002). Steroids are typically released in a pulsatile, diurnal pattern, meant to support the daily rhythms of human physiologic states (not pathologic). However, the role of cortisol in sustaining metabolic and vascular function through various critical illness states is widely underappreciated. During a critical illness, particularly severe sepsis and multiple organ dysfunction syndrome, it is not uncommon for patients to experience a disturbance of cortisol release, resistance, and/or pituitary dysfunction. This disorder, which is often situational, is termed *relative adrenal insufficiency* and is related to the primary stress condition. Previous observational and controlled studies regarding adrenal insufficiency have yielded more controversy and group discussions rather than actual data. Lack of specific signs and symptoms makes early recognition of acute adrenal insufficiency difficult, although the concept of relative adrenal insufficiency has been at the center of many scientific sessions and research in the last 10 years. Debate continues about what represents relative adrenal insufficiency; however, the single most impor-

11.11	Reasons for HPA Dysfunction

Decreased Production/Transport	Decreased Response
1. The hypothalamic–pituitary– adrenal axis is already profoundly stimulated.	1. Decreased number of receptor availability
2. Pituitary glucocorticoid feedback might be altered.	2. Decreased availability of receptor sites
3. The adrenal glands are already stimulated by the increased secretion of peptides with corticotropin releasing hormone—like activity.	3. Diminished binding sites
4. Adrenal hemorrhage	4. Increased clearance

tant clinical clue in critically patients is *failure to respond to fluid boluses* and/or *vasopressor dependency*.

Adrenal insufficiency may be the result of failure of the adrenal glands caused by autoimmune disease, glaucomatous disease, human immunodeficiency virus (HIV) infection, adrenal hemorrhage, meningococcemia or failure of the hypothalamic/pituitary axis, which may occur secondary to withdrawal from glucocorticoid therapy. In critically ill patients, the most studied cause is severe sepsis. Relative adrenal insufficiency may be exacerbated via a chain of events (Table 11.11).

Measurement Issues

Relative or functional adrenal insufficiency occurs in patients with severe illness when the corticosteroid response is reduced in proportion to the severity of illness. This condition usually reverses with recovery from the illness, but can confound the issues of responsiveness as well as interfere with catecholamine—both endogenous and exogenous—effects on vascular tone. The diagnostic criteria for relative adrenal insufficiency continues to be debated, especially as it relates to patients with septic shock or those requiring vasopressors. Unfortunately, the measurement of total cortisol reflects both cortisol bound to protein, cortisol-binding globulin and albumin, and free cortisol, (physiologically active form). Low serum albumin levels may actually create false alterations in the measured serum cortisol levels, and low serum albumin states are very common in critical illness (Marik & Zaloga, 2003). Clinicians have used low random cortisol concentrations, measuring total rather than free, as well as a decreased response to a short adrenocorticotropic hormone (ACTH) stimulation test (standard one time dose of 250 µg or physiologic 1 µg dose of cosyntropin) to diagnose adrenal insufficiency in critical illness. Issues that surround this method of measurement include the following: (a) diurnal or circadian variations are lost in critical illness; (b) 250 µg of ACTH may be a supraphysiologic stimulation, therefore, yielding an adrenal response when the patient may not have a normal physiologic response: and finally, (c) the method, timing, and delay associated with the evaluation may limit introduction of a life-saving corticosteroid replacement therapy.

Opposing researchers have disagreed on both the methodology of evaluation criteria for adrenal insufficiency as well as the laboratory criteria (Marik & Zaloga, 2003; Annane et al., 2004; Hamrahaim, Osenis, & Arafah, 2004). The disagreement focuses on the basic measures of serum cortisol and the components that generate metabolic activity at the cellular levels. Changes in binding proteins can alter total cortisol levels with or without changes in free cortisol concentrations. Most institutions do not measure the free cortisol. Circulating free cortisol measures evaluate cortisol availability as well as cellular uptake.

In this case, therapeutic intervention may be the most important clinical clue. Prompt improvement in the hemodynamic status (particularly blood pressure) of the patient when 100 µg hydrocortisone intravenous (IV) bolus is given may be the most important physiologic indicator of a relative or proportional insufficiency.

In critically ill patients with possible situational or relative adrenal insufficiency, suggestive laboratory findings include hyponatremia, hyperkalemia, persistent acidosis, relative hypoglycemia, in addition to refractory hypotension (pressure not responsive to fluid resuscitation and vasopressor administration). Generally, patients will also present with persistent tachycardia, which may be a clinical differential for acute hypothyroidism. The additional findings that should arouse suspicion of relative adrenal insufficiency in a critically ill patient include fever without an apparent source, or fever that is unresponsive to antibiotics, as well as discrepancy between the expected disease severity and the actual clinical status of the patient.

Emergent treatment may be indicated in these patients, even if the diagnosis is not established. Sprung and colleagues (1984) randomized patients with septic shock in three groups including (a) methylprednisolone 30 mg/kg for one to two doses, (b) dexamethasone 6 mg for one to two doses, or (c) placebo. The overall mortality rate for the entire study period was not different among the groups; however, the mortality rate at 133–150 hours after treatment was significantly lower in the steroid (40%) versus placebo (69%) groups. In addition, shock reversal within 24 hours of randomization was significantly improved in the steroid-treated group. Most recently, the CORTICUS trial (Lipiner–Friedman et al., 2007), the largest to date study on the role of relative adrenal insufficiency in severe sepsis provided the following three confirmations as well as one unexpected result: (a) the defined value of baseline and ACTH stimulated cortisol levels in relation to mortality from severe sepsis or septic shock, (b) delta cortisol, (change occurring when ACTH-stimulated cortisol minus baseline cortisol) should be 9 mg or more. This delta event was more predictive of clinical outcomes than the basal cortisol level, (c) physicians should be aware that etomidate influences ACTH test results and clinical outcome. Importantly, in this large trial, In addition, no survival benefits were evident.

The SCCM guidelines support the intuitive and assumptive use of hydrocortisone in patients with sepsis and/or acute respiratory distress syndrome who present with hypotension that remains refractory to appropriate volume resuscitation and vasopressor management. Other suggestions for management are based on the data from a wide variety of studies.

When Dexmethasone is used initially for emergent steroid replacement, a short ACTH stimulation test can be performed for diagnosis after resuscitative therapy is instituted as Dexmethasone does not interfere with the serum cortisol assay and therefore response.

Vasopressin Abnormalities

Vasopressin is produced in the hypothalamus and released directly from the pituitary gland. The effects of vasopressin depend on the receptor site affinity as well as site activity. Activation of V1

Exhibit

11.4 The Vasopressor Receptors and Their Purpose

Vasopressin Receptors

Two principal types of receptors, V_1 and V_2.
V_1 receptors have been sub classified further as V_{1a} and V_{1b}.
Typical G-protein coupled.

- V_{1a} receptor found in vascular smooth muscle, myometrium, the bladder, platelets, renal medullary interstitial cells, vasa recta in the renal microcirculation, epithelial cells in the renal cortical collecting duct, spleen, testis, and in many CNS structures.
- V_{1b} receptors only in the anterior pituitary
- V_2 receptors are predominantly located in principal cells of the renal collecting duct system.

receptor, which reside on vascular smooth muscle is responsible for vasoconstriction. Activation of V2 receptors on renal tubules is responsible for water reabsorption, reflecting vasopressin's antidiuretic effect (Exhibit 11.4). V3 pituitary receptors have more central effects, such as increasing adrenocorticotrophic hormone production in response to o the V3 receptor sites (Holmes, Landry, & Granton, 2003, 2004). Vasopressin increases the passive water permeability of the cell membrane of the nephron-collecting ducts. It is a potent vasoconstrictor as well as a neurotransmitter, regulating the secretion of ACTH and effects the cardiovascular system, temperature, and other visceral functions. In addition, vasopressin promotes hemostasis as well as stimulating the release of endothelial coagulation factors therefore increasing platelet aggregation.

Loss of Vascular Tone

From the time of Landry's sentinel publication in 1997, several studies have shown that in patients with advanced shock and refractory hypotension there is evidence for low serum concentrations of vasopressin, also known as antidiuretic hormone (ADH). In recent studies, plasma vasopressin levels were almost always increased at the initial phase of septic shock and decreased during the later stages. In fact, Vasopressin deficiency was evaluated in one third of patients with late septic shock (Malay, Ashton, Landry, & Townsend, 1999; Patel, Chittock, Russel, & Walley, 2002). Unfortunately, the appropriate circulating levels of vasopressin in critical illness have not been confirmed; however, measured vasopressin deficiency can be considered as relative at <30 mcg/ml or absolute when <10 mcg/ml.

When patients require catecholamine vasopressors to maintain their systolic blood pressure >90 mmHg, there should always be suspicion of vasopressin deficiency. In this case, vasopressin replacement at a continuous fixed dose (0.01–0.04 units/min IV) can be used to supplement catecholamine infusions. Patients with acute myocardial infarction, acute bowel infarction, or ischemic gangrene of the distal extremities may have worsening ischemia if vasopressin therapy is applied.

Multiple studies have shown that infusion of low-dose vasopressin decreases the norepinephrine dose, maintains blood pressure and cardiac output, decreases pulmonary vascular resistance, and increases urine output in this patient population (Malay et al., 1999; Patel et al., 2002). The introduction of vasopressin must be cautiously approached as vasopressin is linked to vasospasm of both the coronary arteries and the gastric vasculature. When critically ill patients, particularly those in severe sepsis, present with refractory hypotension and require increasing vasopressors support, consider cortisol 100 mg IV bolus, followed by 50–75 mg every 6 hours for 7–10 days and/or initiation of a vasopressin drip at 0.1–0.4 units/min.

Inability to Regulate Vasopressin (ADH) Hormone

The renal regulation of sodium is partially controlled by the expression of ADH or vasopressin, which then affects water conservation or loss. The essential body water, both intracellular and extracellular, must be stable to allow normal cellular functions (dependent on ionic concentration gradients) to take place. Small changes in blood solute concentration (plasma osmolality) regulate vasopressin release. When vasopressin is released in response to the osmolar signal, this directly affects (in physiologic states) the distal tubules of the kidney. The release of vasopressin is primarily related to the serum osmolality and to the volume load, and at very low levels, vasopressin may also decrease portal pressures (Oliver et al., 2007). Together with the renal countercurrent regulation mechanism, the effect is to keep sodium in a content range of 138–142 mmol/L, which then, of course, reflects serum osmolarity. Alterations in sodium and water regulation potentiate a series of life-threatening events.

SIADH: Syndrome of Inappropriate Antidiuretic Hormone. SIADH is a rare but well-recognized disorder, and the clinical diagnosis is based on features first proposed by Bartter and Schwartz in 1967. The syndrome of inappropriate antidiuretic hormone (SIADH) secretion presents with an inappropriately elevated serum ADH level relative to serum osmolality and hypervolemia. Despite a low serum sodium concentration, the patient is not effectively diuresing water to bring concentrations back to a normal range. This disorder can be considered as a failure to **excrete** excessive water appropriately. Urine output may be adequate, but the amount of water to sodium waste is out of proportion.

Causes of SIADH are many and can be generated by a single problem or combination of events (Table 11.12).

Once suspected, SIADH requires careful management with water restriction and occasionally (in severe hyponatremic/hypervolemic states) aggressive salt retaining and diuresis must be applied. When evaluating sodium concentration and content states, attention must be paid to other variables that affect cellular hydration or dehydration.) Hyperglycemia accounts for 15% of hyponatremia in inpatients. Serum Na^+ falls by 1.6 mmol/L for every 100 mg/dl (5.6 mmol/L) increase in plasma glucose (Kumar, 1998).

11.12 Causes of SIADH

Disease States	Pharmacologic States
Acute and chronic pulmonary disease	Phenothiazines
Central nervous system disorders	Vincristine
Acute psychosis	Thiazides
Surgical stress	Morphine
Malignancies	Carbamazepine
Genetic	Vasopressin
HIV–AIDS	Antipsychotic agents

11.13 Differentiating Low Sodium Disturbances

Types	Total Sodium	Total Water	Cause
Hyponatremic Hypovolemia	↓↓↓ total body sodium	↓ total body water	Diuresis (loop) Mineralcorticoid deficiency cerebral salt wasting
Hyponatremic Hypervolemia	normal or ↑ total body sodium	↑↑↑ total body water	Heart, liver, renal failures
Hyponatremic Hypervolemia	Normal total body sodium	Total body water	SIADH

When evaluating patients for hyponatremia, all possible causes must be considered (Table 11.13). The first component of evaluation includes the following four essentials for definitive diagnosis: (a) the effective serum osmolality must be below 270 mOsm/kg water; (b) the urine concentration (>100 mOsm/kg) is inappropriately high related to the dilute serum; (c) the urine sodium is >20 mEq/L in a none salt-wasting state (no diuretic administration, no abnormal salt intake); and (d) adrenal, thyroid, pituitary disease, renal insufficiency cannot be present.

In general, patients with SIADH cannot excrete a solute-free urine, and do not regulate the water-sodium in proportion, giving rise to moderate nonedematous volume expansion and dilutional hyponatraemia. Symptoms depend on the level of hyponatremia and the rate at which it develops. Above 125 mmol/L, symptoms are rare; in the range of 125–130 mmol/L, the predominant symptoms are gastrointestinal. When the serum sodium falls below 125 mmol/L, the patient may present with severe neurological symptoms and this calls for immediate treatment. Signs and symptoms associated with significant hyponatraemia are nausea and vomiting, muscular weakness, headache, lethargy, reversible ataxia, and psychosis and, in severe cerebral edema, respiratory depression, increased intracerebral pressure, seizures, coma, and even tentorial herniation. The presence of symptoms and the duration of the hyponatremic state are key factors which will guide the treatment decisions, as noted in Table 11.14. Hyponatre-

11.14 — Therapies for Acute or Chronic SIADH

	Acute SIADH <48 hours duration	Chronic SIADH >48 hours duration
Risk of cerebral edema	High	Low
Risk of central pontine myelinolysis	Low	High
Neurologic symptoms	Present	Present
Rate of Na+ increase sodium measurement	▓ 2 mmol/hr until symptoms resolve ▓ May then discontinue or return to normal levels	▓ Immediate: 10% replacement (10 mmol/L) ▓ Continuous: 1.0–1.5 mmol/hr
fluid administration rate of 3% sodium chloride	$1–2\ ml \cdot kg^{-1} \cdot hr^{-1}$	$0.5–1.0\ ml \cdot kg^{-1} \cdot hr^{-1}$
fluid administration rate of 3% sodium chloride if symptoms include seizures, obtunded, coma	$4–6\ ml \cdot kg^{-1} \cdot hr^{-1}$	NA

mia developing rapidly over 48 hours or less carries a greater risk of permanent neurological disorders related to cerebral edema unless the serum sodium is corrected. However, patients with chronic hyponatremia are at greater risk of osmotic demyelination if the correction is excessive or too rapid. In addition to sodium replacement, the patient must be fluid restricted.

The use of common pharmacologic agents, such as the selective serotonin re-uptake inhibitors is associated with disruption of antidiuretic hormone action. SIADH is more likely in some populations, including people who are elderly or who take diuretics. Serum sodium levels should be monitored closely in those at higher risk (Rottmann, 2007).

Diabetes Insipidus. The role of the kidney is to maintain a perfectly balanced serum as it relates to Na+ and water. The essential evaluation of this property requires the comparative analysis of the serum sodium (135–145 mmol/dl) to urine sodium (<20 mEq/dl) and the serum osmolality (275–295 mOsm/L) to urine osmolality (50–1000 mOsm/L). When the serum is concentrated, urine should be concentrated; when serum is dilute, urine should be more dilute. The renal mechanisms provide a first line of defense to hypo and hypervolemia as well as hypo and hyperosmolarity. An increase in plasma osmolality, usually indicating a loss of extracellular water, normally stimulates vasopressin secretion (antidiuresis) which promotes fluid conservation and a decreased urine output, and conversely, a decrease in plasma osmolality inhibits vasopressin release into the systemic circulation and promotes more fluid wasting (increased urine output). When vasopressin is released, its primary action will be to stimulate the V2 receptors found in the renal collecting duct (Robertson et al., 1976). The serum osmolality signal, the pituitary release of vasopressin, and the renal response should facilitate urine concentrations that are in the same direction as the serum concentration (if serum is concentrated, urine should be concentrated and sparse, if serum is dilute, urine should be dilute and proportionately plentiful). Finally, the thirst stimulant, which is as important as vasopressin release, is the third regulator of serum osmolality. Polyuric disorders can be caused by any alteration in the three mechanisms (Table 11.15).

The renal losses of water that lead to euvolemic hypernatremia (inability to conserve water) are a consequence of either a defect in vasopressin production and/or release (central diabetes insipidus) or failure of the collecting duct to respond to the hormone (nephrogenic). Common features of both types of diabetes insipidus include polyuria, polydipsia, hypernatremia, and elevated serum osmolality. The diagnostics should be firmly based on the patient's serum sodium/urine sodium levels and even more importantly the serum concentration/urine concentration relationships.

Glucose is a hyperosmolar molecule and, in the insulinopenic state, does not cross the cell wall. By its presence in the extracellular fluid (ECF), the concentration gradient pulls water from the cell (intracellular) to the extracellular space, leading to cellular dehydration, which is one of the reasons hypotonic solution may be needed for *cellular fluid* resuscitation. The lowering of measured serum (Na^+) in this situation is not related to the actual sodium content, but to the *concentration* of sodium in the translocation of fluid from the intracellular to the extracellular compartment. $Na+$ measures in a hyperglycemic state may underpredict the patient's volume status and fluid loss. There-

11.15   Causes of Polyuria

Causes of Polyuria	Symptoms	Urine Output/ Urine Osmolality	Serum Sodium/ Serum Osmolality
Deficiency of osmoregulated vasopressin Central DI/Neurogenic	Polyuria, polydipsia nocturia, signs of severe hypovolemia	↑↑↑ increase ↑↑↑ increase	↑↑↑ increase ↑↑↑ increase RESPONDS to vasopressin administration (11.14)
Reduced renal response to adequate vasopressin Nephrogenic DI	Polyuria, polydipsia, nocturia, signs of severe hypovolemia, often hyperglycemic	↑↑↑ increase ↑↑↑ increase	↑↑↑ increase ↑↑↑ increase DOES NOT RESPOND to vasopressin administration (11.14)
Excessive persistent fluid intake		Variable Serum K+ is low	↑↑ increase ↑↑ increase

fore, total body water has not increased, simply shifted because of the concentration gradient.

The patient with DI has an inability to conserve water The symptoms associated with either central or nephrogenic diabetes insipidus are primarily neurologic. Hypovolemic signs and symptoms as well as altered mental status, lethargy, seizures, hyperreflexia, irritability, and restlessness are common presentations for both types.

The administration of a water deprivation period (2 hours) followed by the administration of aqueous vasopressin differentiates the type of diabetes insipidus (Table 11.14 on page 435). Once definitive diagnosis has been made, therapy will be designed for the problem. Central DI, is treated with fluid resuscitation and the exogenous desmopressin (vasopressin) will be titrated to achieve normal serum–urine relationships. Dosing (0.1–1.1 µg intravenously) will depend on what is required to reverse the osmolalities. Administration of exogenous vasopressin replaces what the pituitary has limited. Unless the problem is congenital, the probability is that the patient will eventually restore normal regulation relationships without the additional vasopressin. Nephrogenic DI must be evaluated first for cause whether it is metabolic or pharmacologic. Following that, salt restriction and salt-wasting diuretics will be administered to increase the urine output and decrease the serum osmolality. Potassium-sparing diuretics may be added to the mix as well.

Summary

Endocrinopathy during critical illness can manifest as hyperglycemia and insulin resistance or as insufficient production of either adrenal corticosteroids or vasopressin. The foundation of normal endocrine response may crumble in critical illness, particularly in hyperinflammatory shock. When the foundation begins to dissemble, the vigilant critical care provider may thwart the destruction with rapid and aggressive therapeutic interventions. There are many conditions associated with endocrine dysfunction and a wide variety of organ alterations. Those discussed here are the most commonly known dysfunctions in the critically ill, adult patient.

References

Ali, N. A., O'Brien, J. M., Jr., Dungan, K., Phillips, G., Marsh, C. B., Lemeshow, S., et al. (2007). Glucose variability is independently associated with mortality in patients with sepsis. *Critical Care Medicine, 35*, A924.

AACE Diabetes Mellitus Clinical Practice Guidelines Task Force. American Association of Clinical Endocrinologists medical guidelines for clinical practice for the management of diabetes mellitus. *Endocr Pract* 2007;13(Suppl 1):1–68.

American Diabetes Association. Standards of medical care in diabetes—2008. *Diabetes Care* 2008;31(Suppl 1):S12–54.

Annane, D., Sébille, V., Charpentier, C., Bollaert, P. E., François, B., Korach, J. M., et al. (2002). Effect of treatment with low doses of hydrocortisone and fludrocortisone on mortality in patients with septic shock. *The Journal of the American Medical Association, 288*, 862–871.

Arabi YM, Dabbagh OC, Tamim HM, et al. Intensive versus conventional insulin therapy: A randomized controlled trial in medical and surgical critically ill patients. *Crit Care Med* 2008;36:3190–7.

Bardsley, J. K., & Want, L. L. (2004). Overview of diabetes. *Critical Care Nursing Quarterly, 27*(2), 106–112.

Bartter, F. C., & Schwartz, W. B. (1967). The syndrome of inappropriate secretion of antidiuretic hormone. *American Journal of Medicine, 42*, 790–806.

Brunkhorst, F. M., Engel, C., Bloos, F., Meier–Hellmann, A., Ragaller, M., Weiler, N., et al. (2008). German Competence Network Sepsis (SepNet): Intensive insulin therapy and pentastarch resuscitation in severe sepsis. *The New England Journal of Medicine, 358*(2), 125–139.

Capes SE, Hunt D, Malmberg K, et al. Stress hyperglycemia and prognosis of stroke in nondiabetic and diabetic patients: A systematic overview. *Stroke* 2001;32:2426–32

De Maio, A., Mooney, M. L., Matesic, L. E., Paidas, C. N., & Reeves, R. H. (1998). Genetic component in the inflammatory response induced by bacterial lipopolysaccharide. *Shock, 10*(5), 319–323.

Devos P, Preiser J, Mélot C. (2007). Impact of tight glucose control by intensive insulin therapy on ICU mortality and the rate of hypoglycaemia: final results of the glu-control study. *Intensive Care Med* 2007;33:S189

Docter R., Krenning E. P., de Jong M., & Henneman G. (1993). The sick euthyroid syndrome: changes in thyroid hormone serum parameters and hormone metabolism. *Clinical Endocrinlogy*;39:499–518.

Clerici, C., & Matthay, M. A. (2000). Hypoxia regulates gene expression of alveolar epithelial transport proteins. *Journal of Applied Physiology, 88*(5), 1890–1896.

Devos, P., Preiser, J. C., Mélot, C., on behalf of the Glucontrol Steering Committee. (2007). Impact of tight glucose control by intensive insulin therapy on ICU mortality and the rate of hypoglycaemia: final results of the Glucontrol study [abstract]. *Intensive Care Medicine, 33*, S189.

Egi, M., Bellomo, R., Stachowski, E., French, C. J., & Hart, G. (2006). Variability of blood glucose concentrations and short-term mortality in critically ill patients. *Anesthesiology, 105*(2), 244–252.

Finfer, S, Chittock, D.,Yu-Shuo Su, S., et al. (2009) Intensive versus Conventional Glucose Control in Critically Ill Patients. NEJM. Mar 26;360(13):1283-97.

Garber, A. J., Moghissi, E. S., Bransome, E. D., Jr., Clark, N. G., Clement, S., Cobin, R. H., et al. (2004). American College of Endocrinology position statement on inpatient diabetes and metabolic control. *Endocrine Practice, 10*(Suppl. 2), 4–9.

Griesdale, D., de Souza, R., van Dam, R., et al. (2009). Intensive insulin therapy and mortality among critically ill patients: a meta-analysis including NICE-SUGAR study data. CMAJ 180: 821-827

Hamrahain, A. H., Osenis, T. S., & Arafah, B. M. (2004). Measurements of serum free cortisol in critically ill patients. *The New England Journal of Medicine, 350*, 1629–1638.

Hollowell JG, Staehling NW & Flanders WD, et al. (2002). Serum TSH, T_4, and thyroid antibodies in the United States population (1988 to 1994): National Health and Nutrition Examination Survey (NHANES III). *Journal of Clinical Endocrinology and Metabolism.* 87:489–499.

Holmes, C. L., Landry, D. W., & Granton, J. T. (2003). Science review: Vasopressin and the cardiovascular system part 1: Receptor physiology. *Critical Care, 7*, 427–434.

Holmes, C. L., Landry, D. W., & Granton, J. T. (2004). Science review: Vasopressin and the cardiovascular system part 2: Clinical physiology. *Critical Care, 8*, 15–23.

Kanji, S., Buffie, J., Hutton, B., Bunting, P. S., Singh, A., McDonald, K.,
    et al. (2005). Reliability of point-of-care testing for glucose mea-
    surement in critically ill adults. *Critical Care Medicine, 33*(12),
    2778–2885.

Krinsley, J. S. (2006). Glycemic control, diabetic status, and mortality in a
    heterogeneous population of critically ill patients before and during
    the era of tight glycemic management: Six and one-half years expe-
    rience at a university-affiliated community hospital. *Seminars in
    Thoracic and Cardiovascular Surgery, 18*(4), 317–325.

Krinsley, J. S. (2008). Glycemic variability: A strong, independent predic-
    tor of mortality in critically ill patients. *Critical Care Medicine, 36*(11),
    3008–3013.

Kumar, S. & Beri, T. (1998). Sodium. *The Lancet. 352*(9123), 220–228.

Landry, D. W., Levin, H. R., & Gallant, E. M., Ashton, R. C., Jr., Seo, S.,
    D'Alessandro, D., et al. (1997).Vasopressin deficiency contributes to
    the vasodilation of septic shock. *Circulation, 95*, 1122–1125.

Landry, D. W., & Oliver, J. A. (2001). The pathogenesis of vasodilatory
    shock. *The New England Journal of Medicine, 345*, 588–595.

Langouche, L.,Vanhorebeek, I.,Vlasselaers, D.,Vander Perre, S.,Wouters,
    P. J., Skogstrand, K., et al. (2005). Intensive insulin therapy protects
    the endothelium of critically ill patients. *The Journal of Clinical
    Investigation, 115*(8), 2277–2286.

Langouche L. & Van den Berghe G. (2006). The dynamic neuroendocrine
    response to critical illness. *Endocrinology & Metabolism Clinics of
    North America. 35(4):777–791.*

Lipiner-Friedman, D., Sprung, C. L., Laterre, P. F., Weiss, Y., Goodman,
    S. V., Vogeser, M., for the Corticus Study Group (2007). Adrenal
    function in sepsis: The retrospective Corticus cohort study. *Critical
    Care Medicine, 35*(4), 1012–1018.

Livingston, D. H., Mosenthal, A. C., & Deitch, E. A. (1995). Sepsis and mul-
    tiple organ dysfunction syndrome: A clinical-mechanistic overview.
    New Horizons, 3(2), 257–266.

Loisa, P., Rinne, T., & Kaukinen, S. (2002). Adrenocortical function and
    multiple organ failure in severe sepsis. *Acta Anesthesiologica Scan-
    dinavica, 46*, 145–151.

Ma, P., Danner, R. L. (2002). The many faces of sepsis-induced vascular
    failure. *Critical Care Medicine, 30*, 947–949.

Malay, M. B., Ashton, R. C. Jr., Landry, D. W., & Townsend, R. N. (1999).
    Low-dose vasopressin in the treatment of vasodilatory septic shock.
    The Journal of Trauma, 47, 699–705.

Marik, P. E., & Zaloga, G. P. (2003). Adrenal insufficiency during septic
    shock. *Critical Care Medicine, 31*(1), 141–145.

Marik, P. E., Pastores, S.; Annane, D. (2006). Corticosteroids in ARDS. *New
    England Journal of Medicine. 355*(3):316–319.

McCowen KC, Malhotra A, Bistrian BR. Stress-induced hyperglycemia.
    Crit Care Clin 2001;17:107–24.

Moshage, H. (1997). Cytokines and the hepatic acute phase response.
    The Journal of Pathology, 181(3), 257–266.

Oliver, J. A., & Landry, D. W. *(2007)*Endogenous and exogenous vasopres-
    sin in shock. *Current Opinion in Critical Care. 13(4):376–382.*

Patel, B. M., Chittock, D. R., Russell, J. A., & Walley, K. R. (2002). Benefi-
    cial effects of short-term vasopressin infusion during severe septic
    shock. *Anesthesiology, 96*, 576–582.

Pruitt, J. H., Copeland, E. M. III, & Moldawer, L. L. (1995). Interleukin-1 and interleukin-1 antagonism in sepsis systemic inflammatory response syndrome and septic shock. *Shock, 3*(4), 235–251.

Rottmann C.N. (2007) SSRIs and the syndrome of inappropriate antidiuretic hormone secretion. *American Journal of Nursing.* 107(1):51–58.

Sánchez–Alvarez, R., Tabernero, A., & Medina, J. M. (2004). Endothelin-1 stimulates the translocation and upregulation of both glucose transporter and hexokinase in astrocytes: Relationship with gap junctional communication. *Journal of Neurochemistry, 89*(3), 703–714.

Selzman, C. H., Shames, B. D., Miller, S. A., Pulido, E. J., Meng, X., McIntyre, R. C., Jr., et al. (1998) Therapeutic implications of interleukin-10 in surgical disease. *Shock, 10*(5), 309–318.

Shimizu, T., Koide, S., Noh J.Y., Sugino, K., Ito, K., Nakazawa, H. (2002). Hyperthyroidism and the management of atrial fibrillation.Thyroid; 12: 489–93.

Sprung, C.L., Caralis, P.V., Marcial, E.H., et al. (1984). The effects of high-dose corticosteroids in patients with septic shock. *The New England Journal of Medicine.* 311:1137–1143.

Surks, M.I., Goswami, G. & Daniels, G.H. (2005) Controversy in Clinical Endocrinology: The thyrotropin reference range should remain unchanged. *Journal of Clinical and Endocrinologic Metabolism,* 90:5489–5496.

Umpierrez, G. E., Khajavi, M., & Kitabchi, A. E. (1996). Review: Diabetic ketoacidosis and hyperglycemic hyperosmolar nonketotic syndrome. *American Journal of Medical Science, 311*(5), 225–233.

Umpierrez, G. E., & Kitabchi, A. E. (2004). ICU care for patients with diabetes. *Current Opinion in Endocrinology and Diabetes. 11*(2), 75–81.

Van den Berghe, G., Wilmer, A., Hermans, G., Meersseman, W., Wouters, P. J., Millants, I., et al. (2006). Intensive insulin therapy in the medical ICU. *The New England Journal of Medicine, 354*(5), 449.

Van den Berghe, G., Wouters, P., Weekers, F., Verwaest, C., Bruyninckx, F., Schetz, M., et al. (2001). Intensive insulin therapy in the critically ill patients. *The New England Journal of Medicine, 345*(19), 1359–1367.

Vriesendorp, T. M., van Santen, S., DeVries, J. H., de Jonge, E., Rosendal, F. R., Schultz, M. J., et al. (2006). Links Predisposing factors for hypoglycemia in the intensive care unit. *Critical Care Medicine, 34*(1), 96–101.

Wartofsky L, Dickey RA. (2005) Controversy in Clinical Endocrinology: The evidence for a narrower thyrotropin reference range is compelling. *Journal of Clinical and Endocrinologic Metabolism,* 90:5483–5488.

Wiener RS, Wiener DC, Larson RJ. Benefits and risks of tight glucose control in critically ill adults: A meta-analysis. *JAMA* 2008;300:933–44.

Williams, G., & Giroir, B. P. (1995). Regulation of cytokine gene expression: tumor–necrosis factor, interleukin-1, and the emerging biology of cytokine receptors. *New Horizons, 3*(2), 276–287.

Suggested Readings

American Diabetes Association. (2001). Hyperglycemic crises in patients with diabetes mellitus. *Diabetes Care, 24*(11), 1988–1996.

American Diabetes Association. (2006). Standards of medical care in diabetes 2006. *Diabetes Care, 29*(Suppl 1), S4–S42.

Andreelli, F., Jacquier, D., & Troy, S. (2006). Molecular aspects of insulin therapy in critically ill patients. *Current Opinion in Clinical Nutrition and Metabolic Care, 9*(2), 124–130.

Bloomgarden, Z. T. (2004). Inpatient diabetes control: Rationale. *Diabetes Care, 27*(8), 2074–2080.

Brenner Z. R. (2006). Management of hyperglycemic emergencies. *AACN Clinical Issues, 17*(1), 56–65.

Brunkhorst FM, Engel C, Bloos F, et al. Intensive insulin therapy and pentastarch resuscitation in severe sepsis. *N Engl J Med* 2008;358:125–39

Das, U. N. (2003). Insulin: An endogenous cardioprotector. *Current Opinion in Critical Care, 9*(5), 375–383.

De La Rosa Gdel D., Donado JH, Restrepo AH, et al. Strict glycaemic control in patients hospitalised in a mixed medical and surgical intensive care unit: a randomised clinical trial. *Crit Care* 2008;12:R120

Eledrisi, M. S., Alshanti, M. S., Shah, M. F., Brolosy, B., & Jaha, N. (2006). Overview of the diagnosis and management of diabetic ketoacidosis. *American Journal of the Medical Sciences, 331*(5), 243–251.

Hansen, K., Thiel, S., Wouters, P. J., Christiansen, J. S., Van den Berghe, G. (2003). Intensive insulin therapy exerts antiinflammatory effects in critically ill patients and counteracts the adverse effect of low mannose-binding lectin levels. *The Journal Clinical Endocrinology and Metabolism, 88*(3), 1082–1088.

Hermayer, K. L. (2006). Strategies for controlling glucose in the intensive care unit. *Clinical Pulmonary Medicine, 13*(6), 332–347.

Malmberg K, Norhammar A, Wedel H, et al. Glycometabolic state at admission: Important risk marker of mortality in conventionally treated patients with diabetes mellitus and acute myocardial infarction: long-term results from the diabetes and insulin-glucose infusion in acute myocardial infarction (DIGAMI) study. *Circulation* 1999;99:2626–32.

Marshall, J. C. (2001). Inflammation, coagulopathy, and the pathogenesis of multiple organ dysfunction syndrome. *Critical Care Medicine, 29*(Suppl. 7), S99–S106.

Sung J, Bochicchio GV, Joshi M, et al. Admission hyperglycemia is predictive of outcome in critically ill trauma patients. *J Trauma* 2005;59:80–3

Terada, L. S. (2002) Oxidative stress and endothelial activation. *Critical Care Medicine, 30*(Suppl. 5), S186–S191.

Turina, M., Fry, D. E., & Polk, H. C. (2005). Acute hyperglycemia and the innate immune system: clinical, cellular, and molecular aspects. *Critical Care Medicine, 33*(7), 1624–1633.

Van den Berghe, G., Wouters, P. J., Bouillon, R., Weekers, F., Verwaest, C., Schetz, M., et al. (2003). Outcome benefit of intensive insulin therapy in the critically ill: Insulin dose versus glycemic control. *Critical Care Medicine, 31*(2), 359–366.

Van den Berghe G, Wilmer A, Hermans G, et al. Intensive insulin therapy in the medical ICU. *N Engl J Med* 2006;354:449–61.

Vanhorebeek, I., Langouche, L., Van den Berghe, G. (2005). Glycemic and nonglycemic effects of insulin: how do they contribute to a better outcome of critical illness? *Current Opinion in Critical Care, 11*(4), 304.

Whitcomb BW, Pradhan EK, Pittas AG, et al. Impact of admission hyperglycemia on hospital mortality in various intensive care unit populations. *Crit Care Med* 2005;33:2772–

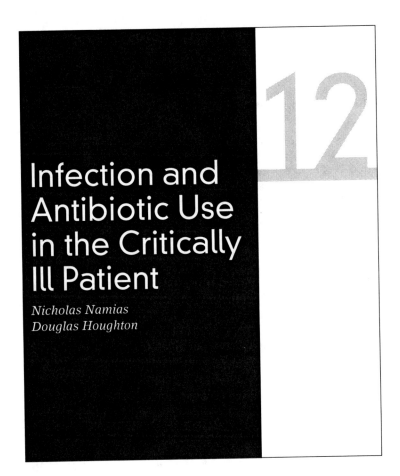

Infection and Antibiotic Use in the Critically Ill Patient

Nicholas Namias
Douglas Houghton

Introduction

The diagnosis and management of infection in the intensive care unit (ICU) affects more than just the individual patient. Whether or not a course of antibiotic therapy is successful for one patient, the bacterial ecology of the unit will be affected in ways that can affect other patients indefinitely. Wise choices can minimize the emergence of resistance, whereas unwise choices and practices can jeopardize the health of many. In this chapter, we will try to explain why patients in the critical care environment are at increased risk for infection, how infection affects patients, and how to diagnose hospital-acquired infections (HAIs) in the critically ill patients. We will then discuss treatment options for infections commonly found in critically ill patients.

Epidemiology

The most common infections in the critical care environment are sinusitis, pneumonia, urinary tract infection (UTI), and catheter-related bloodstream infection (CR-BSI). Most nosocomial infections are subsequent to instrumentation of their respective organ systems. Data from the National Nosocomial Infection Surveillance system (NNIS) demonstrate that 97% of UTI, 83% of nosocomial pneumonia episodes, and 87% of bloodstream infections were associated with indwelling instrumentation of the affected body system (Richards, Edwards, Culver, & Gaynes, 2000). The average added costs for each patient with a health care-associated infection (HAI) were found to be in excess of $8,000 in one recent study (Murphy, Whiting, & Hollenbeak, 2007). Infection-associated mortality rates vary widely across studies and in different patient populations, as well as within these populations due to age, comorbidities, and severity of illness. In the ICU, approximately 30% of patients are affected by HAIs during their stay, with trauma and burn patients having the greatest risk for the development of infection (Vincent, 2003).

Pathophysiology

Treatment in the ICU includes invasion and violation of the most basic bodily defenses against infection. In addition to the breakdown of defenses, the patient care environment is often heavily colonized with the most antibiotic-resistant human pathogens. Other critically ill persons reside close to each other, and many ICUs still retain the design flaw of shared bays, which may contain multiple patients. Patients may be cared for by multiple health care providers who are concurrently caring for other patients with heavy bacterial colonization or active infection.

In critically ill persons, the natural drainage of the sinuses is compromised in patients who are recumbent 24 hours a day. In addition, sedated patients cannot take the normal steps of personal hygiene to keep the upper airways and sinuses clear of secretions. Nasogastric tubes incite inflammation in the nasopharynx and mechanically obstruct their ostia, interfering with drainage. The accumulation of secretions in the sinuses can, and frequently does, become infected. The diagnosis of sinusitis is difficult to make with certainty, and treatment is complicated by the difficulty of draining these bony cavities and the lack of penetration of antibiotics into these virtual abscesses (Stein & Caplan, 2005).

The respiratory system is normally protected by several mechanisms, many of which are routinely compromised in the ICU. Endotracheal intubation bypasses the normal defense of the closed glottis and introduces a foreign body into the trachea. The endotracheal tube incites an inflammatory response, impairs the mucociliary elevator, and provides a surface for the formation of a biofilm. A biofilm is a slippery coating of bacteria that forms quickly and easily on wet environmental surfaces. The biofilm is thought to contain a large proportion of the environmental bacterial biomass and has been linked strongly to the presence of resistant bacteria and recurrent patient infections. These biofilms are inherently resistant to antimicrobial agents through multiple mechanisms; therefore, they provide an ideal nidus for infection in the critically ill patients (Costerton, Stewart, & Greenberg, 1999).

The balloon cuff of the endotracheal tube, contrary to common misconception, does not prevent aspiration of secretions. The cuff also locally injures the epithelial lining of the trachea, allowing for direct invasion of the trachea by bacteria. The lumen of the tube also quickly develops a biofilm, accumulates secretions, and is a direct conduit from the outside world into the lungs. Sedation or paralysis impairs coughing, which is needed to expectorate mucus. Positive pressure ventilation, while lifesaving, does not ventilate all areas of the lung evenly. Portions of the lung can become collapsed, consolidated, and infected if special care is not taken to provide lung recruitment maneuvers with the ventilator (Leong & Huang, 2006) In addition, alkalinization of the stomach from gastric ulcer prophylaxis allows bacterial overgrowth, with potential reflux of this bacteria-laden fluid up an esophagus compromised by a nasogastric tube.

Within the genitourinary system, the urethra serves as the conduit for UTI. Indwelling urinary catheters traverse an orifice normally used only for the release of urine. The urinary catheter locally inflames the urethral epithelium, provides a direct conduit into the bladder from the urine collection bag and provides a nidus for the accumulation of biofilm. Anatomically, the catheter exits the body at a site near the perineum and its attendant frequent soilage, predisposing to ascending infection. Finally, the urinary drainage system may be violated for sampling of urine for laboratory analysis, for pressure measurements, or for routine emptying of the collection bag. Nephrostomy tubes and suprapubic catheters share similar risks to patients (Bagshaw & Laupland, 2006). Urinary tract infections are the most common nosocomial infections in hospitalized patients, likely secondary to the high prevalence of urinary catheters in hospital inpatients (Saint et al., 2008; Vincent, 2003).

Vascular catheters violate the normally closed circulatory system, allow access for bacteria from the skin to the bloodstream, and allow for the formation of biofilm on the catheter. In addition, the catheters are routinely accessed for administration of therapeutic agents, blood sampling, and pressure monitoring. Each time the system is accessed, the opportunity for entry of bacteria exists. The prevention of CR-BSI has spawned an entire industry and science related to its prevention, with anti-infective coated catheters, anti-infective dressings, and protocols for the management of central vascular catheters. (Jones, 2006; Timsit, 2007)

Clinical Manifestations. The manifestations of systemic inflammation and infection mimic each other, as described above. Essentially, all physiologic derangements can be related to either infectious or noninfectious causes. Therefore, localized signs of infection such as purulent sputum or nasal drainage infiltrate on chest radiograph, erythema around a catheter site, or cloudy, foul-smelling urine are of significance when combined with culture data in the critically ill patient. Clinical vigilance and the inclusion of "infection" in the differential diagnosis of each derangement will lead to the prompt and accurate diagnosis of infection (Sprung et al., 2006).

Diagnosis

Diagnosis of infection depends on recognition of clinical signs of infection, appropriate radiologic imaging when indicated, and directed microbiologic sampling. Clinical signs of infection may be difficult to recognize in the ICU. Infection closely mimics the systemic inflammatory response syndrome (SIRS) that can normally be expected in a large percentage of critically ill patients. Fever, tachycardia, tachypnea, and leukocytosis can all be present without an infection, and distinguishing SIRS from sepsis is not always possible. There are no validated criteria by which to differentiate patients with SIRS from those who have an infection, which makes it difficult to determine when to begin antibiotics in patients who are suspected of harboring an infection. Unfortunately, it has been shown that delay of appropriate antibiotic therapy in ICU-related pneumonia and bloodstream infection increases mortality (Iregui, Ward, Sherman, Fraser, & Kollef, 2002; Ibrahim, Sherman, Ward, Fraser, & Kollef, 2000). On the other hand, overuse of antibiotics can lead to resistance, increased cost, and risk of adverse effects. Clinical judgment must be used in each case to decide if an infection is present and if empiric antibiotics should be started.

> Differentiation between infection and SIRS is difficult in patients with critical illness. Correlation of clinical symptomatology, culture results, and clinician judgement is imperative in the diagnosis of infection.

Sinusitis. The diagnosis of sinusitis can be difficult. The intubated and sedated patient usually cannot complain of sinus pain, or pain is masked by the administration of analgesics for other causes. Culture of the sinuses depends on either trans-skeletal aspiration of accessible sinus cavities (not all are accessible) or endoscopic culture, both of which are generally performed only by a trained otolaryngologists or maxillofacial surgeons. Imaging is complicated by the fact that mucosal thickening and accumulation of fluid does not necessarily mean infection is present; both of these findings are possible in the forced recumbency of the critical care environment. The attribution of clinical sepsis to sinusitis is often a diagnosis of exclusion in the absence of direct sampling of the sinus contents.

Pneumonia. The diagnosis of pneumonia in the ICU is complicated by the presence of opacified areas on chest radiograph because of noninfectious entities such as pulmonary contusions, atelectasis, fluid overload, transfusion-related acute lung injury (TRALI), and acute lung injury (ALI) or adult respiratory distress syndrome (ARDS). The Centers for Disease Control (CDC) criteria for the diagnosis of ventilator pneumonia (new or progressing infiltrate on chest x-ray, fever, leukocytosis, and purulent tracheobronchial secretions) are unfortunately nonspecific and can be present in other various conditions. Quantitative clinical assessment tools such as the Clinical Pulmonary Infection Score (CPIS) can aid in the diagnosis through the identification of symptomatic patients who are at higher risk for ventilator-associated pneumonia (VAP) (Luyt, Chastre, & Fagon, 2004; Minei et al., 2006). Microbiologic diagnosis is labor- and resource-intensive and requires a sophisticated microbiology laboratory. Bronchoalveolar lavage, either bronchoscopic or nonbronchoscopic, requires training, sterile technique, and considerable time and expense. Protected specimen brush technique, wherein a protected brush is inserted deep into the airways to collect a specimen, is likewise challenging. Quantitative techniques for culture also demand a high level of resource commitment on the part of an institution. Even with quantitative techniques, there is debate regarding the proper diagnostic cutoff to signify pneumonia and both 10^4 and 10^5 have been commonly used. Nonquantitative techniques do not adequately distinguish between colonization and infection (Rea-Neto et al., 2008).

Urinary Tract Infection. Like all other ICU-associated infections, the diagnosis is complicated by the fact that patients may be sedated or intubated, and may not be able to complain of pain or other symptoms. Only in advanced cases will there be obvious findings such as purulence from the urethral meatus. Cloudiness of the urine is a nonspecific finding, and only urinalysis and culture of the urine when infection is suspected will lead to accurate diagnosis. These infections are more likely in men than in women and are uncommon early in the ICU stay (Golob et al., 2008).

Catheter-Related Bloodstream Infection. The diagnosis of catheter-related bloodstream infection (CR-BSI) requires the presence of a bloodstream infection and a culture positive segment of a vascular catheter. Many techniques of diagnosis have been discussed, but the most commonly accepted is the Maki roll plate technique. Recognizing that the intracutaneous segment most often represents the conduit by which the bacteria reached the bloodstream, Maki described rolling the ICS on sheep's blood agar and submitting this to the laboratory for semiquantitative culture. Greater than 15 colony-forming units of bacteria signify an infected line and the need to remove the line from the infected site. (Maki, Weise, & Serafin, 1977). CR-BSI is more specific and is differentiated from catheter-associated bloodstream infection (CA-BSI), in which the diagnosis requires only a bloodstream infection and the presence of an indwelling vascular catheter. Although any type of bloodstream infection requires antimicrobial therapy, the cause (infected intravascular catheter) and effect (bloodstream infection) is more closely linked in CR-BSI versus CA-BSI because of the addition of an infected catheter segment that contains the same bacteria found in the bloodstream. CA-BSI is more likely than CR-BSI to reflect a bloodstream infection whose primary source lies elsewhere.

Treatment

Effective treatment of infections depends on the following three factors: source control, physiologic support, and appropriate antimicrobial therapy. All three are essential whenever possible; however, source control is not possible in many ICU infections, where the source is often the pulmonary system.

Effective treatment of infection in patients with critical illness includes the following steps:
1. Identification and removal (if possible) of nidus of infection (abscess, catheter or other indwelling device)
2. Culture of affected site/fluid and identification of causative organism
3. Empiric antimicrobial therapy that is highly likely to cover subsequently identified organism
4. Choosing the narrowest spectrum antimicrobial agent that targets the identified organism and effectively achieves therapeutic levels in the target fluid/organ system

Source control is defined as removing the cause of the infection and any infected material. This is clearly understood in intra-abdominal infection—an appendectomy is a source control for appendicitis. It is also clear that in CR-BSI, the infected catheter must be removed and resited in addition to the use of appropriate antimicrobial therapy. In other clinical infections, there are few data with which to define source control.

Physiologic support can be optimized in the ICU patient where most parameters can be controlled to a high degree through medical or nursing interventions. Respiratory failure secondary to infection may require mechanical ventilation, or increased support settings for those patients already receiving mechanical ventilation. Circulatory failure (distributive shock) because of sepsis usually requires intervention with intravenous fluid boluses and not infrequent vasopressor support.

Finally, antibiotic stewardship is critical. There are two phases of the antibiotic treatment. The first is the empiric phase, during which time patients have met clinical criteria for pneumonia, but culture results are not yet available. It is crucial that appropriate empiric antibiotic therapy is started early. Delay in initiation of appropriate empiric antibiotics has been shown to be an independent predictor of mortality in pneumonia (Iregui et al., 2002). Ideally, the antibiotics should be chosen on the basis of an ICU-specific antibiogram. The antibiogram varies between units in a single hospital, and what may be appropriate empiric therapy in one ICU may be entirely inappropriate in another (Namias et al., 2000). Based on the known pathogens in an ICU, appropriately broad empiric therapy should be started. However, this does not imply that the broad spectrum coverage should be continued indefinitely. One approach has been to administer broad spectrum therapy for 72 hours or until final culture results are available, whichever comes first, and then to narrow the empiric coverage down to the least expensive, narrowest spectrum agent with activity against the recovered organism. In this way, patients can benefit from appropriate coverage and the bacterial ecology of the ICU does not have to suffer, because the broad spectrum antibiotics are limited in duration (Namias et al., 2008).

Choice of antibiotics depends entirely on the suspected organism. Published choices for community acquired pneumonia focus on *Streptococcus pneumoniae*, whereas recommendations for hospital-acquired or ventilator-associated pneumonia emphasize coverage for *Pseudomonas aeruginosa*. In addition, methicillin resistant *Staphylococcus aureus* (MRSA) has become so prevalent in ICU that consideration must be given to empiric coverage of MRSA with vancomycin or linezolid. There are controversial data to show the superiority of one agent over another, but it is true that linezolid achieves higher tissue concentrations in the lung than vancomycin at standard doses. Some have suggested that it may be necessary to achieve trough levels of 20 μg/ml of vancomycin to effectively treat MRSA pneumonia (Lam & Wunderink, 2006). Extended-spectrum β-lactamase (ESBL)- producing organisms have made it necessary to use carbapenems more frequently, because these agents are less susceptible to hydrolysis by ESBLs than other agents. However, the next generation of resistant organisms, the *Klebsiella pneumoniae* carbapenemase-producing organisms, are threatening the utility of the carbapenems in North America at this time. These organisms can be resistant to all antibiotics at our disposal (Pitout & Laupland, 2008). *Acinetobacter baumannii* represents another vexing challenge in the treatment of pneumonia. This organism has become highly resistant to most, if not all, common antimicrobials in many inpatient settings (Trottier, Namias, et al., 2007; Trottier, Segura, et al., 2007). A newer agent with activity against *Acinetobacter* is tigecycline. Unfortunately, standard susceptibility breakpoints for tigecycline against *Acinetobacter* do not exist yet, so there is uncertainty in the use of this agent for *Acinetobacter* pneumonia at this time (Karageorgopoulos, Kelesidis, Kelesidis, & Falagas, 2008). Another agent that has been resurrected for *Acinetobacter* is colistimethate, a polymixin analog. This agent is highly nephrotoxic but retains activity against *Acinetobacter* and other Gram-negative organisms such as *Pseudomonas* species.

Treatment of Sinusitis. Treatment of sinusitis is complicated by the difficulty of diagnosis and source control, as mentioned earlier. The health care provider is usually left to make the diagnosis using clinical criteria, as culture techniques that are invasive (endoscopy or trans-skeletal tap) may be deemed of more risk than benefit, and radiologic imaging is nonspecific for infection. Initial management should be directed toward improving drainage by removing any indwelling tubes that block the ostia of the sinuses. Antibiotic therapy is limited by the fact that undrained sinus cavities will be poorly perfused, and antibiotics are therefore unlikely to penetrate the collection. Sinusitis in the ICU should not be treated like sinusitis in the community; appropriate antibiotic choices include ceftazidime, cefepime, piperacillin plus an aminoglycoside, or imipenem (Gilbert, Moellering, Eliopoulos, Sadle, & Chambers, 2008). In severe refractory cases, surgical debridement of the sinuses by an otolaryngologist may become necessary.

Treatment of Ventilator-Associated Pneumonia. Pneumonia is particularly a difficult problem in critically ill patients. A combination of pain, inflammation, recumbency, and sedation all conspire to keep patients from taking maximal inspirations or clearing the airways with an effective cough, and these factors may lead to aspiration of food or oropharyngeal fluids. Once the diagnosis is made, treatment choices must be made. The treatment of pneumonia is with antibiotics specific to the causative organism. The attendant physiologic support is discussed in further details in other chapters.

Colistimethate (colistin) fell out of clinical favor as a result of a high incidence of associated nephrotoxicity with intravenous use; therefore, to avoid systemic toxicity, the nebulized drug has been used in some centers to treat VAP caused by antibiotic-resistant bacteria such as *Acinetobacter*. There are published series of the use of nebulized colistimethate being used to treat VAP with good outcomes. Nebulized tobramycin has also been used for the treatment of *Acinetobacter* and *Pseudomonas* pneumonia, drawing on the extensive experience with the use of nebulized tobramycin in cystic fibrosis patients (Trottier, Namias, et al., 2007; Trottier, Segura, et al., 2007). The primary advantage of nebulized antibiotic use is that the delivery is local (intrapulmonary) and the drug is not systemically absorbed. Therefore, the attendant side effects of intravenous use of the drugs are not experienced by patients. Unfortunately, some patients experience local adverse effects such as bronchospasm with nebulized administration, but these side effects are usually manageable with bronchodilator use.

Duration of therapy for VAP is one of the few cases of antibiotic management where prospective randomized data exist. Chastre et al., (2003) showed that 8 days of therapy yields outcomes equivalent to 15 days of therapy, with the caveat that for certain pneumonias, particularly *Pseudomonas* species, longer courses of therapy may be needed.

Treatment of Urinary Tract Infection. Urosepsis can result from infected calculi or obstruction of urinary outflow, and ultrasound to rule out calculi or hydronephrosis are appropriate in the evaluation of serious UTI. If either of these are found, urologic consultation is mandatory. The critical care practitioner should obtain urine for urinalysis and culture, and immediately begin empiric antibiotics directed at suspected pathogens. Whenever possible, the unit experience with causative organisms for UTI should direct antimicrobial therapy. In the absence of such information, *Escherichia coli*, *Proteus* species, *Enterobacter* species, and *Klebsiella* species are the usual organisms. *Pseudomonas* species should be considered in the ICU setting. Susceptibility reports may be less important in UTI than in other areas, because most of the antibiotics are renally excreted, and are therefore present in concentrations in the urine that can exceed minimum inhibitory concentrations by hundreds of times. Removal of biofilm-bearing catheters is important, because the MIC of organisms in the biofilm may be elevated several hundred fold (Wagenlehner, Weidner, & Naber, 2007). By the time culture results are available, it is likely that the empiric regimen chosen at the outset based on the unit-specific antibiogram will have treated the infection. If symptoms persist and antibiotics are to be continued, they should be narrowed in focus to the identified organism.

Treatment of Catheter-Related Bloodstream Infection. The mainstay of treatment of CR-BSI is removal of the infected catheter. It is the rare exception where the importance of the infected line is so high that it is worth the risk of death to leave it in place with attempts at antibiotic sterilization rather than removing the line. There are no prospective randomized data to direct the duration of treatment of CR-BSI. Certainly, antibiotics should be continued until clinical symptoms have resolved and blood cultures have cleared. Short courses (< 10 days) of antibiotics for *S. aureus* infections have been associated with recurrent septicemia (Raad & Sabbagh, 1992).

Prognosis and Outcomes

Outcomes from infection in the ICU are confounded by the underlying morbidity of patients. It is frequently asked whether a patient died *of* an infection or *with* an infection. Mortality estimates exist for each of the infections discussed herein, which are highly variable according to the patient population and individual patient severity of illness. These estimates are aggregates and do not contribute to the clinical management of patients with these infections. Regardless, mortality rates from HAIs are unacceptably high, and these infections will therefore likely receive increasing scrutiny from payors, the public, and the health care community (Kollef et al., 2006; Vincent, 2003).

Preventive Measures

Excessive costs, decreasing reimbursement, and wide recognition of the significant morbidity and mortality resulting from nosocomial infection has prompted interest in management strategies and products that may decrease rates of HAIs. Many strategies that have been shown to decrease rates of infection are nearly cost-free, but require provider effort and frequently behavioral change for those who have less than admirable adherence rates to practice recommendations. The most obvious example of this kind is handwashing, which is almost cost-free, simple, and has been demonstrated to provide dramatic results in decreasing rates of infection and antimicrobial resistance rates in health care settings (see Exhibit 12.1).

12.1 Evidence-Based Practice Guidelines

Recommendations to Decrease Hospital-Acquired Infections

Prevention of sinusitis

- Remove any indwelling tubes from nares; use orogastric tube, oral endotracheal intubation instead.
- Maintain elevation of head of bed at least 30 degrees to 45 degrees unless contraindicated.
- If sinusitis is suspected, initiate medication to improve drainage such as pseudoephedrine or anti-inflammatory nasal sprays (as tolerated by patient condition).

Prevention of UTI

- Remove indwelling urinary catheters as soon as clinically feasible.
- Consider the use of indwelling urinary catheters with antimicrobial impregnation.
- Assure adequate hydration and dependent gravitational urinary flow.

Prevention of VAP

- Minimize chemical paralysis and sedation use; employ a daily "sedation vacation" as tolerated by the patient's condition.
- Consider endotracheal tubes with subglottic suction port to decrease pooling of secretions on endotracheal tube cuff and subsequent aspiration.
- Oral hygiene and pharyngeal suctioning at least every 4 hours in the intubated patient; consider the use of chlorhexidine oral rinse.
- Do not routinely instill normal saline with endotracheal suctioning.
- Use respiratory care practitioner-driven weaning protocols and facilitate prompt extubation of patients.

Prevention of CR-BSI

- Minimize the use of central venous catheters (CVC); subclavian site preferred if needed CVC.
- Assess need for CVC daily and remove promptly when no longer needed.
- Use antimicrobial-impregnated intravenous catheters.
- Choose the catheter with the fewest number of lumens necessary for patient care.
- Employ chlorhexidine-impregnated disks (Biopatch®) to encircle CVC insertion site
- Assure that an occlusive dressing is covering the insertion site at all times; change when loose or visibly soiled.

Summary

Infection presents a serious problem in the ICU. The diagnosis of infection in critically ill patients is confounded by the presence of SIRS. When uncertainty exists, empiric antibiotics should be judiciously employed while awaiting culture and susceptibility results. ICU-specific antibiograms should be used to direct empiric therapy if they are available, and therapy should be narrowed to the appropriate spectrum when culture results are available. Antibiotic stewardship is critical to mitigate the problem of antimicrobial resistance. The ACNP is uniquely positioned to coordinate the care of critically ill patients in the ICU and to provide longitudinal consistency.

Online Resources

http://www.cdc.gov (Centers for Disease Control and Prevention)
http://www.idsociety.org/Content.aspx?id=9088 (Infectious Diseases Society of America's Clinical Practice Guidelines)
http://www.sisna.org (Surgical Infection Society)
http://www.thoracic.org/sections/publications/statements/index .html (American Thoracic Society Guidelines)
http://www.learnicu.org/SiteCollectionDocuments/NewFever.pdf (Guidelines for Evaluation of New Fever in Critically Ill Adults)

References

Bagshaw, S. M., & Laupland, K. B. (2006). Epidemiology of intensive care unit-acquired urinary tract infections. *Current Opinion in Infectious Disease, 19*(1), 67–71.

Chastre, J., Wolff, M., Fagon, J. Y., Chevret, S., Thomas, F., Wermert, D., et al. (2003). Comparison of 8 versus 15 days of antibiotic therapy for ventilator-associated pneumonia in adults: A randomized trial. *The Journal of the American Medical Association, 290*(19), 2588–2598.

Costerton, J. W., Stewart, P. S., & Greenberg, E. P. (1999). Bacterial biofilms: A common cause of persistent infections. *Science, 284*(5418), 1318–1322.

Gilbert, D. N., Moellering, R. C., Jr., Eliopoulos, G. M., Sande, M. A., Chambers, H. F. (2008). *The Sanford Guide To Antimicrobial Therapy* (38th ed.). Hyde Park, VT: Antimicrobial Therapy.

Golob, J. F., Jr., Claridge, J. A., Sando, M. J., Phipps, W. R., Yowler, C. J., Fadlalla, A. M., et al. (2008). Fever and leukocytosis in critically ill trauma patients: It's not the urine. *Surgical Infection, 9*(1), 49–56.

Iregui, M., Ward, S., Sherman, G., Fraser, V. J., & Kollef, M. H. (2002). Clinical importance of delays in the initiation of appropriate antibiotic treatment for ventilator-associated pneumonia. *Chest, 122*(1), 262–268.

Ibrahim, E. H., Sherman, G., Ward, S., Fraser, V. J., & Kollef, M. H. (2000). The influence of inadequate antimicrobial treatment of bloodstream infections on patient outcomes in the ICU setting. *Chest, 118*(1), 146–155.

Jones, C. A. (2006). Central venous catheter infection in adults in acute hospital settings. *British Journal of Nursing, 15*(7), 362, 364–368.

Karageorgopoulos, D. E., Kelesidis, T., Kelesidis, I., & Falagas, M. E. (2008). Tigecycline for the treatment of multidrug-resistant (including carbapenem-resistant) *Acinetobacter* infections: A review of the scientific evidence. *Journal of Antimicrobial Chemotherapy, 62*(1), 45–55.

Kollef, M. H., Morrow, L. E., Niederman, M. S., Leeper, K. V., Anzueto, A., Benz–Scott, L., et al. (2006). Clinical characteristics and treatment patterns among patients with ventilator-associated pneumonia. *Chest, 129*(5), 1210–1218.

Lam, A. P., & Wunderink, R. G. (2006). Methicillin-resistant *S. aureus* ventilator-associated pneumonia: Strategies to prevent and treat. *Seminars in Respiratory Critical Care Medicine, 27*(1), 92–103.

Laupland, K. B., Bagshaw, S. M., Gregson, D. B., Kirkpatrick, A. W., Ross, T., Church, D. L.(2005). Intensive care unit-acquired urinary tract infections in a regional critical care system. *Critical Care, 9*(2), R60–5.

Leong, J. R., & Huang, D. T. (2006). Ventilator-associated pneumonia. *Surgical Clinics of North America, 86*(6), 1409–1429.

Luyt, C. E., Chastre, J., & Fagon, J. Y. (2004). Value of the clinical pulmonary infection score for the identification and management of ventilator-associated pneumonia. *Intensive Care Medicine, 30*(5), 844–852.

Maki, D. G., Weise, C. E., & Sarafin, H. W. (1977). A semiquantitative culture method for identifying intravenous-catheter-related infection. *New England Journal of Medicine, 296*(23), 1305–1309.

Minei, J. P., Nathens, A. B., West, M., Harbrecht, B. G., Moore, E. E., Shapiro, M. B., et al. (2006). Guidelines for the prevention, diagnosis, and treatment of ventilator-associated pneumonia (VAP) in the trauma patient. *The Journal of Trauma, 60*(5), 1106–1113.

Murphy, D., Whiting, J., & Hollenbeak, C. S. (2007). *Dispelling the myths: The true cost of healthcare-associated infections.* Retrieved March 7, 2009, from http://www.sealshield.com/apic.pdf

Namias, N., Samiian, L., Nino, D., Shirazi, E., O'Neill, K., Kett, D. H., et al. (2000). Incidence and susceptibility of pathogenic bacteria vary between intensive care units within a single hospital: implications for empiric antibiotic strategies. *Journal of Trauma, 49*(4), 638–645; discussion 45–6.

Namias, N., Harvill, S., Ball, S., McKenney, M. G., Salomone, J. P., Sleeman, D., et. al (1998). Empiric therapy of sepsis in the surgical intensive care unit with broad-spectrum antibiotics for 72 hours does not lead to the emergence of resistant bacteria. *Journal of Trauma, 45*(5), 887–891.

Pitout, J. D., & Laupland, K. B. (2008). Extended-spectrum beta-lactamase-producing Enterobacteriaceae: An emerging public-health concern. *Lancet Infectious Disease, 8*(3), 159–166.

Raad, I. I., & Sabbagh, M. F. (1992). Optimal duration of therapy for catheter-related *Staphylococcus aureus* bacteremia: A study of 55 cases and review. *Clinical Infectious Disease, 14*(1), 75–82.

Rea-Neto, A., Youssef, N. C., Tuche, F., Brunkhorst, F., Ranieri, V. M., Reinhart, K., et al. (2008). Diagnosis of ventilator-associated pneumonia: A systematic review of the literature. *Critical Care, 12*(2), R56.

Richards, M. J., Edwards, J. R., Culver, D. H., & Gaynes, R. P. (2000). Nosocomial infections in combined medical–surgical intensive care units in the United States. *Infection Control and Hospital Epidemiology, 21,* 510–515.

Saint, S., Kowalski, C. P., Kaufman, S. R., Hofer, T. P., Kauffman, C. A., Olmsted, R. N., et al. (2008). Preventing hospital-acquired urinary tract infection in the United States: A national study. *Clinical Infectious Diseases, 46,* 243–250.

Sprung, C. L., Sakr, Y., Vincent, J. L., Le Gall, J. R., Reinhart, K., Ranieri, V. M., et al. (2006). An evaluation of systemic inflammatory response syndrome signs in the Sepsis Occurrence In Acutely Ill Patients (SOAP) study. *Intensive Care Medicine, 32*(3), 421–427.

Stein, M., & Caplan E. S. (2005). Nosocomial sinusitis: A unique subset of sinusitis. *Current Opinion in Infectious Disease, 18*(2), 147–150.

Timsit, J. F. (2007). Diagnosis and prevention of catheter-related infections. *Current Opinion on Critical Care, 13*(5), 563–571.

Trottier, V., Namias, N., Pust, D. G., Nuwayhid, Z., Manning, R., Marttos, A. C., Jr., et al. (2007). Outcomes of *Acinetobacter baumannii* infection in critically ill surgical patients. *Surgical Infection, 8*(4), 437–443.

Trottier, V., Segura, P. G., Namias, N., King, D., Pizano, L. R., & Schulman, C. I. (2007). Outcomes of *Acinetobacter baumannii* infection in critically ill burned patients. *Journal of Burn Care Research, 28*(2), 248–254.

Vincent, J. L. (2003). Nosocomial infections in adult intensive-care units. *Lancet, 361,* (9374), 2068–2077.

Wagenlehner, F. M., Weidner, W., & Naber, K. G. (2007). Pharmacokinetic characteristics of antimicrobials and optimal treatment of urosepsis. *Clinical Pharmacokinetics, 46*(4), 291–305.

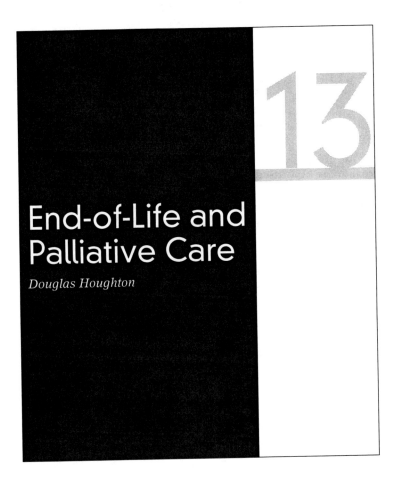

End-of-Life and Palliative Care

Douglas Houghton

Introduction

Technology development and increased knowledge have dramatically improved outcomes in critically ill patients during the past 2 decades. The appropriate and ethical use of expensive resources required to achieve this improved outcome have sparked frequent and sometimes dramatic debate around the world (Bloche, 2005; Ditto, 2006). Fortunately, it is evident that there is increasing interest among critical care clinicians in improving end-of-life and palliative care. With that interest has come the realization that such care requires as much knowledge, skill, and dedication as the intensive preservation of life and restoration of health in critically ill persons (Truog et al., 2008). Research in the area of end-of-life care has matured significantly during the past 2 decades and is gradually progressing from descriptive, observational studies to more advanced trials of clinical interventions to improve the quality of dying and palliative care (Levy & McBride, 2006). Providing comprehensive end-of-life and palliative care requires the dedication of significant resources and the efforts of a multidisciplinary team which includes (at minimum) nursing, medicine, social work, and pastoral care participants. The acute care nurse practitioner (ACNP) can take a leading role in the multidisciplinary team providing palliative and end-of-life care services in various clinical settings. Advanced practice nurses have developed and pioneered models of care suitable for various types of institutions and patient populations, providing benefit to the patient, family, and the primary health care team. These services have often demonstrated a financial benefit to the institutions as well (Emnett, Byock, & Twohig, 2002).

Epidemiology of Death and Dying

Death is an inevitable finale to the life cycle, with more than 70% of deaths occurring in persons older than the age of 65 years. Approximately 2.5 million Americans died in 2006, with the majority of deaths resulting from heart disease, cancer, and stroke (National Center for Health Statistics). Although it is clearly documented in multiple studies that most Americans would prefer to die in the comfort of their home environment, the available data demonstrate that just over half of deaths occur in an acute care environment, with the remaining half fairly evenly divided between home and nursing home deaths (Field & Cassel, 1997; Gruneir et al., 2007). Geographic location and number of available acute care beds are factors that influence the place of death, with urban and developed areas having a higher percentage of in-hospital deaths (Beccaro et al., 2006; Gruneir et al.; Yun, Lim, Choi, & Rhee, 2006). More than 20% of deaths in the United States occur in the intensive care unit, although the number of acute care deaths has decreased during the past 2 decades. This fact is likely a result of increased public awareness and more frequent planning of end-of-life care, as well as patient preferences (Angus et al., 2004).

Ethical and Legal Issues

Medical ethics is a continually evolving area of study. However, certain broad principles are well established in health care and should be applied to all situations when addressing decision making at the end of life. These principles are the following:

- Autonomy—the principle that individuals should be self-determining and that providers have a duty to respect the choices of patients.
- Nonmaleficence—first do no harm; i.e., medical treatment should help patients and not hurt them.
- Beneficence—taking positive steps to actively help patients.
- Justice—fair and equitable treatment, even distribution of resources and opportunities (Beauchamp & Childress, 2001; Thompson, 2007).

At face value, these concepts are easy to understand and appear almost common sense; however, the interpretation of these concepts and their application to clinical situations involving human emotion and unclear patient outcomes is often complex. Providers, families, and patients may become personally invested in specific outcomes for reasons other than the above mentioned. When this is suspected or apparent, the input of an institutional ethics committee to provide a thoughtful and more impartial view of the situation may be helpful and may prevent conflicts. Proactive (anticipatory) ethics consultations were found to be helpful, informative, supportive, fair, and respectful of personal values by both health care providers and family members in a recent study (Cohn, Goodman-Crews, Rudman, Schneiderman, & Waldman, 2007).

Who Makes Decisions at the End of Life? The ethical right of patients to make autonomous decisions and the obligation of health care providers to respect these decisions is well affirmed by medical ethicists (Beauchamp & Childress, 2001). Advance directives are legally recognized by both statutory and common law precedents in 48 states and the District of Columbia, and all states recognize the validity of surrogate decision makers for incompetent patients (Emanuel, Hauser, & Emanuel, 2008). In addition, health care facilities are mandated to inquire about and provide opportunity for persons admitted to the facility to complete an advance directive, as mandated in the United States by the Patient Self-Determination Act (1990). Although as many as 80% of Americans endorse and support the idea of advance directives, only approximately 20% of the population has prepared such a document (Hampson & Emanuel, 2005). Multiple factors including culture, geographic location, and level of education have been described as influencing the completion of advance directives. In addition, in one study, the existence of these documents led to a greater percentage of do-not-resuscitate (DNR) orders and decreased use of cardiopulmonary resuscitation (CPR), but did not affect the use of invasive technologies such as mechanical ventilation (Houghton, 2009).

Because most patients have not completed clear advance directives and many are unable to communicate their wishes in a situation, the use of a durable power of attorney for health care has become common and accepted in the medical community (Arnold & Kellum, 2003; Thompson, 2007; Tonelli, 2005; White et al., 2007). These surrogates may also be known as a health care "proxy," and the process of choosing and appointing this individual may follow specific guidelines according to state law. The ability of these persons to make complex decisions that mirror the patient's actual wishes is a matter of some debate because multiple factors may be involved in the decision-making process that may influence surrogate decisions (Ditto, 2006; Kressel & Chapman, 2007; Limerick, 2007; Lewis et al., 2006; Shalowitz, Garrett–Mayer, & Wendler, 2006; Nelson & Lindemann, 2007). Nonetheless, legal authority to make end-of-life decisions commonly rests with these individuals. The responsibility of the health care provider is to ascertain that these decisions are informed and freely made without undue influences and reflect, to the extent possible, the known or potential wishes of the patient.

In cases where there is no available surrogate for an incapacitated patient, the question of "who decides?" is a matter of debate (White, Curtis, Lo, & Luce, 2006). One recent study found that 1 in 20 ICU deaths occurred in patients without a surrogate or advance directive. In this study, most of these decisions were made by health care providers without judiciary or ethics committee review and were in conflict with the recommendations of both the American College of Physicians and the American Medical Association (White et al., 2007).

Dimensions of End-of-Life Care

End-of-life care can be conceptualized and implemented within five broad dimensions. These dimensions of care consist of communication and conflict resolution; alleviation of distressing symptoms (palliation); withdrawal, limiting, or withholding of therapy; emotional/psychological care of the patient and family; and caregiver organizational support (Houghton, 2009). These represent a fluid conceptual framework for providing care, and clinical situations will vary widely in what is required within each dimension.

Communication and Conflict Resolution

Perhaps the most difficult conversations occurring between health care providers, patients, and families involve the discussion of when it is appropriate to transition from a curative goal to a more supportive "comfort" approach. The primary purpose of critical care units is to save lives and restore health, and this focus is integrated in the culture of critical care providers. Multiple factors have been demonstrated to influence the continued provision of aggressive care in the face of a poor or futile prognosis (Nelson et al., 2006; Robichaux & Clark, 2006; Sibbald, Downar, & Hawryluck, 2007). The lack of availability of accurate tools to predict treatment failure and/ or death often makes the recognition of futile care unclear and subjective, further complicating the decision-making process (Bernat, 2005; Lamont, 2005). In addition, discussing the fact that a given person has failed to respond to a trial of aggressive medical intervention is often difficult for providers and may represent personal failure or defeat to the clinician (Dracup & Bryan-Brown, 2006; Kaufman, 2005). Defining medical futility for a specific treatment in an individual patient is problematic, but a widely recognized definition is care that, in the experience of the provider(s) or on the basis of research evidence, has failed to provide benefit for the last 100 similar patients (Emanuel, Hauser, & Emanuel, 2008). Discussing a poor prognosis with a patient and/or family should be done in a private, unhurried fashion and requires empathy, skill, and listening on the part of the provider. Differences of opinion and conflicting feelings or beliefs about what is best for the patient will often arise. Fortunately, most conflicts involving end-of-life decisions among patients, families, and

providers can be resolved through frequent and open communication on both sides, with the input of an ethics consult if "impartial" input is desired (Bloche, 2005; Cohn et al.,
2007; Lautrette et al., 2007; Lautrette, Ciroldi, Ksibi, & Azoulay,
2006). Discussions in which the patient's terminal status is
clearly presented more often result in decisions to alter the
course of care toward a less aggressive mode (Aldridge &
Barton, 2007). Therefore, if the patient is clearly in the dying
process, this needs to be communicated and may need to be
repeated to the family and the patient (when appropriate).
Although most end-of-life decisions are made by consensus, a
small minority of cases proceed to become public and highly
sensationalized (Bloche, 2005). These unfortunate and often
tragic cases have lead to significant public debate and have
prompted legal action and even court intervention in the
decision-making process. Fear of being embroiled in a similar
situation may drive health care providers to offer alternatives
and provide care they otherwise might view to be futile or not
in the patient's best interest.

The communication process in critical care should be
dynamic and ongoing, because clear and honest communication between members of the health care team and the
patient and/or family has been identified as a key factor in
quality care at the end of life (Truog et al., 2008). The message
from the health care team to the family should be consistent
and presented in nonmedical terms. Family members need
to be given ample time to express themselves and ask questions, as this has been demonstrated to increase satisfaction
with care and decrease dysfunctional bereavement patterns
after the patient's death. The plan of care should be based on
the known or perceived preferences of the patient whenever
possible, and it is important to convey to the family that nei-
ther they nor the patient will receive *less* care if the decision
is reached to withhold, limit, or withdraw therapy (Lautrette
et al., 2007; McDonagh et al., 2004; Weissman, 2004; West,
Engelberg, Wenrich, & Curtis, 2005; White & Curtis, 2006).

Palliative Care within the Critical Care Environment

Palliation is the provision of care with the intent of relieving
distressing symptoms of an illness or injury that may negatively
influence the quality of life of the patient or family (Medina
& Puntillo, 2006; Mosenthal & Murphy, 2006). Palliative care

should be an integral part of the health care of all patients today in any setting, because it is well documented that persons with chronic or acute illness/injury may experience and suffer with a wide range of disease-related symptoms. However, the focus on palliation in the critical care unit is recent and not well integrated into the culture of most units. Palliative care is often overlooked by many critical care clinicians and may be viewed by providers, patients, and families as "giving up" on any hope of cure. Such care need not be in opposition with lifesaving, curative care and should be viewed as a necessary part of humane, patient-focused health care (Mularski et al., 2006).

Some of the most commonly experienced symptoms by critically ill or injured persons include pain, nausea, vomiting, hunger and thirst, diarrhea, confusion, agitation and delirium, anxiety, depression, and sleep disturbance. All of these symptoms are amenable to amelioration with medical and nursing interventions. Palliative care consults have been demonstrated to decrease hospital lengths of stay and resource utilization while improving multiple patient and family-centered outcomes (Campbell, 2006; Curtis, 2005; Medina & Puntillo, 2006; Treece et al., 2006; Twaddle et al., 2007). A multidisciplinary approach to treatment that includes both pharmacological and nonpharmacological interventions is recommended (Qaseem et al., 2008).

Assessment of distressing symptoms of illness/injury or hospitalization must be ongoing, so that the effectiveness of treatments implemented may be objectively measured and treatment tailored to patient response. Clinical tools to assess the severity of patient symptoms should be utilized whenever possible, although in the critical care environment, the patient condition often obviates the use of patient symptom self-reporting tools. When patient condition permits, it is preferable that these assessment tools be completed by the patient or family member rather than by the health care provider. Multiple symptom assessment tools can be found online and can be downloaded free of charge (see Online Resources). Recommendations for pharmacological and nonpharmacological interventions for symptoms commonly distressing to terminally ill patients are provided in Table 13.1 on page 466.

Pain is the symptom experienced by most patients, and the assessment of pain is familiar to most clinicians in all specialty areas. The use of a 0–10 scale for the assessment of pain is commonly practiced, is easy to understand, and is familiar to many patients. Pain rating should be assessed regularly,

13.1 Interventions for Common Distressing Symptoms

Symptom	Pharmacological Treatment	Nonpharmacological Treatment
Anxiety	Benzodiazepines (alprazolam, lorazepam, midazolam, clonazepam)	Patient reorientation, reassurance, explanation of medical/nursing care, quiet environment, guided imagery, music therapy, family presence
Depression	Serotonin reuptake inhibitors (SSRI) (slow onset of action, only available by mouth)	Clear communication of plan of care, psychotherapy, social support systems, pastoral care/spiritual support
Delirium	Antipsychotic agents (haloperidol, olanzapine, risperidone)	Explain to family that delirium is common at the end of life; reduce stimulation; assure patient safety
Dyspnea	Opiates, anxiolytics, diuretics if fluid overload is a concern, bronchodilators if wheezing is present	Optimal positioning, oxygen, minimize activity and physiologic demands (i.e., fever), titration of ventilator
Diarrhea	Loperamide, bismuth subsalicylate (Pepto Bismol), attapulgite (Kaopectate, diphenoxylate & atropine (Lomotil), tincture of opium; treat infectious causes	Identify causative infectious agents or medications, maintain hydration (if deemed beneficial to patient), Fecal Management System (FMS), or other incontinence (if deemed beneficial to patient); management system to minimize patient distress, skin breakdown, and discomfort
Nausea/ vomiting	Metoclopramide (prokinetic) ondansetron, promethazine (anticholinergic)	Quiet environment, head of bed elevated, nasogastric suctioning, review of medications, aromatherapy
Pain	Nonsteroidals (NSAIDS), opioids, tricyclic antidepressants, gabapentin, pregabalin, anesthetics (local/topical or injected), nerve blockade (see Chapter 14)	Assessment and identification of precipitating factors, positioning, distraction, cognitive/behavioral therapy, palliative surgery, others

because some patients are unable or unwilling to communicate their pain to health care providers. When medication or comfort measures such as positioning are implemented, the pain rating should be reassessed within a short time to evaluate effectiveness. Under-treatment of pain is unacceptable, and medication dosages must be titrated upward as necessary to provide the patient with adequate relief; generally, a pain rating of < 2 should be achieved. Chronic pain is not easily relieved with routine analgesics, a more in-depth assessment of the pain can be achieved through the use of the McGill Pain Questionnaire or another standardized instrument (Institute for Clinical Systems Improvement, 2008). Identifying and eliminating the source of the pain (when possible) is vital to effective treatment. Additional means of assessing the source of pain and treating common types of pain identified in clinical settings is provided in Table 13.2 on page 468.

Withdrawing or Withholding Life-Sustaining Interventions

The vast majority of deaths in the critical care unit are preceded by some type of withholding, limiting, or withdrawal of medical therapy, although the public and many health care providers do not seem to be aware of this fact (Sprung et al., 2008; White, Engelberg, Wenrich, Lo, & Curtis, 2007). Emphasis should be noted that actual legal statutes governing the withholding or withdrawal care are rare (with the exception of euthanasia). Therefore, the clinician's actions must be based on the highest ethical principles, institutional or professional guidelines, and most importantly, the perceived or stated wishes of the patient. Most decisions to limit, withhold, or withdraw care are the result of consensus and do not prompt legal intervention or dramatic publicity. As described previously, a surrogate decision maker is common in critical care situations, as the illness of the person usually preempts their active participation in care decisions.

The overriding ethical and legal principle guiding withdrawal or limitation of therapy is the concept of whether or not a treatment or medication is of benefit to the patient (Foster & Carpenter, 2007; Gavrin, 2007; Wainwright & Gallagher, 2007). If there is no foreseen benefit to the patient, then the therapy is futile and can ethically be withdrawn (see Exhibit 13.1 on page 469). Commonly withheld or withdrawn

13.2 Assistive Tool for Determining Type of Pain

	Type of Pain		
	Somatic Pain	Visceral Pain	Neuropathic Pain
Location	Localized	Generalized	Radiating or specific
Patient Description	Pinprick, stabbing, or sharp	Ache, pressure, or sharp	Burning, prickling, tingling, electric shock like, or lancinating
Mechanism of Pain	A-delta fiber activity, located in the periphery	C-fiber activity, involved deeper innervation	Dermatomal (peripheral) or nondermatomal (central)
Clinical Examples	▨ Superficial laceration ▨ Superficial burns ▨ Intramuscular injections, venous access ▨ Otitis media ▨ Stomatitis ▨ Extensive abrasion	▨ Periosteum, joints, muscles ▨ Colic and muscle spasm pain ▨ Sickle cell ▨ Appendicitis ▨ Kidney stone	▨ Trigeminal ▨ Avulsion neuralgia ▨ Posttraumatic neuralgia ▨ Peripheral neuropathy (diabetes, HIV) ▨ Limb amputation ▨ Herpetic
Most Responsive Treatments	▨ Acetaminophen ▨ Cold packs ▨ Corticosteroids ▨ Local anesthetic either topically or by infiltration ▨ Nonsteroidal anti-inflammatory drugs (NSAIDs) ▨ Opioids ▨ Tactile stimulation	▨ Corticosteroids ▨ Intraspinal local anesthetic agents ▨ NSAIDs ▨ Opioid via any route	▨ Anticonvulsants ▨ Corticosteroids ▨ Neural blockade ▨ NSAIDs ▨ Opioids via any route ▨ Tricyclic antidepressants

Source: Institute for Clinical Systems Improvement (ICSI).

Exhibit

13.1 Ethical Principles for Withholding and Withdrawing Life-Sustaining Therapy

1. Death occurs as a consequence of the underlying disease. The goals of care are to relieve suffering and not to hasten death.
2. Withholding life-sustaining treatment is morally and legally equivalent to withdrawing treatment. Both actions require the same degree of active physician/nurse participation as any other procedure.
3. Any treatment can be withdrawn or withheld, including nutrition, fluids, antibiotics, or blood products.
4. Any dose of analgesic or anxiolytic medication may reasonably be used to relieve suffering, even if the medication has the potential to hasten death. Signs of suffering may include dyspnea, tachypnea, diaphoresis, grimacing, accessory muscle use, nasal flaring, and restlessness.
5. Life-sustaining treatment should not be withdrawn while a patient is receiving paralytic agents. After discontinuation of such drugs, the patient must demonstrate sufficient motor activity to allow thorough clinical assessment before withdrawal of support.
6. Cultural and religious views influence the perspectives of patients and family members regarding life-sustaining treatment. These issues should be openly discussed and an effort made to accommodate various perspectives. Pastoral or spiritual care providers may assist in this process.

Adapted from University of Washington/Harborview Medical Center physician orders. Retrieved June 19, 2008, from http://depts.washington.edu/eolcare/instruments/wls-orders2.pdf

therapies include mechanical ventilation, dialysis, vasopressors, antibiotics, and nutritional support. Many institutions will have specific protocols for withdrawal of ventilator or other medical therapies. Clinical protocols for withdrawal of ventilator support (often called *terminal weaning*) are available from professional societies such as the American Association of Critical Care Nurses (AACN) and many large health care institutions (see Online Resources). The process of withdrawal or reduction of ventilator support can be emotionally distressing for both providers and families. Clear communication about the terminal weaning process should be provided to the family, and the clinician should remain immediately available to order medications or other therapies to avoid respiratory distress or patient discomfort.

The practice of terminal weaning is widely variable and could consist of anything from complete extubation to simply decreasing levels of positive end-expiratory pressure (PEEP) or the fraction of inspired oxygen (FiO_2) (Kirchhoff, Palzkill, Kowalkowski, Mork, & Gretarsdottir, 2008; Medina & Puntillo, 2006; Reynolds, Cooper, & McKneally, 2007). Exhibit 13.2 describes common steps in the ventilator removal process.

Exhibit

13.2 Ventilator Removal/Terminal Weaning

Preparation

Meet and discuss options with the family and the patient (when appropriate). Consider:

Does the family want to be present?

Does the family want to spend time with the patient after death?

Is organ donation an option?

When will the process take place?

What method of discontinuation shall be utilized? Options include stepwise reduction of ventilator settings *or* immediate cessation of ventilatory support. The endotracheal tube may be left in place *or* removed if ventilation is completely discontinued.

All conversations must be documented in the patient's medical record.

Procedure

Create the most peaceful environment possible within the area surrounding the patient. Monitors and unnecessary devices should be discontinued, alarms turned off, restraints removed. Provide family visitation access and include chairs, tissues, and privacy.

Educate the family and patient (if appropriate) about the process that will occur and what they may likely experience or witness.

Provide support staff, such as spiritual care providers and social work, and assure adequate nurse availability.

Assure the patient and/or family that all providers will strive to make the patient comfortable during the ventilator withdrawal process, premedicate when appropriate. Ascertain that any neuromuscular blockade effects are gone to avoid the risk of masking patient discomfort.

Adapted from Massachusetts General Hospital Policy and Procedures (n.d.). Limitation of life-sustaining treatment policy: Ventilator withdrawal guidelines.

Making ethical distinctions are important when determining the need for and desired effects of administering medications for pain, anxiety, or respiratory distress symptoms during any withdrawal of care, as euthanasia is illegal in most countries. Because such ethical distinctions are often unclear and context-dependent, clinicians' perception of the situation may vary widely (Rubenfeld & Elliott, 2005; Sprung et al., 2008; Szalados, 2007). Dosages of anxiolytics or opioids are required to assure patient's comfort during the dying process and may far exceed what is commonly administered in clinical practice. Providers are encouraged to administer as much as necessary, keeping in mind the intent is to assure patient comfort and not to hasten the dying process. Specific medications and actions are further discussed in Chapter 14.

Emotional and Psychological Care of the Patient/Family

A recent study demonstrated that severe psychiatric morbidity (major depressive disorder, generalized anxiety disorder, panic disorder, or complicated grief disorder) occurred during the first year after the patient's death in 34% of family members who had served as a surrogate for a relative dying in the intensive care unit (Siegel, Hayes, Venderwerker, Loseth, & Prigerson, 2008). Providing nonjudgmental, emotional, and psychological care to dying patients and their family is probably the most challenging aspect of end-of-life care. Often it requires a great deal of personal strength and ongoing self-care on the part of the clinician to remain emotionally present and authentic in what is likely a difficult situation for the patient's family members (Rushton, Roshi, & Dossey, 2007).

Family-centered care, which emphasizes the importance of the family structure that the patient is a part of, has been identified as the ideal framework for provision of end-of-life care (Truog et al., 2008). With that in mind, it is vital to remember that the patient's family is whomever the patient or family identifies with as being family. This may include nontraditional family structures such as unmarried long-term heterosexual couples, same-sex partners, or other biologically unrelated persons. Emotional and psychological needs of patient and family groups vary widely, and it should never be assumed that all situations call for certain interventions during the dying process. For some families, spiritual support and the presence of a spiritual or religious representative is essential, whereas for other families, the support they require involves good communication and reassurance that can be provided by the clinicians caring for the patient (Cook, Rocker, Giacomini, Sinuff, & Heyland, 2006; Wall, Engelberg, Gries, Glavan, & Curtis, 2007). Some larger institutions now have access to a bereavement team that has expertise in guiding families and professional staff through the withdrawal and dying process.

Maintaining the dignity, privacy, and comfort of the patient and the family during the dying process is essential and often requires more time listening than actually "doing" something. Although the critical care unit is rarely an environment that is conducive to privacy and quiet, every effort needs to be made to allow for family presence and support.

Caregiver Organizational Support

Clinicians caring for dying patients may experience moral distress or "burnout," especially when the dying process involves the withdrawal or withholding of a medical therapy (Badger, 2005; Elpern, Covert, & Kleinpell, 2005; Meltzer & Huckabay, 2004; Rushton, 2006). Experience and education with care of the dying and the withdrawal process may minimize this distress, and both nurses and physicians have strongly identified a need for further and continuing education in care at the end of life (Nelson et al., 2006; Beckstrand, Callister, & Kirchhoff, 2006; Wlody, 2007). Many excellent resources for meeting these educational needs now exist (see Online Resources), but this requires institutional support and provision of adequate time for busy clinicians to attend or complete educational programs. The American Association of College Nursing first made recommendations in 1998 about the inclusion of end-of-life care in nursing curricula, leading to the development of the End-of-Life Nursing Education Consortium (ELNEC). This project, which began in 2000, has since developed six different training programs, one of which focuses specifically on end-of-life

care in the critical care environment (http://www.aacn.nche
.edu/ELNEC/factsheet.htm).

Providing care to dying patients and their families can
be extremely time-intensive, and minimal staffing patterns
may not adequately support this important aspect of patient
care (Beckstrand et al., 2006; Beckstrand & Kirchhoff, 2005;
Nelson, 2006). In addition to supporting nurses and physicians through sufficient staffing resources, other helpful
institutional behaviors include debriefing/support sessions
after the death of a patient, an environment of support
among colleagues, and the availability of persons for discussion of organ donation possibilities (Badger, 2005; Hamric &
Blackhall, 2007; Nelson, 2006; Truog et al., 2008).

Providing Culturally Competent End-of-Life Care

Physicians and nurses frequently believe that they lack
the skills and education to handle difficult end-of-life
issues with critically ill patients and their families (Boyle,
Miller, & Forbes-Thompson, 2005; Nelson et al., 2006).
This discomfort may be magnified when the patient is
from a culture or ethnic background that is different from
that of the provider (Kwak & Haley, 2005; Siriwardena
& Clark, 2004; Valente, 2004). In the United States, this
phenomenon is becoming more and more common as the
nation has become increasingly culturally diverse (U.S.
Census Bureau, 2008). Therefore, it is important to understand how cultural and ethnic differences may influence
the manner in which patients and/or families prefer to
communicate, make decisions, and which care options they
may choose. Acknowledging and embracing these cultural
preferences may improve the quality of the end-of-life
experience for patients, families, and providers (Doolen
& York, 2007; Shrank et al., 2005). Religious beliefs may
also have a profound influence on the patients and their
families' choices for end-of-life care as well as affecting
how providers view these choices. Significant differences
exist *between* and *within* many major religious groups, and
it is important to clarify the beliefs of the patient and family during conversations and family conferences. Insight

on the part of the health care provider into the influence of their own beliefs on end-of-life choices is important in identifying any preexisting value judgments (Dorff, 2005; Johnson, Elbert-Avila, & Tulsky, 2005; Keown, 2005; Markwell, 2005; Sachedina, 2005).

Summary

Providing quality end-of-life care requires significant expertise. Family members will likely remember the manner in which a dying person is treated at the time of death for many years, which may explain why some providers find end-of-life care a very rewarding element of their practice. This is increasingly evident from a growing body of research that specialized in continuing education in this area that is vital for health care providers working in the critical care environment. End-of-life care may be conceptualized and implemented within five domains that include (a) communication and conflict resolution; (b) palliation; (c) withdrawal, limiting, or withholding medical therapy; (d) emotional and psychological care of the patient and family; and (e) caregiver organizational support. Components of important end-of-life interventions are listed in Exhibit 13.3.

Exhibit

13.3 Important Provider Actions for Quality End-of-Life Care

Assess patient and family members' understanding of the condition and prognosis and address any educational needs.

Assure family members that the patient will not suffer or be abandoned and that *care* will continue even if *medical therapy* is withdrawn.

Provide for emotional support and/or spiritual care resources.

Facilitate health care team communication with the family, while respecting cultural preferences for communication and decision making.

Assure that any distressing symptoms shown by the patient are promptly addressed.

Provide for visitation/presence of family and extended family.

Protect patient's privacy and dignity in an environment as peaceful as possible.

Evidence-Based Practice: Palliative Care

Twaddle et al. (2007) reviewed 1,596 health records from 35 academic hospitals across the United States for compliance with 11 key performance measures (KPM) of palliative care. Their objective was to benchmark the quality of palliative care in academic hospitals. The KPM included palliative care activities such as assessment and treatment of pain and dyspnea, psychosocial assessment, communication with patient and/or family, and documentation of prognosis. Compliance with assessment of pain (96.1%) and dyspnea (90.2%) were high, but relief of these problems was lower (73.3% and 77.2%). The overall mortality rate (in hospital) for the sample was 16.8%, demonstrating that the sample was comprised of severely ill patients. Findings demonstrated that compliance with the 11 KPM was associated with improved quality of care, decreased costs, and decreased length of stay.

These findings demonstrate that palliative care is not only humane and in the patient's best interest, but that it makes financial sense as well to integrate comprehensive palliative care into the care of all persons with chronic or acute illness.

Online Resources

http://www.massgeneral.org/palliativecare/WithdrawalProtocol.pdf
http://depts.washington.edu/eolcare/aboutus/index.html (University of Washington/Harborview Medical Center)
http://www.aacn.nche.edu/elnec (American Association of Colleges of Nursing)
http://www.aacn.org/AACN/PalCare.nsf/vwdoc/RWJ (American Assoc. of Critical Care Nurses)
http://www.apa.org/pi/eol/homepage.html (American Psychological Association)
http://www.nlm.nih.gov/medlineplus/endoflifeissues.html (National Library of Medicine)
http://eperc.mcw.edu (Medical College of Wisconsin)
http://www.dyingwell.org (Dr. Ira Byock)
http://www.endoflife.northwestern.edu (Northwestern University)
http://www.nationalconsensusproject.org/Guideline.pdf
http://www.promotingexcellence.org (assessment tools)
http://www.guideline.gov (assessment/treatment guidelines for disease processes/symptoms)

References

Aldridge, M., & Barton, E. (2007). Establishing terminal status in end-of-life discussions. *Qualitative Health Research, 17*(7), 908–918.

American Association of Colleges of Nursing (1998). *End-of-life competency statements for a peaceful death.* Washington, DC: Author.

Angus, D. C., Barnato, A. E., Linde–Zwirble, W. T., Weissfeld, L. A., Watson, S., Rickert, T., et al. on behalf of the Robert Wood Johnson Foundation ICU End-of-life Peer Group (2004). Use of intensive care at the end of life in the United States: An epidemiologic study. *Critical Care Medicine, 32,* 638–643.

Arnold, R. M., & Kellum, J. (2003). Moral justifications for surrogate decision making in the intensive care unit: Implications and limitations. *Critical Care Medicine, 31,* (Suppl. 5), S347–S353.

Badger, J. M. (2005). Factors that enable or complicate end-of-life transitions in critical care. *American Journal of Critical Care, 14,* 513–522.

Beauchamp, T. L., & Childress, J. F. (2001). *Principles of biomedical ethics* (5th ed.). New York: Oxford University Press.

Beccaro, M., Costantini, M., Rossi, P., Miccinesi, G., Grimaldi, M., & Bruzzi, P. (2006). Actual and referred place of death of cancer patients: Results from the Italian survey of the dying of cancer. *Journal of Epidemiology and Community Health, 60*(5), 412–416.

Beckstrand, R. L., Callister, L. C., & Kirchhoff, K. T. (2006). Providing a "good death": Critical care nurses' suggestions for improving end-of-life care. *American Journal of Critical Care, 15*(1), 38–46.

Beckstrand, R. L., & Kirchhoff, K. T. (2005). Providing end-of-life care to patients: Critical care nurses' perceived obstacles and supportive behaviors. *American Journal of Critical Care, 14*(5), 395–403.

Bernat, J. L. (2005). Medical futility: Definition, determination, and disputes in critical care. *Neurocritical Care, 2*(2), 198–205.

Bloche, M. G. (2005). Managing conflict at the end of life. *New England Journal of Medicine, 352*(23), 2371–2373.

Boyle, D. K., Miller, P. A., & Forbes-Thompson, S. A. (2005). Communication and end-of-life care in the intensive care unit: Patient, family, and clinician outcomes. *Critical Care Nursing Quarterly, 28*(4), 302–316.

Campbell, M. L. (2006). Palliative care consultation in the intensive care unit. *Critical Care Medicine, 34*(Suppl. 11), S355–S358.

Cohn, F., Goodman–Crews, P. Rudman, W., Schneiderman, L. J., & Waldman, E. (2007). Proactive ethics consultation in the ICU: A comparison of value perceived by healthcare professionals and recipients. *The Journal of Clinical Ethics, 18*(2), 140–147.

Cook, D., Rocker, G., Giacomini, M., Sinuff, T., & Heyland, D. (2006). Understanding and changing attitudes toward withdrawal and withholding of life support in the intensive care unit. *Critical Care Medicine, 34*(Suppl. 11), S317–S323.

Curtis, J. R. (2005). Interventions to improve care during withdrawal of life-sustaining treatments. *Journal of Palliative Medicine, 8*(Suppl. 1), S116–S131.

Ditto, P. H. (2006). What would Terri want? On the psychological challenges of surrogate decision making. *Death Studies, 30,* 135–148.

Dobbins, E. H. (2007). End-of-life decisions: Influence of advance directives on patient care. *Journal of Gerontological Nursing, 33*(10), 50–56.

Doolen, J, York, N. L. (2007). Cultural differences with end of life care in the critical care unit. *Dimensions of Critical Care Nursing, 26*(5), 194–198.

Dorff, E. N. (2005). End-of-life: Jewish perspectives. *Lancet, 366*, 862–65.

Dracup, K., & Bryan-Brown, C. W. (2005). Dying in the intensive care unit. *American Journal of Critical Care, 14*, 456–458.

Elpern, E. H., Covert, B., & Kleinpell, R. (2005). Moral distress of staff nurses in a medical intensive care unit. *American Journal of Critical Care, 14*, 523–530.

Emanuel, E. J., Hauser, J., & Emanuel, L. L. (2008). Palliative and end-of-life care. In Kasper, Kasper, D. L., Braunwald, E., Fauci, A. S., Longo, D. L., & Jameson, J. L.(Eds.), *Harrison's Principles of Internal Medicine* (17th ed.). New York: McGraw–Hill.

Emnett, J., Byock, I., & Twohig, J. S. (2002). *Advanced practice nursing: Pioneering practices in palliative care*. Missoula, MT: University of Montana.

Field, M. J., & Cassel, C. K. (Eds.)(1997). *Approaching death: Improving care at the end of life*. Washington, DC: National Academy Press (Institute of Medicine). Philadelphia, PA: Lippincott Williams & Wilkins.

Foster, C., & Carpenter, J. (2007). Nutritional support at the end of life: The relevant legal issues. *European Journal of Gastroenterology and Hepatology, 19*(5), 389–393.

Gavrin, J. R. (2007). Ethical considerations at the end of life in the intensive care unit. *Critical Care Medicine, 35*(Suppl. 2), S85–S94.

Gruneir, A., Mor, V., Weitzen, S., Truchill, R., Teno, J., & Roy, J. (2007). Where people die: A multilevel approach to understanding influences on site of death in America. *Medical Care Research and Review, 64*(4), 351–378.

Hampson, L. A., & Emanuel, E. (2005). The prognosis for changes in end-of-life care after the Schiavo case. *Health Affairs (Project Hope), 24*, 972–975.

Hamric, A. B., & Blackhall, L. J. (2007). Nurse–physician perspectives on the care of dying patients in intensive care units: Collaboration, moral distress, and ethical climate. *Critical Care Medicine, 35*(2), 422–429.

Houghton, D. (2009). End-of-life care in the critical care unit. In M.L. Sole, D. Klein, & M. Moseley. (Eds.), *Introduction to Critical Care Nursing* (5th ed., pp. 43–52). New York: Elsevier Saunders.

Institute for Clinical Systems Improvement (ICSI)(2008). Assessment and management of acute pain. Bloomington, MN: Author.

Johnson, K. S., Elbert-Avila, K. I., Tulsky, J. A. (2005). The influence of spiritual beliefs and practices on the treatment preferences of African Americans: A review of the literature. *Journal of the American Geriatrics Society, 53*(4), 711–719.

Kaufman, S. R. (2005). *...And a time to die: How American hospitals shape the end of life*. New York: Simon and Schuster.

Keown, D. (2005). End-of-life: The Buddhist view. *Lancet, 366*, 952–955.

Kirchhoff, K. T., Palzkill, J., Kowalkowski, J., Mork, A., & Gretarsdottir, E. (2008). Preparing families of intensive care patients for withdrawal of life support: A pilot study. *American Journal of Critical Care, 17*(2), 113–121.

Kressel, L. M., & Chapman, G. B. (2007). The default effect in end-of-life treatment preferences. *Medical Decision Making, 27*(3), 299–310.

Kwak, J., & Haley, W. E. (2005). Current research findings on end-of-life decision making among racially or ethnically diverse groups. *The Gerontologist, 45*(5), 634–641.

Lamont, E. B. (2005). A demographic and prognostic approach to defining the end of life. *Journal of Palliative Medicine, 8*(Suppl. 1), S12–S21.

Lautrette, A., Ciroldi, M., Ksibi, H., & Azoulay, E. (2006). End-of-life family conferences. Rooted in the evidence. *Critical Care Medicine, 34*(Suppl. 11), S364–S372.

Lautrette, A., Darmon, M., Megarbane, B., Joly, L. M., Chevret, S., Adrie, C., et al. (2007). A communication strategy and brochure for relatives of patients dying in the ICU. *The New England Journal of Medicine, 365*(5), 469–478.

Levy, M. L., & McBride, D. L. (2006). End-of-life care in the intensive care unit: State of the art in 2006. *Critical Care Medicine, 34*(Suppl. 11), S306–S308.

Lewis, C. L., Hanson, L. C., Golin, C., Garrett, J. M., Cox, C. E., Jackman, A., et al. (2006). Surrogates' perceptions about feeding tube placement decisions. *Patient Education and Counseling, 61*, 246–252.

Limerick, M. H. (2007). The process used by surrogate decision makers to withhold and withdraw life-sustaining measures in an intensive care environment. *Oncology Nursing Forum Online, 34*(2), 331–339.

Markwell, H. (2005). End-of-life: A Catholic view. *Lancet, 366*, 1132–1135.

Massachusetts General Hospital Policy and Procedures (n.d.). *Limitation of life-sustaining treatment policy: Ventilator withdrawal guidelines.* Retrieved July 29, 2008, from http://www.massgeneral.org/palliativecare/WithdrawalProtocol.pdf

McDonagh, J. R., Elliott, T. B., Engelberg, R. A., Treece, P. D., Shannon, S. E., Rubenfeld, G. D., et al. (2004). Family satisfaction with family conferences about end-of-life care in the intensive care unit: Increased proportion of family speech is associated with increased satisfaction. *Critical Care Medicine, 32*(7), 1484–1488.

Medina, J., & Puntillo, K. (Eds.). (2006). AACN Protocols for Practice: Palliative care and end-of-life issues in critical care. Sudbury, MA: Jones and Bartlett.

Meltzer, L. S., & Huckabay, L. M. (2004). Critical care nurses' perceptions of futile care and its effect on burnout. *American Journal of Critical Care, 13*(3), 202–208.

Mosenthal, A. C., & Murphy, P. A. (2006). Interdisciplinary model for palliative care in the trauma and surgical intensive care unit: Robert Wood Johnson Foundation Demonstration Project for Improving Palliative Care in the Intensive Care Unit. *Critical Care Medicine, 34*(Suppl. 11), S399–S403.

Mularski, R. A., Curtis, J. R., Billings, J. A., Burt, R., Byock, I., Fuhrman, C., et al. (2006). Proposed quality measures for palliative care in the critically ill: A consensus from the Robert Wood Johnson Foundation Critical Care Workgroup. *Critical Care Medicine, 34*(Suppl. 11), S404–S411.

National Center for Health Statistics (2008). *U.S. Mortality Drops Sharply in 2006, Latest data show* (press release dated June 11, 2008). Accessed June 20, 2008 at http://www.cdc.gov/nchs/pressroom/08newsreleases/mortality2006.htm

Nelson, J. E. (2006). Identifying and overcoming the barriers to high-quality palliative care in the intensive care unit. *Critical Care Medicine, 34*(Suppl. 11), S324–S331.

Nelson, J. E., Angus, D. C., Weissfeld, L. A., Puntillo, K. A., Danis, M., Deal, D., et al. (2006). End-of-life care for the critically ill: A national intensive care unit survey. *Critical Care Medicine, 34,* 2547–2553.

Nelson, J. L., & Lindemann, H. (2007). What families say about surrogacy: a response to autonomy and the family as (in)appropriate surrogates for DNR decisions. *Journal of Clinical Ethics, 18*(3), 219–226.

Qaseem, A., Snow, V., Shekelle, P., Casey., D. E., Jr., Cross, J. T., Jr., & Owens, D. K., for the Clinical Efficacy Assessment Subcommittee of the American College of Physicians (2008). Evidence-based interventions to improve the palliative care of pain, dyspnea, and depression at the end of life: A clinical practice guideline from the American College of Physicians. *Annals of Internal Medicine, 148,* 141–146.

Reynolds, S., Cooper, A. B., & McKneally, M. (2007). Withdrawing life-sustaining treatment: Ethical considerations. *Surgical Clinics of North America, 87*(4), 919–936.

Robichaux, C. M., & Clark, A. P. (2006). Practice of expert critical care nurses in situations of prognostic conflict at the end of life. *American Journal of Critical Care, 15*(5), 480–489.

Rubenfeld, G. D., & Elliott, M. (2005). Evidence-based ethics? *Current Opinion in Critical Care, 11,* 598–599.

Rushton, C. H. (2006). Defining and addressing moral distress: Tools for critical care nursing leaders. *AACN Advanced Critical Care, 17*(2), 161–168.

Rushton, C. H., Roshi, J. H., & Dossey, B. (2007). Being with dying: Contemplative practices for compassionate end-of-life care. *American Nurse Today, 2*(9), 16–18.

Sachedina, A. (2005). End-of-life: The Islamic view. *Lancet, 366,* 774–779.

Shalowitz, D. I., Garrett–Mayer, E., & Wendler, D. (2006). The accuracy of surrogate decision makers: A systemic review. *Archives of Internal Medicine, 166,* 493–497.

Shrank, W. H., Kutner, J. S., Richardson, T., Mularski, R. A., Fischer, S., & Kagawa–Singer, M. (2005). Focus group findings about the influence of culture on communication preferences in end-of-life care. *Journal of General Internal Medicine, 20,* 703–709.

Sibbald, R., Downar, J., & Hawryluck, L. (2007). Perceptions of "futile care" among caregivers in intensive care units. *Canadian Medical Association Journal, 177*(10), 1201–1208.

Siegel, M. D., Hayes, E., Vanderwerker, L. C., Loseth, D. B., & Prigerson, H. G. (2008). Psychiatric illness in the next of kin of patients who die in the intensive care unit. *Critical Care Medicine, 36*(6), 1722–1728.

Siriwardena, A. N., & Clark, D. H. (2004). End-of-life care for ethnic minority groups. *Clinical Cornerstone, 6*(1), 43–48.

Sprung, C. L., Ledoux, D., Bulow, H. H., Lippert, A., Wennberg, E., Baras, M., et al. (ETHICUS Study Group) (2008). Relieving suffering or intentionally hastening death: Where do you draw the line? *Critical Care Medicine, 36*(1), 8–13.

Szalados, J. E. (2007). Discontinuation of mechanical ventilation at the end-of-life: The ethical and legal boundaries of physician conduct in termination of life support. *Critical Care Clinics, 23*(2), 317–337.

Thompson, D. R. (2007). Principles of ethics: In managing a critical care unit. *Critical Care Medicine, 35*(Suppl. 2), S2–S10.

Tonelli, M. R. (2005). Waking the dying: Must we always attempt to involve critically ill patients in end-of-life decisions? *Chest, 127*(2), 637–642.

Treece, P. D., Engelberg, R. A., Shannon, S. E., Nielsen, E. L., Braungardt, T., Rubenfeld, G. D., et al. (2006). Integrating palliative and critical care: Description of an intervention. *Critical Care Medicine, 34*(Suppl. 11), S380–S387.

Truog, R. D., Campbell, M. L., Curtis, J. L, Haas, C. E., Luce, J. L., Rubenfeld, G.D., et al. (2008). Recommendations for end-of-life care in the intensive care unit: A consensus statement by the American Academy of Critical Care Medicine. *Critical Care Medicine, 36*(3), 953–963.

Twaddle, M. L., Maxwell, T. L., Cassel, J. B., Liao, S., Coyne, P. J., Usher, B. M., et al. (2007). Palliative care benchmarks from academic medical centers. *Journal of Palliative Medicine, 10*(1), 86–98.

U.S. Census Bureau (2008). *Annual estimates of the population by Sex, Race, and Hispanic origin for the United States: April 1, 2000–July 1, 2007*. Retrieved June 20, 2008, from http://www.census.gov/popest/national/asrh/NC-EST2007/NC-EST2007-03.xls

University of Washington/Harborview Medical Center physician orders (2008). Retrieved June 19, 2008, from http://depts.washington.edu/eolcare/instruments/wls-orders2.pdf

Valente, S. M. (2004). End of life and ethnicity. *Journal for Nurses in Staff Development, 20*(6), 285–293.

Wainwright, P., & Gallagher, A., (2007). Ethical aspects of withdrawing and withholding treatment. *Nursing Standard, 21*(33), 46–50.

Wall, R. J., Engelberg, R. A., Gries, C. J., Glavan, B., & Curtis, J. R. (2007). Spiritual care of families in the intensive care unit. *Critical Care Medicine, 35*(4), 1084–1090.

Weissman, D. E. (2004). Decision making at a time of crisis near the end of life. *Journal of the American Medical Association, 292*(14), 1738–1743.

West, H. R., Engelberg, R. A., Wenrich, M. D., & Curtis, J. R. (2005). Expressions of nonabandonment during the intensive care unit family conference. *Journal of Palliative Medicine, 8*(4), 797–807.

White, D. B., & Curtis, J. R. (2006). Establishing an evidence base for physician– family communication and shared decision making in the intensive care unit. *Critical Care Medicine, 34*(9), 2500–2501.

White, D. B., Curtis, J. R., Lo, B., & Luce, J. M. (2006). Decisions to limit life- sustaining treatment for critically ill patients who lack both decision-making capacity and surrogate decision makers. *Critical Care Medicine, 34*(8), 2053–2059.

White, D. B., Curtis, J. R., Wolf, L. E., Prendergast, T. J., Taichman, D. B., Kuniyoshi, G., et al. (2007). Life support for patients without a surrogate decision maker: Who decides? *Annals of Internal Medicine, 147*(1), 34–40.

White, D. B., Engelberg, R. A., Wenrich, M. D., Lo, B., & Curtis, J. R. (2007). Prognostication during physician–family discussions about limiting life support in intensive care units. *Critical Care Medicine, 35*(2), 442–448.

Wlody, G. S (2007). Nursing management and organizational ethics in the intensive care unit. *Critical Care Medicine, 35*(Suppl. 2), S29–S35.

Yun, Y. H., Lim, M. K., Choi, K. S., & Rhee, Y. S. (2006). Predictors associated with place of death in a country with increasing hospital deaths. *Palliative Medicine, 20*(4), 455–461.

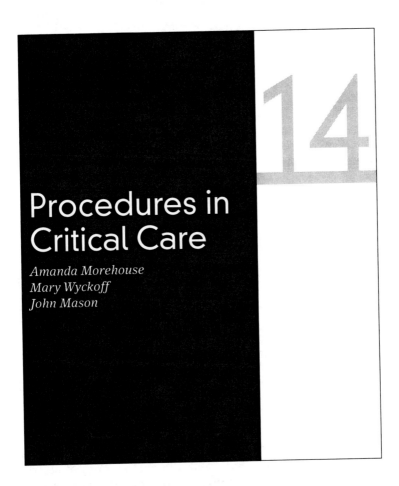

Procedures in Critical Care

Amanda Morehouse
Mary Wyckoff
John Mason

Introduction

Invasive procedures are the mainstay of survival in critical care. Considerations include that these lifesaving interventions are associated with risk and may be as deadly as their potential to resuscitate. How the procedure is performed and how the protective measures are utilized to decrease secondary sequelae may determine the ultimate survival of patients and the success of the procedure. Therefore, education and competency are paramount.

According to the World Health Organization (WHO), 48% of intensive care unit (ICU) patients have central venous catheters and 28,000 ICU patients in the United States of America die each year of central line infections (Berenholtz et al., 2004; WHO, 2007). Therefore, prior to the decision to initiate any invasive procedure, a significant thought process needs to be discussed to determine if the benefit to patients outweighs the potential risks. Patients' physiologic condition and level of stability further needs to be evaluated to determine the likelihood of patient survival should a complication occur.

Preemptive Planning

Preemptive planning may prevent subsequent sequelae. Hemorrhage is a potential risk of most invasive procedures. Therefore, being prepared by knowing the results of recent coagulation profiles, correcting coagulopathies, or considering aborting the procedure based on results may avert a secondary complication. Patients with a prolonged prothrombin time would benefit from a careful thought process regarding whether the intervention would be lifesaving. If there is an alternative intervention, and if the procedure remains the only feasible intervention, then correction of the coagulapathy with fresh frozen plasma should be instituted and ultrasound technology for placement should be considered (Kirkpatrick et al., 2008). Site location for central venous access must be carefully weighed, balancing the risk of infection and venous thrombosis with the potential risk of bleeding. Internal jugular or femoral vein catheterization carry a higher risk of infection, but a lower incidence of hemorrhagic complications upon insertion. The subclavian vein carries a higher risk of hemorrhage from inadvertent subclavian artery puncture, therefore coagulopathy is a relative contraindication to catheterization of this vessel. Health care providers who are capable of intervening in the event of a complication need to be available to intercede if necessary.

Pain Management

Patients' pain and comfort are a priority, and adequate pain control or sedation is crucial to patient and provider safety during invasive procedures. Local anesthesia is essential and may minimize the need for additional medication for analgesia or sedation. Caution should be taken with sedation, particularly in critically ill patients who may have a tenuous respiratory status, inability to protect their airway, or hypotension. The procedural sterile drape should have adequate clear covering so the nurse and ACNP completing the intervention have a clear view of the patient's face, airway, and ventilator apparatus when the patient is artificially ventilated.

Safety

Critically ill patients should be monitored with a cardiorespiratory and oxygen saturation monitoring system. Supplemental oxygen should be provided as indicated while performing the procedure. When the procedure is considered either lifesaving or unavoidable to facilitate recovery and if the patient has tenuous respiratory status, preemptive intubation may be a consideration. As an example, if a central line needs to be placed and the patient would not tolerate Trendelenburg positioning, or if a patient needs a bronchoscopic evaluation and has tenuous respiratory status or respiratory compromise, intubation should be considered as part of the preemptive planning and patient safety.

Observing universal precautions is mandated to protect the patient from serious infectious complications, to inhibit the spread of infectious agents, and also to protect health care providers from exposure to blood and body fluids. Hand washing is the first line of defense to prevent infection. Wash hands for a minimum of 15 seconds with soap and water prior to a procedure and after all patient contact. An alcohol-based product may be utilized appropriately (Boyce and Pittet, 2002).

Skin preparation should be completed with chlorhexidine 2% solution or a combination product with 70% isopropyl alcohol (Chloraprep®). Using sterile gloves, cleansing should be done with a back and forth scrubbing motion around the insertion site, . The area must be allowed to fully dry prior to proceeding (CDC, 2008). Cap, mask with eye protection, gown, and gloves are applied by the inserter and assistants; utilization of strict sterile technique and full body drapes are to be employed for all invasive procedures (Institute of Health Improvement [IHI], 2008). Observers and the patients' bedside nurse should also wear a cap, mask with eye protection, and patient care gown. When the procedure is complete, a Biopatch® (chlorhexidine impregnated dressing), and a sterile, occlusive, transparent dressing or antibiotic-enhanced dressing is placed prior to breaking the sterile field. Bedside procedures are high risk for injury from sharp objects, therefore safety consciousness by monitoring and disposing of all sharps appropriately will prevent secondary injury to the health care providers participating in the care of the patient.

Ultrasound Technology

Ultrasound technology has advanced significantly in the last decade and devices have grown from small 3×3-inch displays to portable machines with large displays and sophisticated capabilities. The use of ultrasound for placing vascular access devices (VADs) and other invasive procedures has become a standard of care and is recommended by the Society of Critical Care Medicine (SCCM). Previously, central lines were placed using landmarks only. With the addition of ultrasound the vessels are able to be visualized, resulting in a higher success rates with fewer attempts and complications. If the arterial system is inadvertently punctured during the placement of a VAD, a hematoma, vascular compromise, compromise of the airway (depending on the site used), blood vessel or other structural damage, and subsequent mortality and morbidity may result. Ultrasound technology minimizes the risks and allows the clinician to use real-time visualization of the needle entering the vessel (Kirkpatrick et al., 2008). The ability to visualize the vessel allows for the appropriate placement of the needle. This should increase patient satisfaction, decrease the number of attempts, and decrease the risk of complications. Evaluation of the vessels depends on the type of procedure that is planned. Education and experience with performing ultrasound are recommended prior to using it for placement of vascular access (Kirkpatrick et al., 2008).

Central venous catheters (CVCs) are typically placed in the internal jugular, femoral, or subclavian veins; ultrasound allows for direct visualization of the vessel. The subclavian vein can be difficult to visualize depending on the size of the patient. The internal jugular, femoral vein, and other venous sites such as the basilic vein for peripherally inserted central venous catheter (PICC) placement are typically easy to visualize using ultrasound, and their large size allows for rapid access.

Utilization of ultrasound guidance for PICC line placement can have multiple benefits. Ultrasound technology facilitates clinicians' ability to evaluate the track of the vein into the axillary and subclavian vein and may also assess malposition of the catheter during the insertion process. After placing the PICC in one of the arm vessels, the internal jugular may be visualized prior to the chest radiograph allowing the clinician to see if the catheter has been inadvertently malpositioned; that is, entering the internal jugular vein instead of the superior vena cava.

There are many different types of ultrasound machines and probes available. The typical requirements for vascular access probe include a length from 25–35 mm and frequency range from 9–14 MHz. The higher probe frequency will provide clearer images but would limit the penetration depth. The lower probe frequency will provide an increased penetration depth but would limit image clarity. Currently, there is no probe that would provide both clarity and good depth penetration; therefore, a machine that can accommodate multiple probes is generally beneficial. This further facilitates the ability to have abdominal and cardiac probes, making the ultrasound multifaceted.

Probe placement during the procedure can be done using two different approaches. The longitudinal approach consists of probe placement parallel to the vessel, facilitating visualization but making vessel access more difficult. The transverse approach provides easy visualization of the vessel and surrounding structures and allows for visualization of the needle puncturing the vessel. The limiting factor can be the ability to follow the needle tip. Once the tip of the needle is past the image area of the probe, it can result in the inappropriate interpretation of the image.

Vascular Access

Central Venous Access

Central venous access indications include invasive monitoring, right atrial/central venous pressure, access for pulmonary artery catheter placement, central venous oxygen saturation, temporary transvenous pacing, administration of resuscitation fluids, and inability to attain peripheral access. Central venous access may be indicated to deliver intravenous fluids, nutrition, or as long-term access. In addition, central catheters are indicated for vasoactive medications, caustic or sclerosing medications, chemotherapy, hyperosmolar solutions, and total parenteral nutrition (TPN), which requires a large, high-flow vein for delivery (Braner, Lai, Erman, Tegtmeyer, 2007). Central venous access may also be used for other procedures such as hemodialysis and plasmaphoresis.

General Technique

The procedure should be explained to the patient or to their health care proxy, including the rationale and potential complications and benefits of the procedure. Written informed consent should be obtained except in the event of a lifesaving emergent intervention, in which case two physicians' consent is obtained. Maintain sterile technique as described previously under the subheading of safety. Place the patient in an approximately 15-degree Trendelenburg position, or flat with lower extremities slightly elevated if Trendelenburg is not tolerated. A shoulder roll may be placed vertically between the patient's scapulae for subclavian vein access, specifically in obese or kyphotic patients. Body positioning will enhance the potential for success.

Identify anatomical landmarks based on site choice and anesthetize the skin at the insertion site with 1% lidocaine. To access the vein, advance the needle bevel up while applying gentle negative pressure on the syringe (see specific section for more details). Once in the vein, the position of the bevel can help direct wire position, for example, inferiorly into the superior vena cava (SVC) for subclavian vein access. Secure the needle with the nondominant hand to prevent needle displacement or vein injury. Evaluate for potential accidental arterial cannulation by observing the color of the blood (least reliable), blood gas analysis (time consuming), and pulsatility of blood return (unreliable in hypotensive patients or patients with right venous pressures). Alternatively, a catheter may be attached to sterile IV tubing and the height of the resulting column of blood may be indicative of relative pressure or pulsatility; the tubing may also be connected to the monitor through a pressure transducer and the waveform observed. Ultrasound may also be employed to visualize the needle, wire, or catheter in vein, except generally in subclavian vein placement. Maintain the open end of the needle completely covered to prevent air emboli especially in hypovolemic or spontaneously breathing patients.

If the vein is not accessed on first attempt, withdraw the needle slowly because the needle may have compressed and subsequently completely penetrated the vein on insertion, particularly in dehydrated patients. Maintain gentle negative pressure on the barrel of the syringe by pulling back on the plunger and the vein may be accessed on withdrawal. Withdraw the needle to skin level before altering the angle; altering the angle with the needle partially inserted may lacerate the vein or accompanying artery. Note that repeated passes of the needle increases the risk of mechanical complications. Remove the needle immediately if the artery is punctured, and compress the vessel for at least 5 minutes if there is no coagulation disorder.

After successful venous catheterization, the J-tipped end of the guidewire is inserted through the needle or wire-guided syringe. Once in place, maintain constant manual control of the guidewire to prevent wire embolization. Monitor continuously for arrhythmias by listening to the heart rate tones on the monitor. As the guidewire is advanced, arrhythmias or ectopy may develop; withdraw wire until the heart resumes previous normal rhythm. The wire should only be inserted to approximately 20 cm depth in most instances to minimize the occurrence of dysrhythmia. Using a scalpel, insert the back of the scalpel along the wire into the skin to make an incision large enough to accommodate the dilator and catheter, approximately 1–2 mm. Insert the dilator just the depth that is required to access the vein. Further advancement of the stiff dilator may cause injury to the wall of the vein and subsequently penetrate the artery. Remove the dilator carefully to avoid displacement of the guidewire. Apply pressure to the skin entry site to control blood loss and prevent air entry in vein. Place the central line catheter over the guidewire while maintaining a portion of the guidewire in hand. The central line catheter must not enter the skin until the guidewire has exited the hub of the catheter, therefore never having the wire out of hand or sight. In general, the right internal jugular (IJ) is placed to approximately 14 cm, right subclavian to 16 cm, left IJ and left subclavian to 18 cm, and femoral to 20 cm. These predetermined lengths will vary based on the size and height of the patient.

Once the catheter is in place, remove the guidewire while keeping all ports of the catheter clamped, covered, or secured with positive or neutral displacement valves. Attain blood return in all ports to the hub of the catheter to prevent air from entering the system, and then flush through the positive displacement valves, confirming that all ports have blood return and flush easily. Suture the catheter to the skin to secure it in position. Clean the skin area around the catheter with 2% chlorhexidine or sterile saline, allow the area to dry, apply skin prep to area around the site, apply antibiotic impregnated transparent dressing or Biopatch® with transparent dressing occlusively to the insertion site (Maki, et al., 2000).

Remove drapes and dispose of sharps and biohazard wastes appropriately. The inserter should clean the area and the tray to avoid injury to others. Obtain a chest x-ray to confirm catheter placement and to evaluate for mechanical complications. The catheter tip should be at the level of the SVC or approximately at the level of the right main stem bronchus on radiograph. Femoral lines do not require radiograph for confirmation of position (see Exhibit 14.1).

Subclavian. The subclavian vein lies under the medial third of the clavicle, superior to the first rib, where it is anterior and inferior to the subclavian artery. The anterior scalene muscle lies between the vein and artery. The vein joins with the internal jugular to become the brachiocephalic vein as it enters the thoracic cavity at the head of the clavicle. Anteriorly, the cupula of the pleura projects the level of the clavicle (Agur & Lee, 1999).

With the subclavian approach, there is an increased risk of pneumothorax as a mechanical complication, particularly in inexperienced practitioners. Other complications include, but are not limited to, hemothorax, air embolism, arterial puncture, tracheal puncture, and aortic perforation (Braner et al., 2007). Bullous emphysema is a relative contraindication for the subclavian approach, as this increases the risk of pneumothorax and spontaneous death. The subclavian artery and vein are difficult to compress; therefore, this approach is also relatively contraindicated in coagulopathic patients. However, the subclavian vein has the lowest risk of infectious complications, possibly because of the ease of site care (IHI, 2008).

Exhibit

14.1 Initial Line Insertion Procedure

Preparation for Initial Insertion Skin
Indications: Central TPN, vancomycin, and poor peripheral access. Minimize use of femoral lines if possible.

Supplies needed at bedside:
- 3 packages 4×4 gauze
- 1 sterile half sheet
- 1 sterile gown, Chlorhexidine solution or Chloraprep® applicator
- 2 pairs sterile gloves
- central line kit, mask, and hat

Procedure:
1. Obtain informed consent from the patient or health care proxy. An experienced practitioner must be present at the bedside to observe or perform line insertion.
2. Put on mask and hat.
3. Don sterile gloves.
4. Prep the catheter insertion site and surrounding skin (approximately 10 inches in diameter) with Chlorhexidine soaked 4×4 gauzes or Chloraprep® applicator. Scrub for 30 seconds minimum in multiple directions. Let Chlorhexidine dry completely.
5. While the Chlorhexidine is drying, remove gloves used during preparation, put on sterile gown and new set of sterile gloves.
6. Proceed with insertion of central venous catheter of the desired type.
7. In cases when the continuous infusion (drip) must be administered through the line just placed, attach a sterile IV extension tubing to the drip, fill the tubing, and attach the sterile end of the extension tubing to the appropriate port of the catheter that will maintain sterility during the remainder of the procedure. This would be the sidearm of the introducer or one of the lumens in the triple-lumen catheter.
8. Suture the introducer in place or, if using a triple-lumen catheter, attach the snap clip.
9. Cover with sterile 4×4 gauze. In the case of a triple-lumen catheter, make sure that the triangle joining the 3 separate lumens is covered by the gauze so that there will be no adhesive adhering to the area that must be cleansed and prepped prior to a guidewire change.
10. Apply Biopatch® and assist the nurse in completing a sterile, occlusive dressing including the time and date of insertion.
11. Document the procedure in the medical record.

The insertion site is approximately one fingerbreadth lateral and one fingerbreadth inferior to the curve of the clavicle in the deltopectoral groove. Insertion occurs at approximately 2 cm lateral and 2 cm caudal to the middle third of the clavicle, advancing the needle into the skin under the clavicle (Braner, et al., 2007). Anesthetize the skin; insert the needle just through the skin and into the subcutaneous tissue. Place the index finger of the nondominant hand at the sternal notch to mark the landmark and help direct the insertion. Use the thumb of the nondominant hand to compress the subcutaneous tissue and needle, to guide the needle under the clavicle while directing the needle toward the sternal notch. Maintain a shallow insertion angle, as close and as parallel to the patient as possible, to avoid causing a pneumothorax. The costoclavicular ligament or head of the first rib or clavicle may be encountered preventing access of the vein. Redirect the angle of the needle if the vein is not accessed by withdrawing the needle and by redirecting the angle slightly cephalad; if still not successful, again withdraw the needle and redirect the angle slightly caudad.

Internal Jugular. The internal jugular vein lies deep to the sternocleidomastoid muscle (SCM), lateral to the carotid artery and continues between the heads of the sternocleidomastoid. The internal jugular vein joins with the subclavian to form the brachiocephalic vein at the head of the clavicle (Agur & Lee, 1999). There is some variability in the position of the internal jugular, making the use of ultrasound beneficial.

Complications include carotid artery puncture, which is potentially avoidable with the use of ultrasound. Should this occur, the needle should be removed immediately and pressure be held. Remember that the pleural cupola extends above the level of the clavicle, making pneumothorax a potential complication. The risk for pneumothorax is lower when a high insertion point is chosen. Infectious complications are higher than the subclavian position, because of the difficulty in maintaining the site and potential for contamination with oral and tracheal secretions.

There are three techniques for cannulation of the internal jugular vein, the anterior, central, and posterior approach as detailed below. For all techniques, turn the patient's head away from the side of insertion. Palpate the carotid artery to obtain landmarks, prior to needle advancement. Palpation of the artery during needle advancement may occlude the lumen of the vein; therefore, use light palpation to avoid occlusion. The vein should be accessed at a 10- to 20-degree angle above the skin to avoid pneumothorax and injury to deep structures in the neck.

Anterior Approach. With the nondominant hand, push the sternal head of the SCM laterally. At the level of the apex of the heads of the SCM, enter the skin medial to the SCM and lateral to the carotid pulse. Direct the needle under the SCM toward the ipsilateral nipple while advancing the needle. Withdraw and redirect the needle medially if the vein is not accessed, but never more medial than the carotid pulse.

Central Approach. At the apex of the heads of the clavicular and sternal heads of the SCM, lateral to the carotid pulse, enter the skin. Direct the needle at an angle of 20 degrees above the coronal plane toward the ipsilateral nipple while advancing the needle (Graham, Ozment, Tegtmeyer, Lai, & Braner, 2007). Withdraw and redirect the needle medially if the vein is not accessed. However, the needle should never be directed more medial than a line parallel with the spinal axis to avoid carotid puncture.

Posterior Approach. At the level of the apex of the heads of the SCM, enter the skin posterior to the dorsal border of the SCM. Direct the needle under the SCM toward the contralateral nipple. Withdraw and redirect laterally if the vein is not accessed. This approach has an increased risk of carotid puncture.

Femoral. The femoral vein lies within the femoral sheath, just medial to the femoral artery. The vein is approximately midway between the anterior superior iliac spine and the pubic tubercle, inferior to the inguinal ligament (Tsui et al., 2008). Femoral access is often obtained as emergency access; it can be placed while chest compressions and intubation are being performed. However, the risk of infectious complications is highest in this position. This is likely because of the frequent emergent placement and also because of the moist groin environment and relative difficulty of site care. There is also a higher risk of thrombosis at the femoral site. The use of ultrasound is recommended to decrease the risk of arterial puncture and potential pseudoaneurysm.

Palpate the femoral artery pulse; if not palpable, the course of the artery may be marked by Doppler signal, but ultrasound should be used if feasible. When placing the catheter under emergent conditions, use the landmarks as described above. Using the location of the femoral artery, enter the skin just medial to the artery. Insert the needle at a 45-degree angle and direct the needle parallel with the course of the artery. Access the vein inferior to the inguinal ligament. Superior to the inguinal ligament, the vessels are not compressible if bleeding should arise or upon removal of the catheter. Redirect the needle if unsuccessful on maintaining palpation of the artery while advancing the needle laterally, closer to the femoral pulse. To guidewire a central venous catheter, see Exhibit 14.2.

Pulmonary Artery Catheter. Indications for pulmonary artery catheter (PAC) placement are controversial, mainly because of the general lack of expertise in interpretation of the data obtained, which may cause more harm than benefit. The insertion of a PAC has not conclusively been shown to affect survivability and other sources may be used to attain similar information. Generally, use is indicated when volume and hemodynamic status cannot accurately be determined by exam and less invasive monitoring (Lefor & Gomella, 2001). Qualified personnel must be available to interpret the data.

Complications occur with insertion, use, and interpretation of data. The incidence of complication varies between 0.05% and 0.2%, but if the complication occurs, the mortality rate is 30% to 50%. With insertion, in addition to complications associated with central venous catheter insertion, complications include dysrhythmias, right bundle branch block, catheter knotting, and pulmonary artery injury or rupture. During use, complications include pulmonary infarction, endocardium or valve injury, cardiac perforation, and catheter balloon rupture (Lefor & Gomella, 2001). Misinterpretation of data may lead to inappropriate interventions, or lack of intervention, and worsening organ system dysfunction.

Placement may be difficult in patients with low cardiac output, pulmonary artery hypertension, dilated right ventricle or atrium, or tricuspid regurgitation. Placement site preference, in terms of ease of placement, is right internal jugular equal to left

Exhibit

14.2 Procedure for Guidewiring an Existing Central Venous Catheter

Supplies needed at bedside:

3 packages of 4×4 gauze mask and hat
1 sterile gown
1 suture removal kit
1 Agar plate or sterile container
Chlorhexidine solution or Chloraprep® applicator

1 sterile drape
2 pairs sterile gloves
1 scalpel
1 catheter insertion kit

1. An experienced practitioner must be present at the bedside to observe or perform the line change.
2. Put on mask and hat. Don gloves.
3. Remove occlusive dressing. Have the 3 lumens capped for ease in preparation. Don sterile gloves. Using chlorhexidine-soaked 4×4 gauze or a Chloraprep® applicator, scrub for 30 seconds minimum in multiple directions. Prep the insertion site surrounding 10-inch area of skin, the external portion of the triple-lumen catheter including the triangle, and the 3 lumens and their corresponding hubs and caps. Place a sterile drape under the catheter and hubs. Let the Chlorhexidine dry completely.
4. Remove the gloves, put on sterile gown and new sterile gloves.
5. With a sterile scalpel, remove the suture holding the catheter; note the centimeter marking at the skin.
6. Insert guidewire through the distal lumen. Optional— using the sterile scalpel, cut the distal lumen near the catheter hub, then thread guidewire.
7. Remove existing catheter over the guidewire; place on sterile tray.
8. Insert the new central venous catheter over the guidewire.
9. Aspirate blood from all ports with sterile syringe, flush with 2–3 cc normal saline. Reposition the catheter as necessary to enable easy aspiration of blood.
10. With sterile forceps, pick up the intra-cutaneous (ICS) segment and cut with sterile scissors both proximally and distally.
11. Exerting downward pressure, roll the ICS back and forth at least four times across the surface of the agar. Gently press the ICS into the agar without breaking its surface. Repeat the process with the catheter tip, placing it on the same agar plate. Alternatively, the catheter ICS and tip may be sent to the laboratory in a sterile specimen cup.
12. Place the clip around the triple-lumen catheter and suture the catheter in place.
13. Assist the nurse in completing a sterile, occlusive dressing including the time and date of insertion.
14. Document the procedure in the medical record.

subclavian, followed by right subclavian, left internal jugular, and lastly, femoral veins, right being easier than left in general.

After placement of an introducer sheath (see central venous catheter placement), sterility is maintained. Sterile gloves are changed and an additional sterile field is applied. The PAC is inspected for bends, kinks, and integrity of the balloon and thermister. The assistant attaches pressure tubing and calibrates the transducer and all lumens are flushed with saline. The pulmonary artery port remains open, and the catheter is moved up and down to show tracing on the monitor.

Place the transducer through a sterile sleeve and lock the proximal end without opening the sleeve. With the balloon deflated, advance the catheter through the introducer sheath to about 20 cm or just through the end of the introducer. Maintain the coil in the catheter in the orientation facilitating that it will "float" through the heart. Inflate the balloon with 1.5 ml of air and slowly advance the catheter while continuously monitoring the pressure tracing and EKG.

Always inflate the balloon when advancing, and deflate the balloon when withdrawing the catheter. Never continue advancing catheter if resistance is met. A central venous pressure tracing will occur until entrance into the right ventricle, which should occur at approximately 35–40 cm from the IJ or 30–40 cm from the subclavian position. A typical ventricle pressure curve will occur with high systolic pressure and low, near zero, diastolic pressure. Quickly advance through the right ventricle to prevent ectopy and catheter coiling.

Entrance into the pulmonary artery is noted by a step up of the diastolic pressure. This should occur within 10 cm after reaching the right ventricle, and if it does not, then the catheter is likely coiling. With the balloon deflated, pull the catheter back, then inflate the balloon and attempt again. When malignant dysrhythmias occur, deflate the balloon and pull the catheter back. After entrance into the pulmonary artery, slowly continue to advance the catheter until a wedged tracing is obtained, and then deflate the balloon and a pulmonary artery pressure should result.

Sometimes the wedge tracing persists and this indicates that the catheter is too deep and should be withdrawn. Reinflate the balloon and if the wedge occurs with less than 1.25 ml, the catheter is too deep and should be repositioned. The presence of mitral regurgitation may make interpretation of wedge tracing difficult, resulting in the placement being wedged in the pulmonary artery. Once the catheter is in appropriate position, then deflate the balloon. The balloon should be left deflated, except when actively checking a wedge pressure for 20 seconds or less to prevent pulmonary infarction and erosion of the pulmonary artery. A pulmonary artery tracing should be continuously observed unless the balloon is inflated. Advance the sleeve to cover the external portion of the catheter and secure with the locking mechanism. Obtain a chest x-ray to confirm placement in proximal branches of the pulmonary arteries, never more than 5 cm from midline. When changing a pulmonary artery catheter to a triple-lumen catheter, follow the central lines guidelines in Exhibit 14.3. For more information on pulmonary

Exhibit

14.3 Central Line Guidelines

Central access will be changed based on following criteria:
Inclusion: Dialysis catheters, triple- and quad-lumen catheters, axilla and femoral arterial lines
Routine guidewire of catheters has __not__ shown a decrease in infection.

Catheter change should occur with symptomatology:

1. Temperature > 38.4 or < 36
   a. Temperature previously stable
   b. Present catheter > 6 days old
   c. Patients on renal replacement therapy with significant change in temperature OR difficulty with blood flow of current catheter.

2. Follow white blood cell count (WBC) and consider all parameters. Isolated increase in WBC has not been correlated with line sepsis.
   a. Consider continuing increase in WBC, if previously stable WBC.
   b. Significant increase in WBC and clinical suspicion of line infection.

3. Patient being transferred out of unit
   a. Consider discontinuation of central access.
   b. Consider change to PICC line if central access still indicated.
   c. Consider need to guidewire catheter if > 14 days old.

Goal:
Discontinue all invasive therapies as soon as feasible.

artery catheter waveform interpretation and troubleshooting, visit the pulmonary artery catheter education project Website (http://www.pacep.org/; Lefor & Gomella, 2001).

Peripherally Inserted Central Line. The indications for a peripherally inserted central venous catheter (PICC) are similar to those for a central line, except a PICC is not an emergency catheter and is not used for rapid resuscitation. A PICC is generally indicated for long-term intravenous needs usually greater than 5–7 days. As technology has advanced, catheter materials have improved, resulting in a wider range of capabilities from long-term antibiotics use to patients requiring critical care. PICC lines now have a range from single lumen to triple lumen and can tolerate the pressure requirement for CT angiography. An alternative to a centrally placed PICC line is a midline catheter, which does not enter the central circulation and may be placed for short-term peripheral therapy. The insertion procedure for the PICC line and midline is the same. A midline is indicated when noncentral therapy is necessary. Total parenteral nutrition (TPN) for example, may be administered through a central PICC, whereas short-term antibiotics could be administered through a midline. Local site hematoma and venous thrombosis are more common than with other central lines, although the risk of either is generally low. Complication rates related to insertion with PICC lines are lower when compared with other catheters. Because the catheter is generally inserted in the basilic vein, the risk of pneumothorax or hemothorax is negligible. A central PICC may be left in place for an indefinite amount of time in the absence of complications. Evaluating a patient for PICC placement requires consideration of the underlying condition. Ultrasound technology should be used to evaluate venous status and availability. Patients who have renal failure may require dialysis access and may not be candidates for upper extremity PICC line placement. Veins above the level of the antecubital fossa should be used, including (in order of preference) the basilic, median cubital, and cephalic veins. The basilic vein is the largest, with the highest flow rate and the most direct course to the superior vena cava. Caution should be used when choosing the cephalic vein, because it will have an increased risk of thrombosis and malposition. Measurement for a PICC line would start from the planned insertion site to the axillary region proceeding to the right clavicular head then down to the third intercostal space. This should place the tip of the catheter in lower superior vena cava (SVC) near the entrance of the right atrium.

The patient should be placed supine with the arm abducted perpendicular to the trunk and the patient's chin turned toward the side of insertion; if this is not possible, then a position of comfort should be selected. Maximum sterile barrier precautions are used for all PICC line placements and may require placing a cap and mask on extubated patients. Prepare the skin by cleaning the area for 30 seconds and then apply sterile barriers as indicated under the subheading of safety. Once the skin cleansing has dried, place the tourniquet, and while using ultrasound guidance with a sterile cover on the ultrasound probe, place a small amount of injectable anesthetic at the proposed insertion site. Once the anesthetic has taken effect, use an appropriate-sized angiocatheter or echogenic needle, based on the wire size contained within the kit in the chosen peripheral vessel. When venous access has been obtained, generally with blood return in the catheter hub, place the guidewire through the intravenous angiocatheter, then remove the angiocatheter and release the tourniquet. The guidewire should slide in smoothly and never be forced.

Using a No. 11 blade scalpel, make a small incision near the guidewire while maintaining control of the guidewire. Prior to making the incision, additional injectable anesthetic may be required at the insertion site. Gently enter the vein with a two-part peel-away dilator, taking care to not rupture the vein or bend the guidewire. Using a sterile measuring tape, verify the catheter length measurement once a definitive insertion site has been obtained and cut the catheter again if indicated. Sterile gloves should be changed at this point if the catheter length needs to be adjusted or additional handling of the catheter is indicated. This should facilitate prevention of site infection and phlebitis. Remove the guidewire and the inner portion of the dilator leaving the peel-away sheath in place. Guide the PICC catheter through the peel-away sheath noting that most catheters have a stylet inside the catheter. Resistance may occur, but do not force the catheter. Reposition or rotate the patient's arm and reattempt passage of the catheter. Once the catheter has advanced past the shoulder into the subclavian vein, remove and take apart the peel-away sheath advancing the catheter completely. While maintaining sterile technique, use the ultrasound sound probe to review and study the internal jugular to evaluate for malposition, because this will be readily visible with the stylet in place. This can decrease the need for repeated radiographs for malposition. Once the catheter is in place, remove the stylet from within the catheter. Check each port for blood return and easy flushing. Securing of the catheter can be done using sutures (not recommended) or an adhesive securing device and place a sterile dressing as indicated in the safety subheading. Obtain a single-view chest radiograph to confirm placement in the superior vena cava. A midline catheter may be placed using the same technique, but with the catheter trimmed such that the final position will rest in the axillary vein, a noncentral location. A chest radiograph is not indicated for a midline catheter.

Complications of Central Venous Catheters

In general, the complications of inserting a central venous catheter are mechanical and infectious. Mechanical complications include pneumothorax, hemothorax, injury to the vein or accompanying artery, thoracic duct injury, wire, catheter or air embolus, venous thrombosis, thrombophlebitis, catheter malposition, and dysrhythmias. Infectious complications include superficial site infection, catheter colonization, and catheter-related or catheter-associated blood stream infections. Infectious complications are reduced with the use of antibiotic impregnated catheters, proper site care, minimizing line access/use, and consideration of site preference with femoral site infection generally greater than internal jugular site infection, which is higher than subclavian site infection (IHI, 2008). In addition, future infection is greatly influenced by maintenance of sterile technique during placement, care, and maintenance of the catheter, dressing, and insertion ports. All catheters should only be opened using strict sterile technique and ports should be entered only after a 15-second scrub of the hub to be accessed with chlorhexidine or alcohol and after allowing the hub to dry (CDC, 2008; IHI, 2008). See Exhibit 14.4 for central catheter guidelines regarding evaluation of infection. All emergently placed catheters should be replaced when the patient stabilizes. All central lines should be removed promptly when they are no longer absolutely needed to minimize infectious complications. This discussion of catheter needs should be addressed daily in rounds and during the evaluation of the patient (IHI, 2008). See Exhibit 14.4 for discontinuation of central venous catheters.

Arterial Line

There are several indications for arterial line placement. Patients with respiratory failure and severe hypoxemia may require frequent blood gases and therefore need access to the arterial system. There are patients who also require beat-to-beat monitoring of blood pressure because of hemodynamic instability that requires titration of vasoactive agents,

Exhibit

14.4 Procedure for Discontinuing a Central Venous Catheter

1. There is no need to routinely culture line segment if it is being discontinued, unless it is desired for confirmation of a diagnosis of line-related bacteremia.
2. If culture is to be formed, don sterile gloves, mask, and hat. Place a small sterile drape.
3. Place patient in Trendelenburg position if line is subclavian or jugular. Remove sutures, securing catheter with sterile scissors or scalpel. With a smooth, swift motion, remove catheter and apply pressure with sterile 4×4s. Place catheter on sterile drape if performing culture.
4. After ensuring hemostasis, apply an occlusive pressure dressing to site.
5. For culture, grasp intracutaneous segment with sterile forceps. Cut a 2–3cm segment and place on agar plate. Roll several times to ensure appropriate inoculation of plate. Only sterile instruments should come in contact with catheter ICS. Repeat the process with the catheter tip placing it on the same agar plate or send in sterile specimen cup.

either for hypotension or hypertension. In addition, patients who will not tolerate variation in blood pressure, for example those with aortic dissection or stroke, are candidates for continuous arterial pressure monitoring.

Contraindications include areas that have compromised circulation such as sites with known deficiencies. Examples include Raynaud syndrome and thromboangitis, including sites with infection or traumatic injury proximal to the area of insertion (Tegtmeyer, Brady, Lai, Hodo, & Braner, 2006). Complications include thrombosis or emboli, which leads to impaired perfusion and potentially limb-threatening ischemia. This risk is minimized with the use of a continuous flush system versus an intermittent flush system. Pseudoaneurysm and hematoma may also occur; this is minimized with adequate compression of the artery upon removal of the catheter. Local site infection or systemic infection occurs similar to central venous catheter; this risk is increased in the axillary or femoral position.

The radial artery is the preferred site followed by the axillary artery. The dorsalis pedis artery should be avoided in diabetic patients or those with peripheral vascular disease. The femoral site is preferred in emergency situations because of the speed and facility of placement, particularly when compressions are being performed. A femoral line should always be placed below the inguinal ligament; where it is compressible should complications arise and upon discontinuation. The brachial artery should be avoided and it is not considered an acceptable site because of the potential embolic and ischemic complications that may occur to the hand.

Radial. The radial artery is located 1–2 cm from the wrist between the bony head of the distal radius and the flexor carpi radialis tendon (Tegtmeyer et al., 2006). Before accessing the radial artery, perform the modified Allen test to confirm collateral flow to the hand from the ulnar artery. Should radial cannulation become complicated, request the patient to make a fist and compress the radial and ulnar arteries. Have the patient release the fist and at this point, release the pressure on the ulnar artery while maintaining pressure on the radial artery. The hand should flush red within 6 seconds if the ulnar artery and palmar arch are patent. The Allen test should determine if the palmer arch is apparently not intact and an alternative location should be considered. Ultrasound may also be used to verify patency, or to guide placement. Place a roll under the patient's wrist to dorsiflex the hand and place the arm on a firm surface, while remembering that excessive dorsiflexion can also cause constriction or occlusion of arterial flow. Consider applying tape to the hand to maintain position. Maintain sterile technique as described under the subheading of safety. Infiltrate a tiny wheal of lidocaine at the insertion site. At approximately 30 to 45-degree angle, insert a 20-gauge 1.5–2-inch angiocatheter or needle toward the pulse until pulsatile blood returns. When using an angiocatheter, flatten the angle to approximately 10 to 15 degrees, and advance the catheter over the needle while holding the needle steady. When using a self-contained over-the-wire catheter, once the artery is accessed, advance the wire followed by placing the catheter over the wire. For the Seldinger technique, once the artery is accessed, thread a guidewire through the needle then remove the needle and then thread a catheter over the wire and remove the wire. For arterial lines placed in the axilla or femoral site, generally a 12 cm catheter is used to lessen the risk of mechanical failure. Flush any entrained air from the system and attach the pressure tubing. Ensure that arterial pressure waveform is obtained. Suture the catheter to the skin and apply a sterile dressing.

For children or smaller patients, a through-and-through technique may be employed. Once the artery is accessed, the catheter and needle are intentionally advanced through the posterior wall of the artery until there is no longer blood return. Slowly withdraw the needle and catheter until a flash of blood occurs, then advance the catheter while removing the needle.

Generally, if the artery is unable to be cannulated, this may be secondary to arterial spasm or the angle of the needle is too acute to access the vessel. Blood return should readily be seen in the hub of the catheter; if this does not occur, the tip of the needle may not be completely in the artery (Tegtmeyer et al., 2006).

Dorsalis Pedis. Use the same technique as for radial artery catheter placement.

Axillary. In preparing the patient as described for all arterial access, abduct and externally rotate the arm. When attempting to access the vessel, enter the axilla as high into the axillary vein as feasible at a downward position while palpating the axillary pulse in the biceps groove. Insert a 20-gauge needle into the axillary artery while using ultrasound guidance if feasible. Place a guidewire through the needle when stabilizing the needle. Remove the needle and insert a 16-cm catheter over the guidewire. Remove the guidewire. Flush the catheter and attach the pressure tubing. Ensure appropriate pressure tracing and then secure the catheter to the skin with suture and apply a sterile dressing.

Femoral. The path of the femoral artery may be marked by Doppler signal or ultrasound may be used for guidance. At least 2 cm below the inguinal ligament, insert a 20-gauge needle at about a 45-degree angle. The skin insertion site should be far enough below the inguinal ligament that the actual arterial puncture occurs below the ligament. Once pulsatile blood return is established, place the guidewire through the needle. Remove the needle and thread a 16-cm catheter over the wire. Remove the wire. Flush and attach pressure tubing. Ensure appropriate pressure tracing. Secure the catheter with suture and place sterile dressing.

Thoracentesis

A thoracentesis may be performed to diagnose the etiology of a pleural effusion, for therapeutic removal of fluid, or for installation of a sclerosing compound for pleurodesis. Analysis of pleural fluid facilitates diagnostic information determining whether the fluid is transudate, which is a product of unbalanced hydrostatic forces, or exudate, which is a product of increased capillary permeability or lymphatic obstruction (Thomsen, DeLaPena, & Setnik, 2006). Some common causes of transudate include congestive heart failure, cirrhosis, nephrotic syndrome, and pulmonary embolism. Common causes of exudate include cancer, pneumonia, trauma, pulmonary embolism, rheumatoid arthritis, and systemic lupus erythematosus (SLE) (Thomsen et al., 2006). Complications of the procedure include pneumothorax, injury to intercostal vessels, hemothorax, visceral puncture, intrabdominal organ injury, air embolism, and bleeding in patients who are anticoagulated secondary to a hypercoagulable state. Vigilance when completing a thoracentesis in ventilated patients should be employed because positive pressure may alter the lungs' anatomy increasing the risk of pneumothorax. Caution must be employed and the approach must be altered with conditions that might elevate the hemidiaphragm including previous lung resection, presence of ascites, or morbid obesity.

Radiographs should be reviewed to evaluate for anatomic variations and size of effusion. When possible, the patient should be seated with legs draped over the edge of the bed, leaning forward, and resting the arms on a bedside table, thus moving the scapulae anterolaterally. When the seated position is not possible, place the patient supine with the arm raised over the head to open the intercostal spaces. Preprocedure imaging and the use of ultrasound technology may guide patient placement and catheter placement location. The level of effusion should also be evaluated by auscultation of diminished or absent breath sounds, dullness to percussion, and decreased or absence of fremitus (Thomsen, DeLaPena, & Setnik, 2006). When the patient is able to sit upright, the parietal pleura is at the level of the 10th vertebra, posteriorly. Staying above the 8th intercostal space should prevent injury to the abdominal viscera. Typically, the 7th intercostal space is used. This is found at the tip of the scapulae in the upright position. This is a sterile procedure, and the patient should be prepared and draped for any invasive procedure.

Initially, use a small 25-gauge needle and 1% lidocaine to anesthetize the skin. Then use a larger needle approximately 22 gauge to anesthetize the subcutaneous tissues and parietal pleura along the superior edge of the ribs. While slowly advancing the needle and injecting the anesthetic, aspirate on the plunger of the syringe to assure that the placement of the needle is not intravascular and to avoid injury to the nerves and vessels. As soon as fluid or air is aspirated, withdraw needle ~2 mm and inject lidocaine. This will inject the lidocaine under the sensitive parietal pleura. Injecting just above the superior edge of the inferior rib will avoid injury to the intercostal neurovascular bundle.

Mark the point on the needle where the depth of fluid or air is aspirated; this is how deep the thoracentesis needle will subsequently need to be inserted. A 20-gauge or larger angiocatheter, with a three-way stopcock attached to a syringe and IV tubing with collection bag is used to enter the pleural space. While aspirating, advance the needle slowly to the previously marked depth. Advance perpendicular to the chest wall to avoid injury to the intercostal neurovascular bundle. When fluid or air is encountered, advance the catheter over the needle into the pleural space and remove the needle. Attain a specimen of fluid (approximately 50 ml) to send for analysis, and then open the stopcock to the collection bag allowing the effusion to drain by gravity. Allowing the effusion to drain by gravity, as opposed to suction, is less painful and has lower risk of reexpansion pulmonary edema. Limiting the drainage to 1,500 ml or less on initial drainage will also diminish the risk of reexpansion injury (Thomsen, DeLaPena, & Setnik, 2006). When drainage is complete, remove the catheter and place an occlusive dressing. Obtain an upright chest radiograph to evaluate for adequacy of drainage and for presence of pneumothorax. Although pneumothorax is rare, if it occurs, the drainage system may be connected to an underwater seal pleurovac to resolve the issue. Send the recovered fluid for laboratory and microbiologic evaluation as indicated.

Chest Tube Thoracostomy

A chest tube thoracostomy may be used to drain traumatic or nontraumatic effusions. Traumatic effusions include pneumothorax, hemothorax, hemopneumothorax, or chylothorax. Nontraumatic effusions include spontaneous pneumothorax, reactive effusion, malignant effusion, empyema, and chylothorax. A chest tube should also be considered in a clinically unstable patient who is unable to be ventilated. Caution should be used in patients with previous thoracic surgery, and potential for complete adherence of the lung to the chest wall, clotting disorders, bullous emphysema, massive hemothorax, and hepatomegaly (Dev, Nascimiento, Simone, & Chien, 2007). Complications include inadequate drainage of the pleural space, bleeding, hemothorax, intercostal artery perforation, perforation of the visceral organs and major vascular structures, subcutaneous emphysema, introduction of bacteria leading to development of empyema, and significant pain if appropriate local anesthesia is not used (Dev et al., 2007).

Select a tube size based on the indication and patient's size. For a nontraumatic pneumothorax, use 18–24 French tube; for a simple effusion, use a 28–32 French tube. For an empyema, chylothorax, hemothorax, or traumatic pneumothorax, a large tube such as 32–40 French tube should be used because of the necessary coexistence of a hemothorax. The use of chest tubes with internal trocars should be avoided to prevent injury to the lungs, mediastinal structures, diaphragm, and abdominal viscera.

Position the patient supine at the edge of the bed, with the ipsilateral arm raised above the head if possible or with the shoulder abducted to expand the intercostal spaces. Use 2% Chlorhexidine solution and sterile gauze to vigorously cleanse the area. Then widely prep and drape the patient such that the anatomic landmarks remain within the sterile field. Most commonly, a chest tube is placed between the fourth and sixth intercostals space in the mid or anterior axillary line when draining a pneumothorax, and in the posterior axillary line for an effusion in a recumbent (bed-bound) patient. The anterior axillary line is marked by the lateral border of the pectoralis muscle. In men, the nipple overlies the fourth intercostal space; in women, the inframammary fold lies at the fifth intercostal space. At the anterior axillary line, the parietal pleural reflection is at the level of the eighth vertebra. A line above the horizontal level of the nipple is often referred to as the "triangle of safety," which is located at the anterior border of the latissimus dorsi, the lateral border of the pectoralis major muscle, and the apex just below the axilla (Dev et al., 2007). Staying above the sixth intercostal space should be low risk for injury to the spleen, liver, or diaphragm. Anesthetize the skin, subcutaneous tissue, and parietal pleura as described. Remember that the intercostal nerves travel from posterior, around the thorax to anterior; therefore, directing the local anesthetic somewhat laterally will provide excellent local anesthesia.

When preparing the thoracotomy tray, set up the chest tube by placing a Kelly clamp on the distal tip of the tube and the proximal end of the tube. Initially use a small 25-gauge needle and 1% lidocaine to anesthetize the skin. Then use a larger needle approximately 21–22 gauge, approximately 10–20 ml of 1% to 2% lidocaine solution to anesthetize the subcutaneous tissues, parietal pleura, and intercostal muscles along the superior edge of the ribs (Dev et al., 2007). While slowly advancing the needle and injecting the anesthetic, aspirate on the plunger of the syringe to assure that the placement of the needle is not intravascular and to avoid injury to the nerves and vessels. After anesthetizing, make a skin incision large enough to admit the index finger over the fifth or sixth rib approximately 1.5–2.0 cm in length parallel to the rib. Use a Kelly clamp to develop a tract that tunnels to the parietal pleura one rib space superior to the incision (Dev et al.). This minimizes air sucking into the chest cavity or pleural fluid leaking out and allows for the subcutaneous tissue to collapse over the hole in the pleura when the chest tube is removed.

Spread the chest wall muscles with a hemostat until the pleura is reached, dissecting through the subcutaneous tissue. With a closed hemostat and your index finger, explore the tract and puncture the pleura in a controlled motion at the superior edge of the rib to prevent injury to the neurovascular bundle. Digitally explore the tract to ensure that there is no lung adhesion to prevent injury, taking caution to prevent personal injury if the patient has rib fractures. Enlarge the hole by opening the hemostat to spread the muscle. A rush of air or fluid should occur. Using the distal tip of the chest tube with the Kelly clamp and the proximal clamp intact, guide the tube through the tract. Once the distal tip has passed through the incision and into the tract, unclamp the Kelly, remove, and then position the tube within the thoracic cavity. To drain an effusion, turn the hemostat posteriorly and toward the mediastinum or diaphragm to guide for posterior placement. The tube may be directed anteriorly and toward the lung apex for a spontaneous pneumothorax. Rotating the tube laterally while advancing the tube will help prevent ineffective placement within the fissure.

Secure the tube and close the incision around the tube with a zero silk suture using a mattress or uninterrupted sutures on both sides of the incision. Use the loose ends of the sutures to wrap around the tube so that when removing the tube, the wound may be closed preventing subsequent pneumothorax and approximating the skin (Dev et al., 2007). Attach the tube to an underwater seal closed drainage system at approximately 20 cm of water. The chest tube should not be reclamped to prevent reaccumulation of pneumothorax. Place an occlusive, absorptive dressing. Obtain an upright chest x-ray to verify tube placement and adequate treatment of the effusion or pneumothorax.

Chest Tube Removal

The removal of the chest tube should occur upon resolution of the reason for initial chest tube placement. A chest tube placed to resolve a pneumothorax should have a chest radiograph to verify that the pneumothorax is resolved. The chest tube should be placed to an underwater seal to assure the lung remains expanded without continuous suction. A repeat chest radiograph should indicate that the lung has remained expanded for approximately 12–24 hours postremoval of suction. A chest tube placed to drain pleural fluid may be removed after resolution of effusion and once drainage is less than 100–200 ml in a 24-hour period. The general expectation would also be that the patient's clinical status has improved.

Instruct the patient to breathe in to total lung capacity after a full expiration of air, or if mechanically ventilated, time the removal to end expiration and quickly remove the tube, pulling the end strings of the sutures together to tie and occlude the site with Vaseline gauze. Using tape and gauze, secure the dressing and evaluate the chest radiograph to ensure that a residual pneumothorax has not occurred.

Paracentesis

A paracentesis is performed to treat symptomatic ascites or to obtain diagnostic fluid. Patients with new onset ascites, should have a sample of the fluid obtained to aid in diagnosis of the etiology. Patients with known ascites, presenting with fever, abdominal pain, hypotension, or encephalopathy should have a sample of fluid evaluated to determine the etiology. A nasogastric tube should be inserted prior to paracentesis for suspected bowel obstruction and a foley should be inserted in the patient with urinary retention, or if feasible, the patient may urinate (Thomsen, Shaffer, et al., 2006). Paracentesis is relatively contraindicated in uncooperative patients and in those with uncorrected coagulopathy, acute surgical abdomen, intra-abdominal adhesions, distended bowel, infections at the puncture site, and in pregnancy. Complications include peritonitis, perforated viscus, hemorrhage, and persistent ascites leak. Oliguria, hypotension, electrolyte abnormalities, and precipitation of hepatic encephalopathy may occur as a result of fluid shifts. The use of ultrasound will enhance the success of the procedure and minimize secondary complications.

Place the patient supine and examine the abdomen to choose a site. Avoid surgical scars and other areas of possible adhesion formation to avoid potential bowel injury. Ultrasound or computed tomography (CT) may be beneficial in selecting a safe window. In the absence of previous abdominal incisions, the preferred site is midway between the umbilicus and anterior superior iliac spine, lateral to the rectus muscle. The needle insertion site is approximately 2 cm below the umbilicus in the midline or in the right or left lower quadrant, 2–4 cm medial and cephalad to the anterior superior iliac spine (Thomsen, Shaffer, White, & Setnik, 2006). Prep and drape the patient in sterile fashion as with any invasive procedure. Anesthetize the skin and subcutaneous tissue down to the level of the peritoneum with 1% lidocaine. Advance a 16–20 gauge angiocatheter while aspirating perpendicular to the abdominal wall then angled to create a "z" track. This helps to prevent persistent ascites leak. Some resistance may be met at the level of the fascia, and a "pop" may be felt when the fascia is traversed. When fluid is encountered, advance the catheter and remove the needle. Attach a stopcock and extension tubing to a closed collection system. Drain the desired amount of fluid while monitoring for hypotension; if a large volume is to be removed, send fluid for analysis. Remove the catheter and place a sterile dressing.

Intubation

In general, indications for endotracheal intubation are airway control and respiratory failure. Intubation may provide patency to an obstructed airway and allow for pulmonary toilet when the patient is unable to clear secretions. In the presence of poor mental status (i.e., Glasgow coma score less than 9) or absent gag or swallow reflex, intubation provides for airway control. Respiratory failure may be a result of hypoxia or inadequate ventilation. Patients may require intubation for acute hypoxia with an arterial partial pressure of oxygen (PaO_2) less than 60 with a fraction-inspired oxygen (FiO_2) more than 0.5, or an alveolar to arterial oxygen gradient greater than 300. Inadequate alveolar ventilation may occur as a result of medications or decreased level of consciousness. It may also result from increased work of breathing or minute ventilation during the bronchoscopy by adjusting mechanical ventilation. Maintaining control of the airway is the lifeline of the patient and decisions regarding the airway should be made with expertise and careful consideration. When in doubt, err on the side of intubation versus loss of an airway and potential patient complications such as cardiorespiratory arrest.

Endotracheal intubation is not a benign procedure, and complications may arise during placement of the tube and from actual endotracheal presence of the tube. During intubation, injury to the lips, teeth, vocal cords, larynx, and cervical spine may occur. Airway bleeding may make intubation difficult. Esophageal intubation, aspiration, arrhythmias, hypotension or hypertension, and laryngospasm are additional risks. Loss of an airway will result in anoxic brain injury. Post intubation, the patient is at risk for tube occlusion, tube migration, ventilator-associated pneumonia, sinusitis, tracheomalacia, and subglottic stenosis.

Experience with airway management should occur in a controlled setting with an individual with experience prior to attempting intubation in emergency conditions. In an emergency, the most experienced person should perform the intubation and always call for backup or additional assistance or a laryngeal mask airway (LMA) placed to maintain the airway. Stay calm and remember to be gentle. Most patients can be bag-mask ventilated until more experienced help arrives if an airway is difficult or unable to be attained. The goal is to avoid emergent intubation by intervening prior to respiratory collapse.

Intubation requires additional personnel to facilitate the procedure by preparing the patient and equipment. Prepare all the equipment necessary, assuring suction and oxygen are readily available. Pre oxygenate the patient using bag, valve, mask (BVM) ventilation. Insert the stylet into the endotracheal tube (ETT) and keep the endotracheal tube sterile until insertion. Pre medicate the patient with appropriate sedative, anxiolytic, narcotic, and/or paralytic medications. Rapid sequence intubation (RSI) may be indicated in cases of potential aspiration, difficult airway, and potential for anoxia. Avoid the use of paralytics unless an experienced provider is available, because the use of paralytics will eliminate the patient's ability to breathe spontaneously. This may be life threatening in the event of a difficult intubation.

Lift the patient's chin and lower jaw and, where able, extend the neck to form a straight path from the mouth to the trachea. Use jaw thrust in a patient with potential cervical spine injury or severe degenerate disease of the spine. Using a curved laryngoscope Macintosh blade, insert the blade on the right side of the mouth, sweeping the tongue to the left as the blade is brought to the midline. As the epiglottis is brought into view, advance the blade into the vallecula. Keep the wrist straight and lift forward and upward because this position prevents the use of the teeth as a fulcrum for leverage. This maneuver stretches the epiglottis upward and exposes the cords. When using a straight Miller blade, advance the blade posterior to the epiglottis and lift upward and forward to expose to cords. Advance the ETT 2–3 cm through the cords, then remove the stylet, and inflate the cuff. Confirm placement with a carbon dioxide detector, observation of chest wall excursion, auscultation over bilateral lung fields and epigastrium, and evaluation of tidal volume return. Obtain a chest x-ray to evaluate correct placement 2–3 cm above the carina.

Common causes of failed intubation include inadequate neck extension, inadequate sedation or muscle relaxation, obscuration of the glottis by the tongue, lack of familiarity with the anatomy, and misplacement of the laryngoscope blade particularly by inserting the laryngoscope too deep resulting in the lifting of the entire larynx such that only the esophagus is visible and accessible. When an attempt at intubation fails, provide BVM to return the patient's oxygen saturation to normal. Attempt again or seek more experienced assistance if available.

Cricothyroidotomy

Cricothyroidotomy is an emergency procedure to secure the airway and is performed when other options are not feasible, secondary to severe oromaxillary facial trauma, or when other options have failed, such as orotracheal or nasotracheal intubation. Even with this invasive approach, failure to secure the airway may still occur. Any bleeding may obscure vision and make completion of the cricothyroidotomy difficult. Injury to the airway, including cords, larynx and trachea, or esophagus may occur. Pneumomediastinum and pneumothorax are additional potential complications and long-term subglottic stenosis may result.

Patients that are able to be ventilated using a BVM should continue to receive oxygen with this intervention throughout the procedure. Unless contraindicated secondary to trauma, hyperextend the patient's neck. Even though a cricothyroidotomy is considered an emergency procedure, prep the skin with chlorhexidine 2% and drape the neck in sterile fashion if feasible. Locate the thyroid cartilage as the most prominent structure in the neck. Moving inferiorly, the cricothyroid membrane will be felt as a space between the thyroid cartilage and the cricoid cartilage. Anesthetize the skin if the patient is conscious and time permits.

Stabilize the trachea with the nondominant hand using the left thumb and middle finger and using the index finger to palpate the thyroid cartilage. Move the index finger down until the cricoid cartilage is palpated and then make a midline, longitudinal 2.5 cm skin incision centered over the cricothyroid membrane; carry the incision through the subcutaneous tissue. An initial transverse incision may incur more bleeding, obscuring visualization and potential injury to the laryngeal nerves (Hsiao & Pacheco-Fowler, 2008). Next, identify the cricothyroid membrane and make a transverse incision in the membrane approximately 1.3 cm in depth to minimize the risk of esophageal perforation (Hsiao & Pacheco-Fowler, 2008). Using a clamp or the scalpel handle, spread the membrane longitudinally to hold the airway open.

Insert an appropriately sized endotracheal tube or tracheostomy tube, usually a 4.0–6.0 mm in an adult, into the trachea while directing the tube caudally. Never let go of the tube until it is secured to prevent accidental dislodgement of the tube and loss of the airway. Inflate the cuff and then connect the bag valve to the endotracheal tube and ventilate with 100% oxygen. Auscultate breath sounds, observe chest rise, and utilize the carbon dioxide detector to confirm placement. Secure tube with suture and tracheostomy ties or tape and place a gauze dressing around the tube. Obtain a chest x-ray to confirm placement. Because of the risk of subglottic stenosis, a cricothyroidotomy will need to be revised to a formal tracheostomy when the patient is stable, usually within 24–72 hours (Hsiao & Pacheco-Fowler, 2008).

In patients under 12 years of age, needle cricothyroidotomy should be the only form of cricothyroidotomy to be performed because of the relatively high risk of subglottic stenosis. Stabilize the trachea with the nondominant hand. Insert a 12- or 14-gauge angiocatheter with syringe attached through the cricothyroid membrane perpendicular to the trachea. When air is aspirated, advance the catheter, direct it caudally and remove the needle. Attach an oxygen source via extension tubing or the bag valve unit. This is a temporary procedure (about 45 min), allowing the patient to be oxygenated until he or she is stable to be transported to a higher level of care.

Bronchoscopy

Bronchoscopy is most commonly used for therapeutic or diagnostic aspiration of the tracheobronchial tree. Bronchoscopy is used to obtain specimens for evaluation and culture in cases of suspected lower respiratory tract infection, to treat major atelectasis resulting from bronchial plugging, and to evaluate and possibly treat hemoptysis. Specifically, trained practitioners may use bronchoscopy for endobronchial or transbronchial biopsies, retrieval of foreign bodies, and to guide intubation for difficult airways. Complications include hypoxia, hypercapnea, barotrauma, hypertension, hypotension, dysrhythmias, aspiration, introduction of infection, hemorrhage, laryngospasm, and elevated intracranial pressure. Contraindications to bronchoscopy in intubated patients include cardiovascular instability despite pharmacologic intervention, hypoxemia despite fraction of inspired oxygen of 100% and severe acid/base or electrolyte abnormalities. Even experienced providers should not perform bronchoscopy in an extubated patient with respiratory distress and hypoxemia, because despite supplemental oxygen by mask, this precludes cooperation or the ability to protect the airway. These patients should be intubated prior to proceeding with bronchoscopy.

While preparing for the procedure, increase the supplemental oxygen to 100%. Hypoxia occurs during bronchoscopy even in healthy patients. Select a bronchoscope size based on size of the endotracheal tube, which will allow for ventilation, typically the inner diameter of the ETT tube must be 2.5 mm larger than the bronchoscope. A pediatric bronchoscope (4 mm) may be used for smaller endotracheal tubes; however, the suctioning ability is limited. A 5 mm scope can be used through an 8 mm or 9 mm endotracheal tube. The patient should be provided with equivalent minute ventilation during the bronchoscopy by adjusting mechanical ventilation. Decrease the flow rate to minimize peak pressures; increase the respiratory rate and tidal volume to compensate for air leak. An assistant should be available to monitor the minute ventilation, pulse oximetry, and vital signs. Provide appropriate analgesia and sedation. Paralytics may be used in intubated patients to protect the patient and the bronchoscope. Make sure to increase the ventilator settings to maximize ventilation until the paralytic agent has reversed. In extubated patients, 1% lidocaine may be applied topically to the airway and used alternatively to control cough.

Place a sterile drape on the patient's chest and wear sterile gloves, hat, and mask with eye protection, to minimize introduction of organisms into the patient's bronchial tree and to protect the provider from the spray of secretions. Place a three-way adapter between the endotracheal tube and ventilator. The port through which the bronchoscope is passed has a rubber diaphragm to minimize air leakage. Have an assistant hold the endotracheal tube to prevent displacement. Lubricate the bronchoscope with water soluble lubricant. Place the bronchoscope through the adaptor and continue through the endotracheal tube. Aspirate upper airway secretions, keeping the suction port off the mucosa. Use the carina and membranous portion of the trachea for orientation. Systematically evaluate the right middle, right lower, right upper, left lower, left upper lobes, and lingula down to the level of the subsegmental bronchi. Make sure not to push the bronchoscope against the mucosa to avoid injury. Aspirate mucus plugs and have the assistant place a collection trap in line with the suction port. Gently wedge the bronchoscope into segmental or subsegmental bronchus in the area of infiltrate seen on chest x-ray. When diffuse infiltrates are seen on radiograph, use a nondependent area like the lingula or right middle lobe to obtain washings. Have the assistant instill 20 ml aliquots of sterile saline to a total of 100 ml. Aspirate each aliquot before installation of the next. Aliquots can be collected and pooled as one specimen. At least 40% of the lavage fluid must be recovered for the sample to be considered adequate. Send the specimen for cell counts, special stains, and cultures (bacterial, mycobacterial, fungal, viral) as indicated.

In cases of major atelectasis with physiologic compromise, bronchoscopy is therapeutic only if the atelectasis is the result of bronchial obstruction. Evaluate the chest radiograph to confirm proper placement of the endotracheal tube. Auscultate breath sounds, and if breath sounds are present over the affected area, the atelectasis is unlikely to be post obstructive and the bronchoscopy will not be therapeutic. In this instance or if physiologic compromise is not present, chest physiotherapy or increasing positive end expiratory pressure (PEEP) are preferred treatments.

Hemoptysis in intubated patients is usually the result of airway trauma from the end of the endotracheal or tracheostomy tube or from suctioning. Hemoptysis resulting from endobronchial lesions, such as tumors, may be treated topically. Occasionally, pulmonary embolus results in hemoptysis, but lesions will not be seen on bronchoscopy. Pneumonia may produce hemoptysis, especially in coagulopathic patients. Rarely, a tracheostomy may erode into the innominate artery resulting in massive hemoptysis, although this may be preceded by a less dramatic, herald bleed. Bleeding from a tracheoinnominate fistula is a surgical emergency, and bronchoscopy is not indicated. The source of a herald bleed is unlikely to be seen by bronchoscopy. Bronchoscopic treatment of hemoptysis includes installation of epinephrine (3–5 ml of 1:10,000 solution) and topical application of thrombin. When bleeding is not controlled with topical measures, a more experienced practitioner may place a balloon-tipped catheter to tamponade the bleeding. In addition, arteriography with embolization or surgical intervention may be indicated.

Percutaneous Tracheostomy

Patients who are anticipated to require long-term airway control are generally considered for tracheostomy. The percutaneous option is available when the surface anatomy is readily identifiable and normal. This is not an emergency airway option. In addition, a percutaneous tracheostomy is not safe in patients who are unable to tolerate bronchoscopy or who require high levels of ventilator support, especially high positive end-expiratory pressure (PEEP). Complications include inadvertent loss of the airway, injury to the trachea, injury to the esophagus, malposition of the tracheostomy tube (i.e., pretracheal space). Long-term complications include tracheoesophageal fistula, tracheoinnominate fistula, tracheal stenosis, and tracheal malacia.

This procedure requires two operators: one to perform the bronchoscopy and one to perform the tracheostomy. Place the patient supine and extend the neck if possible.

Provide the patient with adequate analgesia, sedation, and paralytic. Adjust the ventilator settings to allow adequate oxygenation and ventilation during the procedure. Perform bronchoscopy to identify anatomic landmarks and the anterior portion of the trachea. With the bronchoscope positioned at the end of the endotracheal tube, withdraw the endotracheal tube to the level of the cricothyroid membrane. Take extreme caution not to extubate the patient, and maintain the bronchoscope at the end of the endotracheal tube to allow visualization of the entire trachea. This enables the bronchoscopist to monitor tracheal dilation and subsequent tracheal dilation.

Prep the neck and widely drape as for any invasive procedure. Confirm that the cuff of the tracheostomy tube is functional prior to the start of the procedure. Anesthetize the skin with 1% lidocaine because inadvertent injection into the thyroid leads to rapid absorption of the lidocaine and epinephrine and can lead to hypertension and tachycardia. Identify the larynx and cricoid cartilage, moving caudally, count the tracheal rings. The tracheostomy should be placed between the first and second or second and third tracheal rings. Make a midline, vertical skin incision centered over the second and third tracheal rings just large enough to accommodate the tracheostomy tube. The midline is avascular and less bleeding should be encountered than with a horizontal incision, although a small horizontal incision may be used and is generally more aesthetic.

Use the nondominant hand to stabilize the trachea. Slowly advance the angiocatheter perpendicular to the trachea while aspirating until air returns indicating the position within the airway. Avoid puncture of the posterior, membranous portion of the trachea to avoid injury to the esophagus. The bronchoscopist should confirm if placement is midline and at the correct tracheal ring level also to monitor for potential injury to the membranous portion of the trachea. Advance the angiocatheter caudally and remove the needle. Insert the guidewire through the catheter and remove the catheter. Inserting the wire too deep can cause injury to the lung. From this point, the guidewire is the only thing securing the path to the trachea. Do not remove the wire until final tracheostomy placement is confirmed within the airway. Dilate the subcutaneous tissue and trachea with the smallest dilator placed over the wire, utilizing the Seldinger technique.

Depending on the brand of the kit used, use sequential dilators or tapered dilator to enlarge the tract and hole in the trachea to the size of the tracheostomy tube. While advancing the dilator, maintain its position perpendicular to the trachea following the curve of the dilator. Use only moderate force to prevent injury to the trachea, and if the dilator does not pass easily, return to a smaller dilator. The skin incision may need to be enlarged if the skin creates resistance. Load the tracheostomy tube on the appropriate sized dilator and insert the tracheostomy over the guidewire and into the trachea. Remove the dilator and the wire, never releasing the tracheostomy until it is secured to prevent accidental dislodgement of the tube and resultant loss of the airway. Place the bronchoscope through the tracheostomy to visualize the carina, confirming proper position within the airway. Remove the bronchoscope, inflate the cuff, insert the inner cannula, and attach the ventilator. Confirm placement with carbon dioxide detector, observation of chest rise, auscultation of breath sounds, and return of appropriate tidal volume via the ventilator. Secure the tracheostomy with sutures and tracheostomy ties. Now it is acceptable to remove the endotracheal tube. Obtain a chest x-ray to confirm placement and evaluate for complications.

Recommended References

Abrams, J., Druck, P., & Cerra, F. (Eds.). (2005). *Surgical critical care* (2nd ed.). Taylor & Francis Group: Boca Raton.

Berry, S., et al. (Eds.). (1997). *The Mont Reid surgical handbook,* (4th ed.). Mosby, St. Louis.

Civetta, J., Taylor, R., & Kirby, R. (Eds.). (1997). *Critical Care* (3rd ed.), Lippincott-Raven, Philadelphia.

Nyhus, L., Baker, R., & Fischer, J. (Eds.). (1997). *Mastery of surgery* (3rd ed.). Boston: Little, Brown and Company.

To delve further into the procedures and topics discussed throughout this text, please feel free to access complementary procedural videos from Cook Medical at http://www.cookmedical .com/cc/educationResource.do?id=Educational_Video

References

Agur, A., & Lee, M. (1999). *Grant's atlas of anatomy,* (10th ed.). Lippincott Williams & Wilkins, Philadelphia.

Bach, A., Stubbig, K., & Geiss, H. H. (1992). Infectious risk of replacing venous catheters by the guidewire technique. *Zentralbl Hyg Umweltmed, 193*(2), 150–159.

Berenholtz, S. M., Pronovost, P. J., Lipsett P. A., Hobson, D., Earsing, K., Farley, J. E., et al. (2004). Eliminating catheter-related bloodstream infections in the intensive care unit. *Critical Care Medicine, 32,* 2014–2020.

Boyce, J. M., Pittet, D. (2002). Guidelines for hand hygiene in health care settings: Recommendations of the Healthcare Infection Control Practices Advisory Committee and the HICPAC/SHEA/APIC/IDSA Hand Hygiene Task Force *MMWR Recommendations and reports, 51*(RR16), 1–44.

Braner, D. A., Lai, S., Erman, S., & Tegtmeyer, K. (2007). Central venous catheter-subclavian vein. *New England Journal of Medicine, 357,* e26. Retrieved August 2008, from http://content.nejm.org/misc/videos .shtml?ssource=recentVideos

Center for Disease Control [CDC], (2008). Retrieved August, 2008 from http://www.cdc.gov/ounceofprevention/

Dev, S. P., Nascimiento, B., Simone, C., & Chien, V. (2007). Chest-tube insertion. *New England Journal of Medicine, 357,* e15. Retrieved August 2008, from http://content.nejm.org/misc/videos.shtml ?ssource=recentVideos

Graham, A. S., Ozment, C., Tegtmeyer, K., Lai, S., & Braner, D. (2007). Central venous catheterization. *New England Journal of Medicine, 356,* e21. Retrieved August 2008, from http://content.nejm.org/misc/videos .shtml?ssource=recentVideos

Hsiao, J., & Pacheco-Fowler, V. (2008). Cricothyroidotomy. *New England Journal of Medicine, 358,* e25. Retrieved August, 2008, from http:// content.nejm.org/misc/videos.shtml?ssource=recentVideos

Institute for Health Improvement (IHI). (2008). Retrieved August, 2008, from http://www.ihi.org/IHI/Topics/CriticalCare/IntensiveCare/ Measures/CentralLineBundleComplianceRate.htm

Kirkpatrick, A., Blaivas, M., Sustic, A., Chun, R., Beaulieu, Y., & Breitkreutz, R. (2008). Focused application of ultrasound in critical care medicine. *Critical Care Medicine, 36*(2). 654–655.

Lefor, A., & Gomella, L. (Eds.). (2001). *The pulmonary artery catheter education project.* Retrieved from http://www.pacep.org/ Surgery on call (3rd ed.). McGraw Hill, New York.

Maki, D. G., Mermel, L. A., Kluger, D., Narans, L., Knasinski, V., Parenteau, S., et al. (2000). The efficacy of a chlorhexidine-impregnated sponge (Biopatch) for the prevention of intravascular catheter-related infection—A prospective, randomized, controlled, multicenter study. *Abstract Interscience Conference on Antimicrobial Agents and Chemotherapy, 40,* 422.

Tegtmeyer, K., Brady, G., Lai, S., Hodo, R., & Braner, D. (2006). Placement of an arterial line. *New England Journal of Medicine, 354,* e13. Retrieved August 2008, from http://content.nejm.org/misc/videos .shtml?ssource=recentVideos

Thomsen, T. W., DeLa Pena, J., & Setnik, G. S. (2006). Thoracentesis. *New England Journal of Medicine, 355,* e16. Retrieved August 2008, from http://content.nejm.org/misc/videos.shtml?ssource=recentVideos

Thomsen, T. W., Shaffer, R. W., White, B., & Setnik, G. S. (2006). Paracentesis. *New England Journal of Medicine, 355,* e21. Retrieved August 2008, from http://content.nejm.org/misc/videos.shtml ?ssource=recentVideos

Tsui, J. Y., Collins, A. B., White, D. W., Lai, J., & Tabas, J. (2008). Placement of femoral venous catheter. *New England Journal of Medicine, 358,* e30. Retrieved August 2008, from http://content.nejm.org/misc/videos.shtml?ssource=recentVideos

World Health Organization (WHO). (2007). Improved central line care to prevent health care-associated infections.

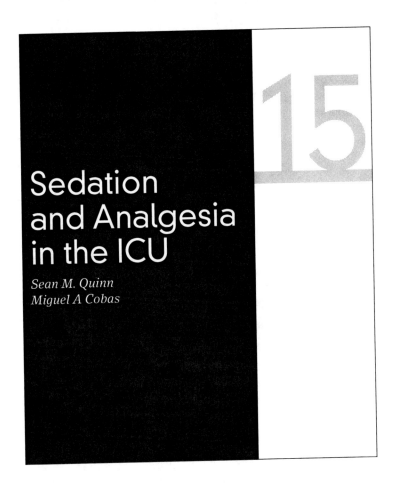

Sedation and Analgesia in the ICU

Sean M. Quinn
Miguel A Cobas

Introduction

In critically ill patients, adequate sedation and analgesia increase patient comfort, reduce the stress response as related to inflammation and trauma, facilitate diagnostic and therapeutic procedures, and enable patients to interact with the environment while being able to endure medical and nursing interventions. Achieving an appropriate level may have a beneficial impact in decreasing morbidity by reducing pulmonary complications and preventing agitation. Although there is no clear consensus on the best evaluation and management of sedation and analgesia in critically ill patients, numerous tools have been devised to help guide clinicians. Regular evaluations of patient sedation and pain requirements are important when setting individual patient-specific goals. This may be guided by standardized protocols to facilitate a balanced sedation and analgesia plan while reducing duration of mechanical ventilation, length of time in the intensive care unit (ICU) setting, and subsequent cost. In this chapter, we address issues pertinent to sedation and analgesia for the ACNP.

Sedation in the ICU

Introduction

Providing adequate sedation for the critically ill patient can be challenging because it is necessary to provide a sufficient level of patient comfort while avoiding the risk of oversedation and its associated complications. Sedation reduces the stress response, provides anxiolysis, controls agitation, aids in mechanical ventilation, provides amnesia during neuromuscular blockade, and helps to facilitate nursing care (Ostermann, Keenan, Seiferling, & Sibbald, 2000; Weissman, 2005). The optimal level of sedation provides relief of anxiety and agitation based on specific goals while still allowing for the patient to comfortably interact with the environment. The sedation goal is patient specific to achieve defined targets, for example, management of a difficult airway or improvement in mechanical ventilation. However, the common principle is to target sedation to a level appropriate for that individual patient and to avoid the excessive use of sedation medications. Because of the lack of analgesic properties of most sedatives, it is necessary to treat pain separately while achieving an adequate level of sedation.

Sedation Therapy

The indications for the use of sedative agents are generally multifactorial and are not well defined. The causes of anxiety in critically ill patients may be caused by the inability to communicate in an environment with continuous noise secondary to monitoring alarms, personnel, continuous ambient lighting, and excessive stimulation from frequent vital signs, motion, and inadequate analgesia (Jacobi et al., 2002). Anxiety, agitation, and delirium are commonly seen in up to 85% of critically ill patients when using validated sedation scales (Ely et al., 2001). Assurance, communication, and information may facilitate calming a patient as an initial intervention, but pharmacological agents are more frequently needed to relieve anxiety in the ICU setting.

Benzodiazepines. The most common intravenous benzodiazepines used in the ICU setting include midazolam, lorazepam, and diazepam, which are an accepted standard of care because of their relative safety, anterograde amnesia, and relative opioid-sparing effects. Medications in this category are lipid-soluble to some degree and are hepatically metabolized and renally excreted. Benzodiazepines generally do not cause respiratory depression in healthy individuals, although an exaggerated response is seen in patients with respiratory, cardiac, or hepatic insufficiency or in the elderly caused by decreased metabolism of benzodiazepines (Barr, Zomorodi, Bertaccini, Shafer, & Geller, 2001). Benzodiazepines differ in their potency, onset of action (generally 2–5 minutes), and duration of action caused by half-life, uptake, distribution, and metabolism. Patient-specific factors such as age, comorbidities, prior alcohol, and drug use affect intensity and duration of action and require individual titration of benzodiazepines.

Midazolam is the benzodiazepine of choice for short-term sedation because of its fast onset, short duration of action, and high lipid solubility. Midazolam is usually administered as a continuous infusion and may generate prolonged sedation because of drug and active metabolite (hydroxymidazolam) accumulation (Fragen, 1997). Lorazepam has the slowest onset of action of the intravenous benzodiazepines, but also has the less potential for drug interactions because of its metabolism via glucuronidation. Although this makes lorazepam a poor drug for initial treatment of agitation, the long half-life is ideal for the continuation of sedation via either intermittent bolus or continuous infusion (Watling, Johnson, & Yanos, 1996). Because of the long elimination timeframe and half-life of 12–15 hours, lorazepam is not a recommended drug when rapid awakening is desired but is more appropriate for long-term ventilated patients.

Diazepam provides rapid onset of sedation and awakening after single dose but produces prolonged sedation after repeated doses because of the accumulation of active metabolites. Although this had been acceptable for providing long-term sedation, diazepam is the least favorable benzodiazepine in the ICU. Also, preparations of lorazepam and diazepam contain the solvents polyethylene glycol and propylene glycol, which have been implicated in reversible acute tubular necrosis and lactic acidosis when used in high doses.

Propofol. Propofol is a unique, rapid-acting sedative-hypnotic drug that is used for induction and maintenance of general anesthesia and for short-term sedation for mechanically ventilated patients in the ICU. Propofol is an extremely lipophilic drug and has rapid onset of action while producing similar degrees of amnesia as benzodiazepines without the analgesic properties. Propofol is redistributed and metabolized by the hepatic conjugation and allows for awakening shortly after discontinuation of the infusion. Propofol is ideal for use during invasive procedures and for sedation <72 hours, although recent evidence suggests that it may also be useful and cost-effective for longer time periods in selected patients (Carson et al., 2006). Propofol is also appropriate for patients with neurological injury, as it will allow for frequent and accurate neurological examinations. Because of the potential for significant respiratory depression, propofol should only be used in mechanically ventilated patients and in controlled airway situations for short procedures. Propofol has a potential to cause profound hypotension, which is more common in patients with hypovolemia, heart failure, and the elderly and is relatively contraindicated in severe hypovolemia or hemorrhagic shock (McKeage & Perry, 2003). Because propofol is suspended in a lipid emulsion and contains 1.1 kcal/ml, these calories should be counted toward the patient's daily nutrition and fat intake. This formulation is also known to cause a transient elevation in triglyceride levels in up to 10% of patients and must be frequently monitored during prolonged infusions. Anaphylactoid reactions to propofol are infrequent but can be severe (Riker & Fraser, 2005). Strict sterile technique must be adhered to as the lipid emulsion promotes bacterial growth and improper technique has been previously attributed to postsurgical infection complications (Bennett, et al., 1995). Propofol infusion syndrome is rare but lethal event that may be seen with high-dose, prolonged infusions characterized by acute onset heart failure, bradycardia, lactic acidosis, hyperlipidemia, and rhabdomyolysis (Kang, 2002).

Dexmedetomidine. Dexmedetomidine is a relatively new, highly selective, centrally acting alpha 2-adrenergic agonist that produces sedation, anxiolysis, mild analgesia, and sympatholysis. The sedation produced with dexmedetomidine allows for patients to be quickly awakened and has minimal effect on respiratory depression. Patients receiving dexmedetomidine infusions are easily aroused, appear calm and comfortable, and will often return to a hypnotic state if not stimulated. Because of the short half-life, dexmedetomidine is usually given by continuous infusion and may be used in nonmechanically ventilated patients or noninvasive positive-pressure ventilation. The unique properties of this drug make it especially useful in patients who are at risk for respiratory depression, such as patients with sleep apnea, patients with chronic obstructive lung disease, and patients with severe alcohol withdrawal. Common adverse reactions to this drug include hypotension and bradycardia, which is usually seen in the elderly and in those with advanced heart block. Currently, dexmedetomidine is approved for <24 hours; however, new data suggests that it may be continued for 5 days and may decrease delirium in critically ill patients (Pandharipande et al., 2007).

Assessment of Sedation

Approximately 80% of all patients in the ICU receive some method of pharmacological sedation (Walder, Frick, Gueg-ueniat, Diby, & Romand, 2002). With the majority of patients receiving sedation, it is surprising that just over half of patients are continually monitored with sedation scales and in even fewer facilities that protocols exist to reach sedation goals to predetermined endpoints. An ideal sedation scale should be easy to use, should quantify behavior, should provide an accurate description of sedation or agitation within a defined category, should aid to guide sedation therapy, and should be validated in an ICU population.

There are more than 20 different scales published, but there is not a single scale that exists that has been accepted as a golden standard (De Jonghe et al., 2000). The Riker Sedation–Agitation Scale categorizes a patient's behavior into seven predetermined groups and was the first scale to be proven effective and validated in critically ill patients

(Riker, Picard, & Fraser, 1999). Today, the most common tools used in the ICU to quantify sedation are the Ramsay Scale, which describes three levels of awake states and three levels of asleep states, and the Richmond Agitation–Sedation Scale (RASS), which defines a numerical score from varying levels of sedation and agitation on a 10-level scale. The RASS has been the most validated scale and arguably, may be the scale of choice to use (Ely et al., 2003).

However, the specific scale chosen appears less important than having a system in place to monitor sedation. An institution-accepted sedation scale will place focus on patient safety and comfort, provide better communication among caregivers, and improve the consistency of medication administration and quality of sedation. Sedation scales facilitate and evaluate trends in patient behavior that may reveal a change in the underlying condition, which allows more precise medication titration. Sedation scales also decrease overall sedative and analgesic drugs while decreasing length of time on mechanical ventilation or need for vasopressor support (Sessler & Varney, 2008).

The value of implementing a sedation and pain scale alone to guide management has also been shown not only to decrease agitation and pain events, but also to dramatically reduce both duration of mechanical ventilation and the rate of nosocomial infection (Chanques et al., 2006). An inherent problem with any scale is the issue of subjectivity of the scoring systems, interindividual rating variability, and lack of continuity of measurements. New objective methods including tracking of heart rate variability, lower esophageal contractility, auditory, and somatosensory have evoked potentials and processed electroencephalography have been suggested, but none have been validated in the ICU.

Sedative Selection

An ideal sedative agent would have rapid onset of action, would be effective at providing adequate sedation, would allow rapid recovery after discontinuation, would be easy to administer, would lack drug accumulation, would have few adverse effects, would interact minimally with other drugs, and would be inexpensive. There is much controversy and conflicting data that exists in the recent literature about the most appropriate selection of sedating agents. The algorithm suggested by the Society of Critical Care Medicine in the last published clinical practice guidelines is a good starting point for the selection of pharmacological agents (Jacobi et al., 2002). The guidelines recommend using sedation scales, set defined treatment goals, and suggest pharmacological agents for use after pain and delirium have been addressed. Midazolam is the preferred drug agent for agitation because of its rapid onset of action. For ongoing sedation, either lorazepam or propofol is suggested as initial therapy. However, except for neurosurgery patients, it is recommended that propofol be converted to lorazepam after 72 hours. Although this is a rational approach to the utilization of sedatives, new data on propofol and dexmedetomidine challenge this view when clinical outcomes are studied.

The effectiveness of both midazolam and propofol are very similar, and a quantitative systemic review of 27 trials failed to show superiority of either drug (Walder, Elia, Henzi, Romand, & Tramèr, 2001). When propofol was compared with intermittent lorazepam for sedation, patients who receive propofol had fewer mechanically ventilated days; however, there was no difference in mortality between groups (Carson et al., 2006). A combination of midazolam–propofol also had no improvement in length of time to wean patients following cardiac surgery (Walder, Borgeat, Suter, & Romand, 2002). In the decision-making process, although the use of dexmedetomidine for sedation in the ICU has been limited to 24 hours previously, recent research has shown efficacy and safety data that extends the use of dexmedetomidine for 5 days and a decreased incidence of delirium when compared to lorazepam, especially in an elderly population (Pandharipande et al., 2007).

Analgesia in the ICU

Introduction

In addition to providing adequate sedation for patients in ICU, it is also imperative to recognize pain as an individual parameter, assess, evaluate, and intervene appropriately to resolve pain. Although the potential of providing excessive amounts of analgesics is always possible, if adequately assessed, the risk of this can be minimized. Most patients receive some form of parenteral analgesic while in the ICU, and over half of patients discharged from the ICU recall pain as their worst experience (Dasta, Fuhrman, & McCandles, 1994).

Analgesics may also have some sedating properties in moderate to high doses, whereas some sedatives will have opioid-sparing effects. However, sedation and analgesia should be seen as two parallel concepts in the ICU and appropriate pharmacologic agents should be chosen to treat each process. Additionally, the appropriate dose of opioid must be administered and titrated to patient response but not to a specific dose or limit. The effective management of pain in the ICU also depends on detecting and quantifying the intensity of pain, optimizing nonpharmacologic measures, and reassessing the daily goals of analgesia.

Treatment of Pain

Although the pain experienced by patients in the ICU originates from many sources, the treatment modalities are in general fairly similar. The first step in the assessment and treatment of pain involves ruling out potentially reversible or treatable etiologies of pain (i.e., surgical intervention) and then targeting the irreversible etiologies of pain. Regional anesthetic techniques (neuraxial or peripheral nerve blocks) should be considered in appropriate patients and can adequately treat pain with local anesthetic and/or opioids while limiting the systemic effects of these agents. These techniques usually achieve patient analgesia goals, some may also benefit by limiting parenteral opioids and allowing for a more rapid postoperative recovery. This idea can be exemplified by the placement and use of a thoracic epidural catheter in a patient after thoracotomy, which allows for excellent pain relief while minimizing splinting and pulmonary complications. However, the large majority of ICU patients will require parenteral opioids as the necessary means of achieving analgesia.

Opiates

Opiates are synthetic substances that produce their effects by stimulating discreet receptors in the central nervous system. Opiates relieve pain and the sensibility to noxious stimuli while also producing sedation and euphoria. Opiates may produce a change in sensorium, especially the more soluble forms such as morphine and hydromorphone (Pasternak, 1993). However, it is important to remember that opioids do not produce amnesia. The risks of opiates include respiratory depression, pruritis, ileus, urinary retention, histamine release, and the potential for accumulation of active or neurotoxic metabolites. Patients may be given parenteral opiates either as *pro re nata* (prn) boluses, intermittent scheduled boluses, continuous infusion, or via patient-controlled analgesia (PCA) through infusion pump. PCA administration of opioids has been associated with improved satisfaction, more effective analgesia, and decreased side effects when compared to intermittent administration of opioids in an appropriate patient population (Liu, Carpenter, & Neal, 1995).

Morphine. Morphine is the most common opioid used in both postoperative and critically ill patients. Typical onset of action is 10–20 minutes, duration is between 2–4 hours, and is hepatically metabolized and renally excreted. Although the relatively long duration of action can be advantageous to limit dosing intervals, morphine has several active metabolites that can potentially accumulate, especially in higher doses and in patients with renal insufficiency. Morphine-6-glucuronide is a more potent active drug, and morphine-3-glucuronide can produce central nervous system excitation with seizures and myoclonus (Smith, 2000). Morphine also causes histamine release and may lead to vasodilatation and hypotension after its administration.

Fentanyl. Fentanyl is a synthetic opioid that has a much shorter onset of 1–2 minutes and duration of 30–60 minutes. Because of these properties, the administration of fentanyl is appropriate for continuous infusion, easily titratable because of its rapid onset of action, and is indicated in mechanically ventilated patients requiring a continuous level of analgesia. Fentanyl is significantly more lipid soluble than morphine and does not cause histamine release, resulting in stable hemodynamic properties. Although fentanyl has no biologically active metabolites, continuous infusions may result in prolonged sedation because the context-sensitive half-life is increased while the drug is deposited into fatty tissue. When appropriately titrated to patient response and comfort level, fentanyl also has a rapid offset to allow for relative ease in evaluating neurological function and daily wake up tests.

Hydromorphone. Hydromorphone is an opioid with an onset of action from 5–15 minutes and duration of 2–3 hours. Hydromorphone is approximately five times as potent as morphine, is frequently used when pain is not well controlled by morphine, and may be given by intermittent bolus, continuous infusion, or PCA. The advantage is a decreased side effect profile without histamine release or hypotension and is an alternative when morphine is not well tolerated. Although it has active metabolites, dosing adjustment is not indicated for renal impairment.

Nonopioid Analgesics. Kertorolac is currently the only parenterally administered nonsteroidal anti-inflammatory drug. This nonspecific cyclooxygenase inhibitor has moderate analgesic and anti-inflammatory activity. The analgesic properties of ketorlac can be seen within 30 minutes and last up to approximately 6 hours after administration. Ketorlac is usually administered with an opioid and used for its opioid-sparing effects. Although ketorlac is partially metabolized in liver and renally excreted, it should not be administered for >5 days because of the increased risk of gastrointestinal and operative site bleeding. There is also a risk of renal function impairment because it inhibits renal prostaglandin synthesis, but this effect is minimal if the drug is not used for >5 days and should not be initiated in preexisting renal impairment.

Assessment of Pain

Although pain is nearly ubiquitous in an ICU setting, the actual assessment of pain is more difficult to discern. Several scales have been well validated in addressing sedation in ICU patients; however, no single method for evaluating pain has been adequately validated for the ICU. Monitoring pain in an awake and interactive patient is best accomplished by directly asking the patient about the intensity, quality, nature, and duration of the pain. The Visual Analogue Scale, Verbal Descriptor Scale, and Numeric Rating Scale are all subjective scales that have been used with varying degrees of success to quantify pain. More objective markers of pain, such as evaluation of vital signs and behavioral responses can also be used to evaluate pain, especially in a patient who is unable to communicate. The Critical Care Pain Observation Tool is a relatively new scale that attempts to objectively quantify pain in critically ill patients. This scale evaluates facial expression, body movement, muscle tension, and ventilator compliance, and assigns a value of 0–2 for each parameter (Gélinas & Johnston, 2007). The benefit of this type of scale is that it allows a reproducible objective measure of pain that can be followed, even if the patient cannot identify a specific level of discomfort. This tool facilitates objective communication among health care providers regarding levels of pain and can assist with assessments evaluating that the goals of analgesia are achieved. Although there is no ideal scale for the quantification of pain, it is imperative that pain be evaluated frequently by a consistent measure, which can then help guide the treatment of pain in ICU patients.

Summary

The understanding, assessment, and treatment of anxiety, pain, and agitation in the ICU is essential to providing care to critically ill patients. Although nearly all patients will experience anxiety and pain in the ICU, the actual detection and quantification of these constructs are challenging. The use of adequate scales and scoring systems can assist clinicians to consistently document the level of sedation or pain, which will help to guide specific patient therapy. Although numerous pharmacological agents are currently in our armamentarium to provide analgesia and sedation to patients, it is often not clear which agent is the best in a specific patient scenario, especially with new emerging studies and drugs challenging older paradigms of sedation. The crucial event is to integrate specific sedation and analgesia assessment scales and protocols into daily ICU practice to provide the best care possible and ultimately improve patient outcomes.

References

Barr, J., Zomorodi, K., Bertaccini, E. J., Shafer S. L., & Geller E. (2001). A double-blind, randomized comparison of i.v. lorazepam versus midazolam for sedation of ICU patients via a pharmacologic model. *Anesthesiology, 95,* 286–298.

Bennett, S. N., McNeil, M. M., Bland, L. A., Arduino M. J., Villarino M. E., Perrotta D., et al. (1995). Postoperative infections traced to contamination of an intravenous anesthetic, propofol. *New England Journal of Medicine, 333,* 147–154.

Carson, S. S., Kress, J. P., Rodgers, J. E., Vinayak A., Campbell-Bright S., Levitt J. (2006). A randomized trial of intermittent lorazepam versus propofol with daily interruption in mechanically ventilated patients. *Critical Care Medicine, 34,* 1326–32.

Chanques, G., Jaber, S., Barbotte, E., Violet S., Sebbane M., Perrigault P. F., et al. (2006). Impact of systematic evaluation of pain and agitation in an intensive care unit. *Critical Care Medicine, 34,* 1691–1699.

Dasta, J. F., Fuhrman, T. M., & McCandles, C. (1994). Patterns of prescribing and administering drugs for agitation and pain in patients in a surgical intensive care unit. *Critical Care Medicine, 22,* 974–980.

De Jonghe, B., Cook, D., Appere-De-Vecchi, C., Guyatt G., Meade M., & Outin H. (2000). Using and understanding sedation scoring systems: A systematic review. *Intensive Care Medicine, 226,* 275.

Ely, E. W., Inouye, S. K., Bernard, G. R., Gordon S., Francis J., May L., et al. (2001). Delirium in mechanically ventilated patients: validity and reliability of the confusion assessment method for the intensive care unit (CAM-ICU). *Journal of American Medical Association, 286,* 2703–2710.

Ely, E. W., Truman, B., Shintani, A., Thomason J. W., Wheeler A. P., Gordon S., et al. (2003). Monitoring sedation status over time in ICU patients: reliability and validity of the Richmond Agitation-Sedation Scale (RASS). *Journal of American Medical Association, 289,* 2983–2991.

Fragen, R. J. (1997). Pharmacokinetics and pharmacodynamics of midazolam given via continuous intravenous infusion in intensive care units. *Clinical Therapy,19,* 405–419.

Gélinas, C., & Johnston, C. (2007). Pain assessment in the critically ill ventilated adult: Validation of the Critical-Care Pain Observation Tool and Physiologic Indicators. *Clinical Journal of Pain, 23*(6), 497–505.

Jacobi, J., Fraser, J. L., Coursin, B. D., Riker R. R., Fontaine D., Wittbrodt E. T. et al. (2002). Clinical practice guidelines for the sustained use of sedatives and analgesics in the critically ill adult. *Critical Care Medicine; 30,* 119–141.

Kang, T. M. (2002). Propofol infusion syndrome in critically ill patients. *Annals of Pharmacotherapy, 36,* 1453–1456.

Liu, S., Carpenter, R. L., & Neal, J. M. (1995). Epidural anesthesia and analgesia. Their role in postoperative outcome. *Anesthesiology, 82,* 1474–1506.

McKeage, K., & Perry, C. M. (2003). Propofol: A review of its use in intensive care sedation of adults. *CNS Neuroscience and Therapeutics, 17,* 235–272.

Ostermann, M. E., Keenan, S. P., Seiferling, R. A., & Sibbald W. J. (2000). Sedation in the intensive care unit: A systematic review. *Journal of American Medical Association, 283,* 1451–1459.

Pasternak, G. W. (1993). Pharmacological mechanisms of opioid analgesics. *Clinical Neuropharmacology,*16, 1–18.

Pandharipande, P. P., Pun, B. T., Herr, D. L., Maze M., Girard T. D., Miller R. R., et al. (2007). Effect of sedation with dexmedetomidine vs. lorazepam on acute brain dysfunction in mechanically ventilated patients: the MENDS randomized controlled trial. *Journal of American Medical Association, 298,* 2644–2653.

Riker, R. R., & Fraser, G. L. (2005). Adverse events associated with sedatives, analgesics, and other drugs that provide patient comfort in the intensive care unit. *Pharmacotherapy, 25,* 8S–18S.

Riker, R. R., Picard, J. T., Fraser, G. L. (1999). Prospective evaluation of the Sedation-Agitation Scale for adult critically ill patients. *Critical Care Medicine, 27,* 1325–1329.

Sessler, C. N., & Varney, K. (2008). Patient-focused sedation and analgesia in the ICU. *Chest, 133,* 552–565.

Smith, M. T. (2000). Neuroexcitatory effects of morphine and hydromorphone: Evidence implicating the 3-glucuronide metabolites. *Clinical Experience Pharmacology Physiology, 27,* 524–528.

Walder, B., Borgeat, A., Suter, P. M., & Romand, J. A. (2002). Propofol and midazolam versus propofol alone for sedation following coronary artery bypass grafting: A randomized, placebo-controlled trial. *Anaesthesia Intensive Care, 30,* 171–178.

Walder, B., Elia, N., Henzi, I., Romand J. R, & Tramèr M. R. (2001). A lack of evidence of superiority of propofol versus midazolam for sedation in mechanically ventilated critically ill patients: a qualitative and quantitative systematic review. *Anesthesia Analog, 92,* 975–983.

Walder, B., Frick, S., Guegueniat, S., Diby, M., & Romand, J. A. (2002). Pain following cardiac surgery is present for at least one month. *Intensive Care Medicine,* 28–S109.

Watling, S. M., Johnson, M., & Yanos, J. (1996). A method to produce sedation in critically ill patients. *Annals of Pharmacotherapy, 30,* 1227–1231.

Weissman, C. (2005). Sedation and neuromuscular blockade in the ICU. *Chest, 128,* 477–479.

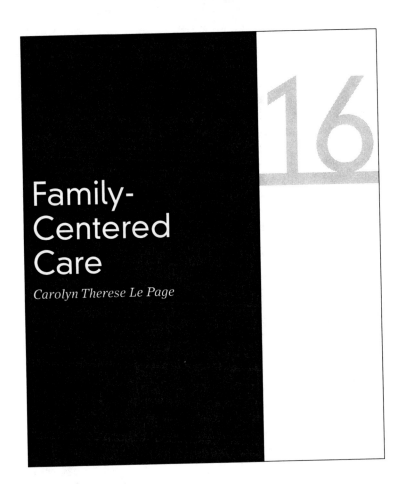

Family-Centered Care

Carolyn Therese Le Page

Family-Centered Critical Care

While walking to get his morning coffee, Julio, a 69-year-old Hispanic man, was struck by a motor vehicle. He was critically injured and entered the health care system. Unconscious and badly injured, he was not carrying any license or identification. He was evacuated to the nearest trauma center. Hours later, the police located Julio's family and they drove 2 hours to reach him, unaware of just what they would find. . .

This scenario is too familiar to critical care professionals. An injured patient typically requiring an entire team to provide immediate life-saving measures "hits the door." The adrenaline of the team is palpable as the art and science of nursing and medicine merge to address the complex needs of the victim. Trauma, resuscitation, and intensive care are cutting edge and highly specialized services, and the experienced health care professional views the process as orchestral, whereas the novice views it as fast paced and overwhelming. The goals of the team are to prevent the loss of life and maximize quality of life. The central focus is clear: the patient.

Patients typically have minimal recall of the most acute aspects of their hospitalization following illness, injury, or surgical intervention. They surrender control (voluntarily or involuntarily) to highly trained and competent providers. They designate their loved ones to advocate on their behalf. Most are unaware of the enormity of the task of being a family member of a critical care patient. The emotional effects can seem insurmountable.

The needs and expectations of the family of critically ill patients are replete in the literature. Family members typically want health professionals to supply clear information about their loved one, provide pertinent education, and offer realistic guidance and support during the process. However, these are typically secondary to the need to be near their loved one. Most families articulate the importance of trust and sensitive interactions among the health care team. The value of compassion and effective communication are essential to family adjustment regardless of patient outcome. Research underscores the value of family and friends in the critical care experience. However, many facilities are unwilling or unable to bridge the gap between traditional critical care paradigms and the needs of patients and families.

Julio's wife, adult daughter, brother, and sister-in-law arrive to the critical care unit. What will they encounter? How will those providing care to the family members integrate them into the plan of care? Will they be met with a traditional and exclusively patient-dominated culture? Will the team be open to accept the family as part of the critical care process?

Dodek et al., (2004) reiterated two decades of data to support that improvement of the quality of care in intensive care units (ICUs) requires the measurement and utilization of family satisfaction data in a manner that reflects active translation into unit-based quality improvement initiatives. They further added that acutely ill, hospitalized individuals require holistic care that includes family-centeredness as a dimension of health care quality. Hanson, Danis, and Garrett (1997) and Malacrida et al., (1998) offered initial studies on measuring family satisfaction in the critical care setting and provided evidence suggesting that several key factors related to communication, ICU staff courtesy, and compassion were critical factors. Heyland et al., (2003) added the importance of family respect and an emphasis on information provided to loved ones as central to family-centered care. Azoulay et al., (2004) cited the level of health care received by patients as significant predictors of overall family satisfaction. The Joint Commission on Accreditation of Healthcare Organizations (JACHO) and the U.S. Institute of Medicine identify family centeredness as one of the key dimensions of health care quality and being safe and secure in the hospital environment.

Empirical data on family satisfaction in intensive care has shed some light on the importance of effective communication with family and support systems. Families need compassion and empathy, polite professional encounters, comprehensive educational information, and high-quality care targeted to the patient as well as the individuals supporting the patient. Dodek and colleagues (2004) iterated that excellence in critical care necessitates the measurement and utilization of family satisfaction data in quality initiatives. This is only possible when direct and ongoing communication is evident.

The satisfaction of the family is no longer a secondary gain or an optional nursing intervention. To meet the standards of optimal care to critically ill patients, there must be data that can be translated into a measure of family-centered care. Even though the patient is at the core of any care model, it is essential that effective contemporary models of acute care include the family as a direct extension of the patient. The JACHO holds institutions accountable in fostering a family-centered approach to care. Evidentiary support to illustrate each facility's perspective is reviewed on a regular interval. The day-to-day challenges remain at the hands of the direct care nursing team.

Family-centered care must carry more than a theoretical connotation. This is an organized and intentional way of providing critical care governing standards of care across the country and requires a team approach. There is no single element that transcends a unit to "family-centered care." Family-centered care requires a philosophical commitment and a genuine desire to negate traditional approaches.

The Philosophy of Family-Centered Care

A family-centered care concept views a patient's family as a unit to be cared for and organizes care delivery around the patient's family, as opposed to the more traditional patient centered model (see Table 16.1). The philosophy should lend itself easily to the mission and vision of the institution while maintaining harmony with the theory that guides nursing practice. Family centered care demands a collaborative approach to care in which *all* members of the team identify the significance of this philosophy and regard family as an essential part of the practice of critical care. There is an inherent duty to ensure that the family needs are met when the loved one is critically ill.

Hennemen and Cardin (2002) noted that the commonalities of organizations providing family-centered care typically include strong evidence of leadership, caring nursing personnel, and the support of a committed multidisciplinary team. This painstaking process and typically those hesitant to recreating a family-centered paradigm have strong personal beliefs and attitudes supporting their reality. Proponents of quality critical care advocate for a holistic approach to the patient and are readily able to embrace the family as part of the whole picture.

Barriers to family-centered care have included nurse's perceptions that patients suffer physiologic stressors secondary to visitors; nurses may have identified a desire to limit caregiver stress and exhaustion as rationale to maintain antiquated policies and procedures. Some team members perceive that meeting family needs will detract from the time with the patient. As health care is more consumer-driven and judged by aspects of patient and family satisfaction, the evolution of family-centered care becomes more of an expectation than an exception. Family members are more likely to be involved in determining where and how the patient's care

16.1 Comparison of Traditional Patient-Centered Model versus Family-Centered Critical Care Model

	Traditional Patient-Centered Model	Family-Centered Unit Model
Entry	Families seek permission to enter. Uncertainty of the ability to see their loved one is common.	An individual who is aware of the general status of the family member greets and welcomes the family.
Access	Visiting hours are clearly defined. If it is not a "visiting time," an exception may be made this time to appease family (two at a time). No furniture is near the bedside or a chair must be obtained from outside the patient's bedside perimeter.	The family is escorted to the bedside and introduced to the nurse and team as available. A chair is available for the family to sit close to their loved one. There is "time" to acclimate to the surroundings.
Immediate Information	Initial information by a designated team member/ unit clerk Phone numbers to unit and/ or physician Visiting hours	Information from direct care provider regarding environment, patient status, and current level of care
Education	Episodic and prospective approach Referred predominantly to medical provider	Proactive team approach Information regarding daily family rounds Invitation to attend daily rounds
Evaluation	Patient focused	Patient and family provide input.

will progress. The practicality of keeping the family within the confines of a waiting room is outdated and unacceptable. Partnership with family serves to promote a holistic approach to the care of patients with critical illness.

Synergy Model for Patient Care

The American Association of Critical Care Nurses reconceptualized the synergy model to form their *AACN Synergy Model for Patient Care* to address the needs of critically ill patients (Hardin & Kaplow, 2005). The model centers on the concept that the needs or characteristics of patients and families influence and drive the characteristics or competencies of nurses. Synergy results when the needs and characteristics of a patient and clinical unit or system are matched with a nurse's competencies.

The continuum of health to illness necessitates a wide range of needs for patients. Individuals who are acutely ill have more severe or complex requirements. The dimensions of nursing practice are driven by the needs of patients and their family. Therefore, nurses must be capable of providing care in multiple dimensions along the continuum. The fundamental tenet of synergy is that when the nurse's competencies arise from patient needs, then characteristics of the nurse and the patient synergize, and optimal patient outcomes can result.

The synergy model is reflective of the ideal that each patient and family and clinical unit and system is unique, with a varying capacity for health and vulnerability to illness. Each one brings a set of unique characteristics to the care situation. These characteristics span the health–illness continuum. Some of the key components are delineated in Table 16.2.

The synergy model emphasizes that nursing care is reflective of the integration of knowledge, skills, experience, and attitudes needed to meet the needs of patients and families. Specific areas of competence are defined in Table 16.3, on page 540. Just as the continuum of patient care is dynamic, the continuum of nursing characteristics are derived from patient needs. The levels of expertise ranging from competent to expert are further explored in the model, which may be viewed at the AACN Website.

The AACN synergy model assumes that the needs of the patient and the competencies of the nurse are viewed in context. The patient is seen as a part of both family and community, and the nurse must be cognizant of this relationship in enacting a plan of care. To guide the model, there are

16.2 Characteristics of Patients, Clinical Units and Systems of Concern to Nurses

Resiliency	The capacity to return to a restorative level of functioning, using compensatory mechanisms; the ability to bounce back quickly after an insult
Vulnerability	Susceptibility to actual or potential stressors that may adversely affect patient outcomes
Stability	The ability to maintain a steady-state equilibrium
Complexity	The intricate entanglement of two or more systems (i.e., family, therapies)
Resource availability	Extent of resources (technical, fiscal, personnel)
Participation in care	Extent to which patient/family engages in aspects of care
Participation in decision making	Extent to which patient/family engage in decision making
Predictability	A characteristic that allows one to expect a certain course of events or illness

Adapted from the AACN Synergy Model for Patient Care (http://www.aacn.org/WD/Certifications/Content/synmodel.pcms?mid=2869&menu=#Patient)

five assumptions regarding patients, nurses, and families. These are the following:

- Patients are biological, psychological, social, and spiritual entities who present at a particular developmental stage. The whole patient (body, mind, and spirit) must be considered.
- The patient, family, and community all contribute to providing a context for the nurse–patient relationship.
- Patients can be described by several characteristics. All characteristics are connected and contribute to each other. Characteristics cannot be looked at in isolation.
- Similarly, nurses can be described on several dimensions. The interrelated dimensions paint a profile of the nurse.
- A goal of nursing is to restore a patient to an optimal level of wellness as defined by the patient. Death can be an acceptable outcome, in which the goal of nursing care is to move a patient toward a peaceful death.

16.3	Nurse Competencies of Concern to Patients, Clinical Units and Systems
Clinical Judgment	Clinical reasoning, which includes clinical decision making, critical thinking, and a global grasp of the situation, coupled with nursing skills acquired through a process of integrating formal and informal experiential knowledge and evidence-based guidelines
Advocacy and Moral Agency	Concerns of the patient/family and nursing staff; serving as a moral agent in identifying and helping to resolve ethical and clinical concerns within and outside the clinical setting
Caring Practices	Nursing activities that create a compassionate, supportive, and therapeutic environment for patients and staff, with the aim of promoting comfort and healing and preventing unnecessary suffering

Includes, but is not limited to, vigilance, engagement, and responsiveness of caregivers, including family and health care personnel |
| Collaboration | Working with others (e.g., patients, families, health care providers) in a way that promotes/encourages each person's contributions towards achieving optimal/realistic patient/family goals

Involves intradisciplinary and interdisciplinary work with colleagues and community |
| Systems Thinking | Body of knowledge and tools that allow the nurse to manage whatever environmental and system resources exist for the patient/family and staff, within or across health care and non-health care systems |
| Response to Diversity | The sensitivity to recognize, appreciate, and incorporate differences into the provision of care

Differences may include, but are not limited to, cultural differences, spiritual beliefs, gender, race, ethnicity, lifestyle, socioeconomic status, age, and values. |
| Facilitation of Learning | The ability to facilitate learning for patients/families, nursing staff, other members of the health care team, and community

Includes both formal and informal facilitation of learning |
| Clinical Inquiry (Innovator/ Evaluator) | The ongoing process of questioning and evaluating practice and providing informed practice

Creating practice changes through research utilization and experiential learning |

Adapted from the AACN Synergy Model for Patient Care (http://www.aacn.org/WD/Certifications/Content/synmodel.pcms?mid=2869&menu=#Nurse)

Implementation toward a Family-Centered Approach

Family-Centered Care. Implicit in the synergy model, family-centered care is not easily defined. There is no universal meaning of family-centered care. A generalized concept of policy, belief, and action by a team is necessary to develop a family-centered model. This is not an isolated activity and should not be confused with open visitation. Adding a chair to the bedside is only a minor adaptation. Instead, family-centered care is best understood as a philosophical commitment to acknowledge the needs of the patients' family as well as the vital role that family brings to the health and well-being of patients.

Some patients may require the presence of a supportive loved one to achieve stability. However, enabling a spouse to remain at the bedside 24 hours a day should not be translated into effectively meeting the needs of the family. Just as the care of the patient is driven by the uniqueness of circumstance, so should the care of the family. Effective communication strategies enhance the ability of patient and family to determine the level of family inclusion in the critical care process.

Misconceptions exist regarding how family-centered care may impact the ability of nurses to provide optimal care. Clarification of the goals and purpose of family-centered care will enable the team to explore, discuss, and allay fears regarding this philosophy. Ultimately, the family-centered care approach supports a patient's right to a safe and supportive critical care experience. Whenever possible, patients should be allowed to direct the quantity of inclusion or exclusion of family participation with respect for care and the extent of information that they wish to be provided to their family. The needs of patients are always held paramount even in a family-centered care approach.

Policies, procedures, and educational materials that provide for the care and safety of patients and family in critical care are typically viewed as positive and essential to navigate the system (AACN, 2007). They can help staff to streamline key issues while promoting a positive first impression. An orientation to the unit and preprinted information should focus on open and effective relationships with the patients and their family. Unit-specific information may offer the family insight into the philosophy of caring within the ICU setting (AACN, 2007). This is an ideal moment for staff to convey key procedures necessary in providing structure consistent with the patient needs while still finding consistency in family-centered critical care practices.

> What would Julio's family see and hear when they enter the critical care area? Will they perceive a welcoming presence? Will there be any doubt that they are part of their loved one's plan of care?

Understanding Family Needs

Families of critically ill patients need to be assured that they will receive current and accurate information about their loved one, afforded comfort and support, guided in appropriate decision making, and given the opportunity to remain close to the patient. Although this may appear to be a simple strategy, it is evident through research that this is not consistently offered to families. There are existing tools and guides to enable adequate assessment of family needs (AACN, 2007).

Nurses are viewed as primary resources for relaying information about the patients' current condition and updates on critical elements of care. Nurses have traditionally functioned as liaisons between the medical team and families. Nurses are very effective in conveying changes in condition, and families have relayed confidence and satisfaction with nurses' ability to keep them informed.

Nurses, families, and other members of the health care team may interpret issues from alternative view points. Cultural determinants, familial roles, and existing family dynamics may enhance or aggravate the health and well-being of the patient. Realistic expectations are necessary to identify that the desires of the patient in family-centered care may necessitate restrictions for some family members. Because of individual circumstances, the critical illness or injury of a loved one may necessitate a referral for intensive counseling or spiritual support.

The ability of the nurse to provide for the needs of the patients and their family is evident in the ongoing care, communication, and support provided at the bedside. Strategies that target the needs of the family include promoting a caring perspective in all interactions, engaging with the patient and family, and offering practical, realistic, and truthful support while providing encouragement. These strategies are incorporated into a family center concept and the establishment of flexible visiting schedules. Nurses are inescapably linked to the caring perspective of healing in critical care.

Discussion Questions

Establishing a family-centered approach must start with the fundamental question: Who is the patient's family? Once the health care team is aware who the patient considers family, then the additional dialogue is necessary to extend an optimal level of nursing care, which is the hallmark of advanced practice in critical care.

The following is a series of questions that place in perspective the currency of family-centered care in an institution. Taken in the context of the discussion presented in this chapter, responding to these questions can help in defining how to proceed in securing and enhancing procedures in terms of such care.

- What practices currently exist that may be viewed as family friendly?
- What practices may display a sense that family is unwelcomed or unwanted in the critical care area?
- How effective is your team in keeping the family current on information?
- What strategies are employed to offer consistent comfort and support?
- Are there resources that may be included beyond the critical care unit?
- How does the team guide the patient and family in appropriate decision making?
- What do you and your teams do specifically to ensure that the family can remain close to the patient?
- Does a family educational guide exist to facilitate understanding of the concepts of the ICU?

How will the needs of Julio and his family be addressed by the health care team? What strategies can be employed to orient them to the situation, establish an open and working relationship, and maintain communication?

Adapting Existing Policy

Once the multidisciplinary team defines the concept of family-centered care, the process of transition can begin. The team needs to determine the presence or absence of policies and procedures that support the proactive beliefs of family centeredness. Multidisciplinary presence will be critical to the creation of effective practices. The team may include representatives from nursing, medicine, administration, ancillary services, security, social work, volunteer services, education, and former patient and family representatives (most facilities have committees with former patient and family advocates volunteering ideas).

Typically, visitation is one area that needs to be adapted to enable effective family-centered care. There are dual reasons that presence at the bedside enhances the needs of patients and their loved ones. Successful visitation protocols offer the family the opportunity to see firsthand the high-quality critical care that a unit offers to the critically ill. Staff may need to be reoriented to the perspective that the family seeing them in action may allay fears that their loved one is in good hands when they are not present. A family-centered care approach should be visible in all areas of the unit. Upon entry, the family should be able to sense a welcoming perspective. This may be achieved by colorful signs or posters identifying the connection between patient, family, and staff. Patient and family educational aids should support the philosophical approach. Staff areas should foster a positive reminder of the importance of an open approach to family communications.

Orientation for new employees should foster the concept of family-centered care and delineate the unit practices that are essential to enact it. Quality improvement measures should include aspects of family satisfaction, and continuous recognition of effective team members will underscore the value of the family-centered approach. During transitioning or improving family-centered protocols, the role of education cannot be minimized. Unit conferences and staff development offerings should include clear and concise interventions that demonstrate family-centered ideals. Spiritual support personnel, social workers, and counselors may provide reassurance and support especially in times when nursing personnel may be engaged in direct care with the patient.

An ongoing and proactive approach to the family ensures attention to patient care and may prevent conflict or crisis during periods of high family stress. The family should feel appreciated and welcomed into the critical care environment. Maintaining an effective unit structure, attention to detail, and education regarding the specific unit protocol promotes safety and security. As an example, each visitor must present photo identification and receive a badge according to hospital policy. Some units request family to remain at the bedside or in the waiting area during change of shift to protect patients' privacy.

Discussion Questions

The following discussion questions will also help in clarifying the status of family-centered care in an institution.

- Who is currently involved in patient and family care?
- Who should be included in employing, improving, and maintaining family-centered care strategies?
- What policies and procedures embrace the family-centered philosophy?
- Which practices negate the concept of family-centered care?

How will Julio's wishes, condition, and family presence be incorporated in his plan of care while maintaining a safe and effective unit operation?

The Dynamics of Ongoing Quality Family-Centered Critical Care

The commitment to family-centered care is complex and requires consistency. Families must be assured that they have access to information and the ability to see their loved one regularly. Inconsistency creates a sense of frustration, lack of trust, and a loss of control in families who are already distraught. This may trigger thoughts of how patient care practices may be applied among varied providers. Overt variations to policy can also create a sense of partiality and negativity among team members. No one wishes to be perceived as a non caring provider by asking the family to limit visiting time when in actuality, they are upholding existing guidelines. Establishing guidelines to partner with families influences the ability of the caregiver to consistently achieve mutual goals.

The road to family-centered care will contain many twists and turns. With a commitment to success, a desire to optimize care, and provision of a supportive environment, no goal is insurmountable. Open communication among staff, administration, and advocacy teams will allow for review of ongoing improvement. The learning curve must be recognized and staff will require mentorship, positive reinforcement, and feedback to change philosophy and engage in regular family-centered care practices. The extreme situations in which difficult family dynamics or problem family members will not dissipate with family centered care. However, it is reasonable to believe that they will be the exceptions to the rule and staff may be more able to preempt aggressive or ineffective interactions by identifying red flags early in family assessment.

Ensuring that a family oriented critical care philosophy and standards of care are upheld by the governing bodies of the unit and health care facility is essential to patient, family, and team satisfaction. Growth and success of the staff, in accordance with the creation of a positive and effective culture centered on quality outcomes, is paramount. Implementing a family-centered approach to care is only the beginning of an ongoing institutional commitment (Table 16.4).

Family-centered care is a reality in today's health care climate. Patients and their families have basic needs that must be met if health care institutions are to be successful in addressing clients' needs and providing holistic care.

Discussion Questions

Additional discussion questions include:

- How can the ICU implement proactive strategies to maintain a family-centered approach?
- How do patients, families, and health care providers define successful family-centered care?
- How do health professionals define successful family-centered care?

■ How do we establish quality measures for improvement and benchmarking?

What will Julio's family tell you about their experience? Would they want to return to your unit if circumstanced required critical care? Are they interested in being ambassadors for future families?

16.4 Considerations in Adopting a Family-Centered Critical Care Approach

Patient-Specific Consideration	Unit-Specific Aspects
Who does the patient define as family? Does the patient wish to limit family visitation? How does the patient prefer information to be communicated to the family? Is there a primary contact person? How does the patient wish to include family in their plan of care? Will family presence facilitate healing? Will family presence offer reassurance? What is important for staff to know in caring for the patient and his/her family while the patient is in the critical care area? Will the family be able to see the patient? How will the family know that the patients is okay? What if something bad happens to the patient?	How do we identify a patient's family? Where is the information documented? How do we approach the patient about family-centered care practices? How do we approach the family about unit practices to support the patient? Are there any specific needs or issues that must be addressed to provide optimal care? Does the unit reflect an openness to encourage family presence? How will communication be maintained when family presence is not possible? How will the staff maintain continuity of FCCC practices despite varied attitudes and beliefs? Who should be included in the planning, implementation, and evaluation of the process?

Advancing Practices in Family-Centered Care

Family Presence during Resuscitation. Duran et al., (2007) defined family presence as the attendance of patients' family members during resuscitation and/or invasive procedures that have a place in the context of family-centered care. The goals of family-centered care do not become negated during the most critical moments of care. The health care team must make every effort to meet the needs of patients' families, including their requests for information, support, and the ability to remain close to the patient even during resuscitation. Research (Duran, 2007) supports that the patients' families have certain needs during a health-related crisis. They may be met through observation of clinical staff and support of team efforts during a code scenario. Protocols should designate an individual to maintain honest, consistent, and thorough communication with the family. This team member should remain in close proximity of the codes and emotionally connected to the patient. Families can then witness providers caring for the patient and have access to see for themselves the status of their loved one. Family presence during resuscitation and/or invasive procedures may enable the family to gain perspective that is otherwise impossible to achieve.

Traditional obstacles to family presence have centered on professional and litigious perceptions. There is little data to support an increase in litigation. Most anecdotal discussion centers on nurses and physicians fear of upsetting or offending family. There is concern that families are incapable of handling the stress of the situation, others offered concerns for staff pressure and most related concerns that family may distract or impede efforts aimed at the patient.

The Emergency Nurses Association (ENA, 2001) offered the first research studies to explore family presence during resuscitation. Findings supported that families viewed this as positive in addressing their needs (ENA, 2001). Providers described increases in locus of control, understanding of the reality of their family member's situation, and improved education. Subsequent studies by the American Association for the Surgery of Trauma (AAST) and the ENA to determine the members' opinions on family presence during trauma resuscitation revealed nurses more open to family presence than trauma physicians. More recent data supports this trend (Moreland, 2005, Sachetti, Paston, & Carraccio, 2005).

The American Nurses Association (ANA) Code of Ethics (ANA, 2000) addresses nurses' primary responsibility to recognize the "patient's place in the family or networks of relationship" reference. Protocols for family presence are included in many specialty organizations including AACN and ENA. The National Association of Emergency Medical Technicians, the National Association of Social Workers, and The American Heart Association endorse family presence policies.

Studies addressing patients and family member's perceptions during resuscitation largely support the option of allowing family to be present (reference). Most family cited that being near the patient enabled them to comprehend the reality of the situation, process grief responses, and demonstrate beyond a doubt that everything had been done to resuscitate their loved one. To date, no study has found that keeping family away from the bedside during treatment or CPR benefits anyone (Mason, 2004). In fact, families may suffer emotional turmoil including anxiety, depression, helplessness, and guilt if excluded from resuscitation efforts (Marrone & Fogg, 2005). As family presence becomes a more accepted practice, health care providers will need to accommodate families at the bedside and address unit and system specific barriers.

Discussion Questions

- Is our unit presently promoting family presence?
- What would be needed to facilitate this action?
- How would the patient and family perception of health care be impacted by the promotion of family presence policies and procedures?

Online Resources

American Association of Critical care Nurses
  http://www.aacn.org/
American Hospital Association
  http://www.aha.org/aha/issues/Quality-and-Patient-Safety
  /strategies-patientcentered.html
Institute for Family Centered Care
  http://www.familycenteredcare.org/advance/orglm-links.html

Institute for Healthcare Improvement
   http://www.ihi.org/ihi
Institute of Medicine
   http://www.iom.edu/
Joint Commission Accreditation
   http://www.jointcommission.org/

References

American Nurses Association. (ANA). (2000). *Code of Ethics for Nurses With Interpretive Statements.* Silver Spring, MD.

Azoulay, E., Sprung CL. (2004). Family-physician interactions in the intensive care unit. *Critical Care Medicine, 32*(11), 2323–2328.

Dodek, P. M., Heyland, D. K., Rocker, G. M., & Cook, D. J. (2004). Translating family satisfaction data into quality improvement. *Critical Care Medicine, 32,* 1922–1927.

Duran, C. R., Oman, K. S., Abel, J. J., Koziel, V. M., & Szymanski, D. (2007). Attitudes toward and beliefs about family presence: A survey of healthcare providers, patients' families, and patients. *American Journal of Critical Care, 16*(3), 270–279.

Emergency Nurses Association. (2001). *Presenting the option for family presence.* (2nd ed.). Bedford Park, IL.

Hanson L. C., Danis, M., & Garrett, J. (1997). What is wrong with end-of-life care? Opinions of bereaved family members. *Journal of the American Geriatric Society, 45,* 1339–1344.

Hardin, S. R., & Kaplow, R. (2005) *Synergy for Clinical Excellence: The AACN Synergy Model for Patient Care.* Boston: Jones & Bartlett.

Henneman, E. A., & Cardin, S. (2002). Family-centered critical care: A practical approach to making it happen. *Critical Care Nurse, 22,* 12–19.

Heyland D. K., Rocker, G. M., O'Callaghan, C. J., Dodek, P. M., & Cook, D. J. (2003) Dying in the ICU: Perspectives of family members. *Chest, 124,* 392–397.

Malacrida, R., Bettelini, C. M., Degrate, A., Martinez, M., Badia, F., Piazza, J., et al. (1998) Reasons for dissatisfaction: A survey of relatives of intensive care unit patients who died. *Critical Care Medicine, 26,* 1187–1193.

Marrone, L., & Fogg, C. (2005). Family presence during resuscitation: Are policies allowing family into the trauma room humane and necessary—or just asking for trouble? *Nursing 35*(8) ED Insider Suppl., 21–22.

Mason, D. (2004). Family presence. *NSO Risk Advisor – Fall 2004.* Retrieved May 1, 2009 from http://www.nso.com/newsletters/advisor/2004_fall/

Moreland, P. (2005). Family presence during invasive procedures and resuscitation in the emergency department: A review of the literature. *Journal of Emergency Nursing, 31*(1), 58–72.

Piazza, J. et al. (1998) Reasons for dissatisfaction: A survey of relatives of intensive care patients who died. *Critical Care Medicine, 26,* 1187–1193.

Sacchetti, A., Paston, C., & Carraccio, C. (2005). Family members do not disrupt care when present during invasive procedures. *Academic Emergency Medicine, 12,* 477–479.

INDEX

G

H

M

N